Problem Solving in

If to be human is to be limited, then the role of caring professions and institutions – from surgeons to nursing homes – ought to be aiding people in their struggle with those limits. Sometimes we can offer a cure, sometimes only a salve, sometimes not even that. But whatever we can offer, our interventions, and the risks and sacrifices they entail, are justified only if they serve the larger aims of a person's life. When we forget that, the suffering we inflict can be barbaric. When we remember it the good we do can be breathtaking.

Atul Gawande
Being Mortal: Medicine and What Matters in the End, 2014

Problem Solving in
Older Cancer Patients

Edited by

Alistair Ring, MD, MA, FRCP
Consultant Medical Oncologist, Royal Marsden NHS Foundation Trust, London, UK

Danielle Harari, MBBS, FRCP
Consultant Geriatrician, Guy's and St Thomas' NHS Foundation Trust, London, UK;
Division of Health and Social Care Research, King's College London, London, UK

Tania Kalsi, MBBS, MRCP
Consultant Geriatrician, Guy's and St Thomas' NHS Foundation Trust, London, UK;
Division of Health and Social Care Research, King's College London, London, UK

Janine Mansi, MD, FRCP
Consultant Medical Oncologist, Guy's and St Thomas' NHS Foundation Trust, London, UK;
Biomedical Research Centre, King's College London, London, UK

Peter Selby, CBE, MD, MA, DSc, FRCP, FRCR, FMedSci
Professor of Cancer Medicine, Leeds Cancer Centre, St James's University Hospital, Leeds,
UK; honorary president of the Association of Cancer Physicians and of the European
Cancer Concord

**Published in association with the Association of Cancer Physicians and
the British Geriatrics Society**

CLINICAL PUBLISHING

OXFORD

CLINICAL PUBLISHING
an imprint of Atlas Medical Publishing Ltd
110 Innovation House, Parkway Court
Oxford Business Park South, Oxford OX4 0JY, UK

Tel: +44 1865 811116
Email: info@clinicalpublishing.co.uk

Web: www.clinicalpublishing.co.uk

Distributed worldwide by:
Marston Book Services Ltd
160 Eastern Avenue
Milton Park
Abingdon
Oxon OX14 4SB UK
Tel: +44 1235 465500
Fax: +44 1235 465555
Email: trade.orders@marston.co.uk

A catalogue record for this book is available from the British Library.

ISBN 13   978 1 84692 110 0
ISBN e-book 978 1 84692 650 5

Series design by Pete Russell Typographic Design, Faringdon, Oxon, UK
Typeset by Ian Winter Design, Ramsden, Oxon, UK
Printed by Latimer Trend and Company Ltd, Plymouth, UK

Contents

Contributors

Dr Lucy Adkinson, Specialist Registrar in Palliative Medicine, Yorkshire and Humber Deanery, Leeds

Dr Stephen Alcorn, Specialist Registrar in Anaesthesia, Western General Hospital, Edinburgh

Dr Doraid Alrifai, Speciality Registrar in Medical Oncology, Guy's and St Thomas' NHS Foundation Trust, London; Biomedical Research Centre, King's College London, London

Dr Alan Anthoney, Consultant Medical Oncologist, Leeds Cancer Centre, St James's University Hospital, Leeds

Dr Matthew Appleby, Core Psychiatry Trainee, Camden and Islington Foundation Trust, London

Dr Edward Armstrong, Specialist Registrar in Medical Oncology, Royal Marsden Hospital NHS Foundation Trust, London

Professor Riccardo Audisio, Professor of Surgical Oncology, University of Liverpool, Liverpool; Consultant Surgical Oncologist, St Helens and Knowsley Teaching Hospitals NHS Trust, St Helens

Dr Susana Banerjee, Consultant Medical Oncologist, Gynaecological Cancers Research Lead, Royal Marsden Hospital NHS Foundation Trust, London

Dr Emily Bart-Smith, Specialist Registrar in Haematology, Brighton and Sussex University Hospitals NHS Trust, Brighton

Professor Michael Bennett, St Gemma's Professor of Palliative Medicine, St Gemma's Hospice, Leeds

Dr Shree Bhide, Consultant Clinical Oncologist, Royal Marsden Hospital NHS Foundation Trust, London

Dr Rebecca Birch, Research Fellow, Cancer Epidemiology Group, Section of Epidemiology and Biostatistics, Leeds Institute of Cancer and Pathology, University of Leeds, Leeds

Dr Jonathan Birns, Consultant in Stroke Medicine, Geriatrics and General Medicine, Guy's and St Thomas' NHS Foundation Trust, London

Mr Mike Birtwistle, Founding Partner, Incisive Health, London

Dr Etienne Brain, Medical Oncologist, Hôpital René Huguenin/Institut Curie, Saint-Cloud, Paris; President of the International Society of Geriatric Oncology (SIOG)

Dr Eileen Burns, Consultant in Elderly Medicine, Leeds Teaching Hospitals NHS Trust, Leeds

Dr Ian Chau, Consultant Medical Oncologist, Royal Marsden NHS Foundation Trust, London

Dr Vinton Cheng, Specialist Registrar in Medical Oncology, Leeds Cancer Centre, St James's University Hospital, Leeds

Dr Timothy Chevassut, Senior Lecturer in Haematology, Brighton and Sussex Medical School, Brighton

Dr Ruhe Chowdhury, Specialist Registrar in Medical Oncology, Guy's and St Thomas' NHS Foundation Trust, London; Dimbleby Cancer Research Centre, King's College London, London

Dr Andrew Clegg, Consultant Geriatrician, Bradford Teaching Hospitals NHS Foundation Trust, Bradford

Mr William Cross, Consultant Urological Surgeon, St James's University Hospital, Leeds

Dr Denis Curtin, Specialist Registrar in Geriatric Medicine, Cork University Hospital, Cork

Dr Iva Damyanova, Specialty Registrar in Medical Oncology, Leeds Cancer Centre, St James's University Hospital, Leeds

Dr Michael Davidson, Specialist Registrar in Medical Oncology, Royal Marsden Hospital NHS Foundation Trust, London

Dr Peter Diem, Consultant in Geriatric Medicine, Guy's and St Thomas' NHS Foundation Trust, London

Dr Natalie Doyle, Nurse Consultant, Living With and Beyond Cancer, Royal Marsden NHS Foundation Trust, London

Dr Emma Drasar, Specialist Registrar in Haematology, King's College Hospital, London

Professor Sean Duffy, National Clinical Director for Cancer, NHS England, Leeds

Dr Lucy Dumas, Specialist Registrar in Medical Oncology, Royal Marsden Hospital NHS Foundation Trust, London

Professor Paul Finan, Professor of Colorectal Surgery, Cancer Research UK Cancer Epidemiology Unit, St James's University Hospital, Leeds

Dr James Fleet, Registrar in Geriatric, Stroke and General Internal Medicine, Guy's and St Thomas' NHS Foundation Trust, London

Dr Irwin Foo, Consultant Anaesthetist, Western General Hospital, Edinburgh

Dr Paul Gallagher, Consultant Physician in Geriatric Medicine, Cork University Hospital, Cork

Dr Sharmistha Ghosh, Clinical Fellow in Medical Oncology, Guy's and St Thomas' NHS Foundation Trust, London; Biomedical Research Centre, King's College London, London

Dr Jacqueline Gilbert, Specialist Registrar in Geriatric and General Internal Medicine, Queen Elizabeth the Queen Mother Hospital, Margate

Professor Margot Gosney, Professor of Elderly Care Medicine, Royal Berkshire NHS Foundation Trust, Reading

Dr Emily Grist, Specialist Registrar in Medical Oncology, Royal Marsden NHS Foundation Trust, London

Dr Geoff Hall, Consultant Medical Oncologist, Leeds Cancer Centre, St James's University Hospital, Leeds

Dr Peter Hall, Consultant Medical Oncologist, Edinburgh Cancer Research Centre, Edinburgh

Professor Freddie Hamdy, Nuffield Professor of Surgery, University of Oxford, Oxford; Honorary Consultant Surgeon, John Radcliffe Hospital, Oxford

Dr Joanna Hampton, Consultant in Elderly Care Medicine, Addenbrooke's Hospital, Cambridge

Dr Catherine Handforth, Academic Clinical Fellow in Medical Oncology, Leeds Cancer Centre, St James's University Hospital, Leeds

Dr Danielle Harari, Consultant Geriatrician, Guy's and St Thomas' NHS Foundation Trust, London; Division of Health and Social Care Research, King's College London, London

Dr Joanna Hardwick, Specialist Registrar in Geriatrics and General Internal Medicine, Guy's and St Thomas' NHS Foundation Trust, London

Ms Anita Hargreaves, Specialty Training Registrar in Breast and General Surgery, Royal Liverpool and Broadgreen University Hospitals NHS Trust, Liverpool

Ms Karen Hargreaves, Macmillan Occupational Therapist, Comprehensive Care for Older People with Cancer Team, Reading

Dr Mark Harries, Consultant Medical Oncologist, Guy's and St Thomas' NHS Foundation Trust, London; Biomedical Research Centre, King's College London, London

Dr Ann Henry, Consultant Clinical Oncologist, Leeds Cancer Centre, St James's University Hospital, Leeds

Mr Richard Henry, Lecturer in Cancer Nursing, Queens University, Belfast

Dr Jane Hook, Specialty Registrar in Medical Oncology, Leeds Cancer Centre, St James's University Hospital, Leeds

Dr Nicola Hughes, Academic Clinical Fellow in Medical Oncology, Leeds Cancer Centre, St James's University Hospital, Leeds

Dr David Jackson, Consultant Medical Oncologist, Leeds Cancer Centre, St James's University Hospital, Leeds

Dr Satinder Jagdev, Consultant Medical Oncologist, Leeds Cancer Centre, St James's University Hospital, Leeds

Dr Adam Januszewski, Academic Clinical Fellow in Medical Oncology, London

Dr Adel Jebar, Academic Clinical Lecturer in Medical Oncology, Leeds Cancer Centre, St James's University Hospital, Leeds

Professor Peter Johnson, Chief Clinician, Cancer Research UK; Professor of Medical Oncology, University of Southampton, Southampton

Dr Debra Josephs, Academic Clinical Lecturer, Guy's and St Thomas' NHS Foundation Trust, London; Biomedical Research Centre, King's College London, London

Dr Tania Kalsi, Consultant Geriatrician, Guy's and St Thomas' NHS Foundation Trust, London; Division of Health and Social Care Research, King's College London, London

Dr Ingrid Kane, Consultant Stroke Physician, Brighton and Sussex University Hospitals NHS Trust, Brighton

Dr Eleni Karapanagiotou, Consultant Medical Oncologist, Guy's and St Thomas' NHS Foundation Trust, London; Biomedical Research Centre, King's College London, London

Miss Sonali Kaushik, Consultant in Gynaecological Oncology, Brighton and Sussex University Hospitals NHS Trust, Brighton

Dr Samantha Keeling, Specialist Registrar and Honorary Clinical Lecturer in Geriatric Medicine, St George's University Hospitals NHS Foundation Trust, London; St George's, University of London, London

Dr Khurum Khan, Clinical Research Fellow, Royal Marsden NHS Foundation Trust, London

Dr Mark Kinirons, Consultant Geriatrician, Guy's and St Thomas' NHS Foundation Trust, London

Dr Kimberley Kok, Specialty Registrar in Geriatric Medicine, King's College Hospital London, London

Dr Satish Kumar, Consultant Medical Oncologist, Velindre Cancer Centre, Cardiff

Dr Winnie Kwan, General Practitioner and Clinical Lead for End of Life Care and Cancer, Bexley Clinical Commissioning Group, Bexleyheath

Dr Kate Lankester, Consultant Clinical Oncologist, Brighton and Sussex University Hospitals NHS Trust, Brighton

Dr James Larkin, Consultant Medical Oncologist, Royal Marsden Hospital NHS Foundation Trust, London

Professor Mark Lawler, Professor of Translational Cancer Genomics, Queen's University, Belfast

Dr Daniel Lee, Consultant Medical Oncologist, Airedale General Hospital, Keighley

Professor Bob Leonard, Professor of Medical Oncology, Imperial College London, London

Dr Cressida Lorimer, Clinical Research Fellow in Neuro-Oncology, Brighton and Sussex University Hospitals NHS Trust, Brighton

Dr Hazel Lote, Specialist Registrar in Medical Oncology, Royal Marsden NHS Foundation Trust, London

Professor Jane Maher, Joint Chief Medical Officer, Macmillan Cancer Support; Consultant Oncologist, Mount Vernon Cancer Centre, Northwood, Middlesex

Dr Janine Mansi, Consultant Medical Oncologist, Guy's and St Thomas' NHS Foundation Trust, London; Biomedical Research Centre, King's College London, London

Dr Maria Marples, Consultant Medical Oncologist, Leeds Cancer Centre, St James's University Hospital, Leeds

Professor Finbarr Martin, Consultant Geriatrician, Guy's and St Thomas' NHS Foundation Trust, London; Division of Health and Social Care Research, King's College London, London

Dr Fionna Martin, Specialist Registrar in Geriatric and General Medicine, Lewisham and Greenwich NHS Trust, London

Professor Malcolm Mason, Cancer Research Wales Professor of Clinical Oncology, Cardiff University, Cardiff

Dr Kathryn Mitchell, Specialist Registrar in Clinical Oncology, Bristol Haematology and Oncology Centre, Bristol

Dr Ana Montes, Consultant Medical Oncologist, Guy's and St Thomas' NHS Foundation Trust, London; Biomedical Research Centre, King's College London, London

Dr Jenna Morgan, Specialist Registrar in Surgery and Research Fellow, University of Sheffield, Sheffield

Dr Eva Morris, Principal Research Fellow, Cancer Epidemiology Group, Section of Epidemiology and Biostatistics, Leeds Institute of Cancer and Pathology, University of Leeds, Leeds

Dr Vidhya Nair, Consultant in Elderly Medicine, Pinderfields General Hospital, Wakefield

Dr Kate Newbold, Consultant Clinical Oncologist, Royal Marsden NHS Foundation Trust, London

Dr Sarah Ngan, Consultant Medical Oncologist, Guy's and St Thomas' NHS Foundation Trust, London; Biomedical Research Centre, King's College London, London

Dr Mary O'Brien, Consultant Medical Oncologist, Royal Marsden NHS Foundation Trust, London

Dr Alicia Okines, Specialist Registrar in Medical Oncology, Royal Marsden NHS Foundation Trust, London

Dr Sasi Pathmanathan, Specialist Registrar in Geriatrics and General Internal Medicine, Guy's and St Thomas' NHS Foundation Trust, London

Dr Sarah Payne, Fellow in Medical Oncology, Guy's and St Thomas' NHS Foundation Trust, London

Dr Alexandra Pender, Specialist Registrar in Medical Oncology, Royal Marsden NHS Foundation Trust, London

Professor Tim Perren, Professor of Cancer Medicine, Leeds Cancer Centre, St James's University Hospital, Leeds

Dr Lisa Pickering, Consultant Medical Oncologist, St George's University Hospitals NHS Foundation Trust, London

Dr Vijay Bhagawati-Prasad, Specialty Registrar in Medical Oncology, York Hospital, York

Professor Allan Price, Consultant Clinical Oncologist, Edinburgh Cancer Centre, Edinburgh; Honorary Professor of Radiation Oncology University of Edinburgh, Edinburgh

Dr Christy Ralph, Consultant Medical Oncologist, Leeds Cancer Centre, St James's University Hospital, Leeds

Professor Malcolm Reed, Brighton and Sussex Medical School, Brighton; Dean and Honorary Consultant Surgeon, Brighton and Sussex University Hospitals NHS Trust, Brighton

Dr Dimitra Repana, Clinical Fellow in Medical Oncology, Guy's and St Thomas' NHS Foundation Trust, London; Biomedical Research Centre, King's College London, London

Dr Alistair Ring, Consultant Medical Oncologist, Royal Marsden NHS Foundation Trust, London

Dr Paul Ross, Consultant Medical Oncologist, Guy's and St Thomas' NHS Foundation Trust, London; Biomedical Research Centre, King's College London

Dr Sarah Rudman, Consultant Medical Oncologist, Guy's and St Thomas' NHS Foundation Trust, London; Biomedical Research Centre, King's College London, London

Dr Debashis Sarker, Senior Lecturer and Consultant Medical Oncologist, Guy's and St Thomas' NHS Foundation Trust, London; Biomedical Research Centre, King's College London, London

Dr Zuzanna Sawicka, Consultant in Elderly Medicine, Pinderfields Hospital, Wakefield

Dr Claire Scampion, Consultant in Elderly Medicine, Leeds Teaching Hospitals NHS Trust, Leeds

Dr Pamela Seenan, Consultant Physician, Gartnavel General Hospital, Glasgow

Professor Peter Selby, Professor of Cancer Medicine, Leeds Cancer Centre, St James's University Hospital, Leeds

Dr Jenny Seligmann, Clinical Lecturer in Medical Oncology, Leeds Cancer Centre, St James's University Hospital, Leeds

Mr Thangaraj Senniappan, Honorary Occupational Therapist, Royal Berkshire NHS Foundation Trust, Reading

Professor Matthew Seymour, Professor of Gastrointestinal Cancer Medicine, Leeds Cancer Centre, St James's University Hospital, Leeds

Dr Gulnaz Shah, Specialist Registrar in Haematology, Brighton and Sussex University Hospitals NHS Trust, Brighton

Dr Adam Sharp, Specialist Registrar in Medical Oncology, Royal Marsden Hospital NHS Foundation Trust, London

Dr David Shipway, Consultant Physician and Geriatrician, Comprehensive Onco-Geriatric Surgery Service, St Mary's Hospital, Imperial College Healthcare NHS Trust, London

Professor Susan Short, Professor of Clinical Oncology, Leeds Cancer Centre, St James's University Hospital, Leeds

Dr Jacqueline Simms, Specialist Registrar in Geriatrics and General Internal Medicine, Guy's and St Thomas' NHS Foundation Trust, London

Dr Aspasia Soultati, Clinical Fellow in Medical Oncology, Guy's and St Thomas' NHS Foundation Trust, London; Biomedical Research Centre, King's College London, London

Dr Katie Spencer, Specialist Registrar in Clinical Oncology, Leeds Cancer Centre, St James's University Hospital, Leeds

Dr Edward Spilg, Assistant Professor, Division of Geriatric Medicine, Ottawa Hospital, Ottawa

Dr Naureen Starling, Consultant Medical Oncologist, Royal Marsden NHS Foundation Trust, London

Dr Matt Sweeting, Consultant Physician and Geriatrician, Broomfield Hospital, Mid Essex Hospital Services NHS Trust, Chelmsford

Dr Daniel Swinson, Consultant Medical Oncologist, Leeds Cancer Centre, St James's University Hospital, Leeds

Dr Hannah Taylor, Specialist Registrar in Medical Oncology, Bristol Oncology Centre, Bristol

Dr Kiruthikah Thillai, Specialist Registrar in Medical Oncology, Guy's and St Thomas' NHS Foundation Trust, London; Biomedical Research Centre, King's College London, London

Dr Sebastian Trainor, Specialist Registrar in Medical Oncology, Leeds Cancer Centre, St James's University Hospital, Leeds

Dr Samantha Turnbull, Specialist Registrar in Medical Oncology, Leeds Cancer Centre, St James's University Hospital, Leeds

Dr Nicola Turner, Consultant in Elderly Medicine, Leeds Teaching Hospitals NHS Trust, Leeds

Dr Gordon Urquhart, Specialist Registrar in Medical Oncology, Huddersfield Royal Infirmary, Huddersfield

Dr Naveen Vasudev, Consultant Medical Oncologist, Leeds Cancer Centre, St James's University Hospital, Leeds

Dr David Watkins, Consultant Medical Oncologist, Royal Marsden Hospital NHS Foundation Trust, London

Dr Andrew Webb, Consultant Medical Oncologist, Brighton and Sussex University Hospitals NHS Trust, Brighton

Dr Hans Wildiers, Medical Oncologist, University Hospitals Leuven, Leuven

Dr Kee Howe Wong, Specialist Registrar in Clinical Oncology, Royal Marsden Hospital NHS Foundation Trust, London

Dr Juliet Wright, Senior Lecturer and Honorary Consultant in Elderly Medicine, Brighton and Sussex Medical School, Brighton

Dr Gilbert Zulian, Geriatrician and Medical Oncologist in Palliative Medicine, Geneva University Hospitals, Geneva

Acknowledgements

The editors and authors are grateful to all their patients who have inspired them to prepare this book and to work together to improve their care. The editors warmly acknowledge the support they have received in preparing this book. Nicole Goldman coordinated and oversaw the book's preparation and organization.

We are especially grateful to Cancer Research UK and Macmillan Cancer Support for their sponsorship of the book and the workshop that preceded it, without which the whole project would not have been possible.

The editors, authors and the publisher are most grateful to Professor Johnathan Joffe, chairman of the Association of Cancer Physicians (ACP), and the ACP Executive for their support and advice during the development of this book. They would also like to thank the British Geriatrics Society Executive for their support, including the new formation of a Special Interest Group in Geriatric Oncology.

We are very grateful to Beverley Martin at Clinical Publishing for her expert work, support, goodwill and interest in our purpose in preparing the book.

Dr Ring would like to acknowledge the support of the Royal Marsden National Institute for Health Research Biomedical Research Centre for Cancer. Dr Harari and Dr Kalsi would like to acknowledge the support of Guy's and St Thomas' NHS Foundation Trust, and King's College London Division of Health and Social Care Research. Dr Mansi would like to acknowledge the support of Guy's and St Thomas' NHS Foundation Trust and the Biomedical Research Centre, King's College London. Professor Selby would like to acknowledge the support of the University of Leeds, Leeds Teaching Hospitals NHS Trust, the National Institute for Health Research and the European Research Council.

Preface

The cancer care community of patients, healthcare professionals, scientists, managers and charity workers, as well as the general public, are becoming increasingly aware of how vital it will be to plan thoroughly to meet the needs of the growing number of older people who will be living with cancer now and in the future. Not only will the number of cases increase but it will be essential for healthcare services to ensure that diagnostic approaches, treatments and care are satisfactorily tailored to meet the needs and choices of individuals who are at higher risk of comorbidities and frailty. We must avoid the pitfall of tailoring our approaches to individuals based on their chronological age: our approaches must fit with all the needs of older patients, from their financial outlook through to the support they can or cannot access, as well as their medical fitness.

Macmillan Cancer Support and Cancer Research UK were pleased to support the Association of Cancer Physicians and the British Geriatrics Society in their 2014 workshop held in Manchester and in this publication, *Problem Solving in Older Cancer Patients*. Experts from the UK and abroad have provided perspectives on the important issues and challenges that we face in providing the right approaches to the diagnosis and care of older cancer patients. Importantly, the workshop and book are very patient-centred and focus on over 30 individual cases. The knowledge and skills of oncologists and geriatricians of all professions – established professionals as well as those in training – are brought to bear on individual cases. This integrated approach to the preparation of the book should help to ensure future integrated approaches in clinical care across the UK.

Experts have identified areas where we can learn from other countries, especially those in mainland Europe that have specific initiatives for the care of older cancer patients. The importance of innovation and research to allow us to find better ways of diagnosing and managing cancer in older people has been emphasized and is welcomed. The workshop and the book have highlighted the importance of the many different groups of healthcare professionals who together are responsible for caring for cancer patients and older people. Different professional groups often have different styles and different cultures but they all share the aim of bringing about the best outcomes, the best quality of life and the best experience for their patients. We anticipate that this new text will be a useful contribution to improving planning for the care of cancer patients and the development of clinical care teams from oncology, geriatrics, primary care and many others to deploy their skills for the maximum benefit of this important group of patients.

Alistair Ring, Danielle Harari, Tania Kalsi, Janine Mansi and Peter Selby, Editors
Lynda Thomas, Chief Executive, Macmillan Cancer Support
Harpal Kumar, Chief Executive, Cancer Research UK

Abbreviations

AAA	Abdominal aortic aneurysm	ER	Oestrogen receptor
ACP	Association of Cancer Physicians	ESMO	European Society for Medical Oncology
ADL	Activities of daily living	ETF	Elderly Task Force
ADT	Androgen deprivation therapy	EVAR	Endoscopic repair of abdominal aortic aneurysm
AF	Atrial fibrillation		
AHP	Allied health professional	FIGO	International Federation of Gynecology and Obstetrics
AML	Acute myeloid leukaemia		
ASA	American Society of Anesthesiologists	FOLFIRI	Folinic acid, fluorouracil, irinotecan
BNP	B-type natriuretic peptide	FOLFIRINOX	Folinic acid, fluorouracil, irinotecan, oxaliplatin
BPH	Benign prostatic hypertrophy		
BSC	Best supportive care	FOLFOX	Folinic acid, fluorouracil, oxaliplatin
CAPOX	Capecitabine, oxaliplatin		
CCG	Clinical commissioning group	5-FU	Fluorouracil
CDI	*Clostridium difficile* infection	GCSF	Granulocyte colony-stimulating factor
CGA	Comprehensive Geriatric Assessment		
CHOP	Cyclophosphamide, doxorubicin, vincristine, prednisolone	GFR	Glomerular filtration rate
		GIST	Gastrointestinal stromal tumour
CK	Cytokeratin	GOJ	Gastro-oesophageal junction
CMF	Cyclophosphamide, methotrexate and fluorouracil	GTN	Glyceryl trinitrate
		HER2	Human epidermal growth factor receptor 2
COPD	Chronic obstructive pulmonary disease		
		HNA	Holistic Needs Assessment
CUP	Cancer of unknown primary	IADL	Instrumental activities of daily living
DCIS	Ductal carcinoma *in situ*		
DLBCL	Diffuse large B cell lymphoma	IMCA	Independent mental capacity advocate
DRE	Digital rectal examination		
EBRT	External beam radiation therapy	LDH	Lactate dehydrogenase
ECOG	Eastern Cooperative Oncology Group	LMWH	Low-molecular-weight heparin
		LPA	Lasting Power of Attorney
ECX	Epirubicin, cisplatin, capecitabine	LVEF	Left ventricular ejection fraction
eGFR	Estimated glomerular filtration rate	MCA	Mental Capacity Act 2005
		MDT	Multidisciplinary team
EGFR	Epidermal growth factor receptor	MET	Metabolic equivalent of task
EORTC	European Organisation for Research and Treatment of Cancer	MIBC	Muscle-invasive bladder cancer
		mpMRI	Multiparametric magnetic resonance imaging

mRCC	Metastatic renal cell carcinoma
MUO	Malignancy of unidentified primary origin
NCEI	National Cancer Equality Initiative
NHSCB	NHS Commissioning Board
NSAIDs	Non-steroidal anti-inflammatory drugs
NSCLC	Non-small-cell lung carcinoma
NTproBNP	N-terminal pro-B-type natriuretic peptide
NYHA	New York Heart Association
OAB	Overactive bladder
OH	Orthostatic hypotension
OS	Overall survival
OSA	Obstructive sleep apnoea
PD-1	Programmed cell death protein 1
PFS	Progression-free survival
POI	Pharmaceutical Oncology Initiative
PS	Performance status
PSA	Prostate-specific antigen
PVD	Peripheral vascular disease
R-CHOP	Rituximab, cyclophosphamide, doxorubicin, vincristine, prednisolone
RCT	Randomized controlled trial
RFA	Radiofrequency ablation
R-mini-CHOP	Full-dose rituximab, low-dose cyclophosphamide, doxorubicin, vincristine, prednisolone
ROC	Receiver operating characteristic
SACT	Systemic anticancer therapy
SIOG	International Society of Geriatric Oncology
SNP	Single nucleotide polymorphism
SSRI	Selective serotonin reuptake inhibitor
TIA	Transient ischaemic attack
TKI	Tyrosine kinase inhibitor
TSH	Thyroid-stimulating hormone
TTF	Thyroid transcription factor
UTI	Urinary tract infection
VEGF	Vascular endothelial growth factor
VTE	Venous thromboembolism
XELIRI	Capecitabine, irinotecan

PERSPECTIVE

01 Cancer in Older People: an Overview

Catherine Handforth, Nicola Turner, David Jackson, Andrew Clegg, Peter Hall, Katie Spencer, Geoff Hall, Mark Lawler, Peter Selby

There is increasing discussion about service needs and developments for cancer care for older people. The topic is not new.[1–4] In the USA, the population aged 65 or over will double by 2050, and, in the EU, people over 65 years will outnumber children by 2060.[5,6] In the UK, by 2030, about 70% of cancers will occur in people aged over 65 years.[7] Studies by the International Cancer Benchmarking Partnership and EUROCARE, the European Cancer Registry, suggest that the survival gap is widening between older and younger patients diagnosed with cancer in Europe.[8–10] There are also worrying indications from within these studies that older patients in the UK may be relatively disadvantaged.[8–11]

Improvements in the care of older patients with cancer will ultimately depend on revisiting the biology underlying cancer in older patients. This is because fundamental biological questions about the relationship between ageing and cancer remain poorly understood, requiring a deeper understanding of processes such as cellular senescence, DNA damage and genomic instability, telomere biology, autophagy, and cellular responses to metabolic and oxidative stress.[12–14] Currently at a clinical practice level, however, it is very clear that older patients are disadvantaged in their access to systemic therapy, radiotherapy and surgery: the main modalities of anticancer therapy.

Systemic therapy in the forms of cytotoxic chemotherapy and biological agents has a role to play in most tumour types. Current evidence, however, suggests that older patients are undertreated, as chronological age remains an independent factor for the use of chemotherapy, even when adjustments are made for comorbidity and frailty. This lack of equity in access and uptake of cancer care may lead to worse outcomes in older cancer patients. For example, more than 70% of cancer deaths occur in men aged over 75 with prostate cancer, yet few older patients receive treatment for localized prostate cancer. In the majority of cases, older patients are denied access to chemotherapy for advanced disease, which if carefully selected can confer benefits with avoidable toxicity.[15] Colorectal cancer is another disease of the older adult, yet again the evidence suggests that optimal therapy is not always being provided to these patients.[16] A significant proportion of older women with triple-negative breast cancer receive less chemotherapy than their younger counterparts, despite the available evidence demonstrating its increased efficacy. Older women may also receive less endocrine therapy than their younger counterparts with breast cancer.[17–19] Specifically in the UK, a National Cancer Equality Initiative (NCEI)/Pharmaceutical Oncology Initiative (POI) joint report concluded that 'clinicians may over rely on chronological age as a proxy for other factors, which are often but not necessarily associated with age, e.g. comorbidities, frailty'.[20] An NHS England publication[21] entitled *Are older people receiving cancer drugs?* (published in 2013) demonstrated considerable variation in the use of systemic anticancer therapy in older people and concluded: 'It does not seem plausible that differences in referral patterns or the age profile of populations served by hospitals could alone explain the variation. The reason for this variation requires further exploration. It seems likely that some variation at least will be caused by the use of age as a proxy for clinical factors, rather than differences in patient health status or preference.'

Despite the importance of appropriate radiation treatment in all cancer patients, including older patients, the uptake of this treatment is relatively low.[22] There are relatively few trials specifically conducted in this population; nonetheless, it is clear that any consideration of radiotherapy in older patients must take into account the altered loco-regional tumour behaviour in older patients with several tumour types, the impact of comorbidities and the impact of diminished functional reserve.[22]

Surgery remains the most important curative modality for cancer patients and is appropriate for many older patients. The evidence to support decision making in this age group remains limited, but Korc-Grodzicki and colleagues[23] have emphasized that 'chronological age alone should not be a determinant for treatment decisions'. Older patients benefit from careful preoperative assessment, which should evaluate functional ability, comorbid conditions, polypharmacy, cognition, nutritional status and frailty in order to determine the risk of adverse events. In some situations, a period of multidisciplinary intervention prior to surgery may improve outcomes. This could include medication review, a cardiopulmonary exercise programme, nutritional supplements or physiotherapy assessment.

Recognizing the disparities that exist for cancer care in older people, the European Organisation for Research and Treatment of Cancer (EORTC) established an EORTC Cancer in the Elderly Task Force, with the stated aim of improving access to clinical trials and research in order to deliver optimum standards of care for the geriatric population. A joint position paper between the EORTC, the Alliance for Clinical Trials in Oncology and the International Society of Geriatric Oncology has recently been published, specifying a roadmap for research and clinical trials in older people and emphasizing the absolute requirement for clinical trials to be without an upper age limit, thus removing a critical barrier for the eligible older patient.[24,25] They also recommend the need for standardized approaches to the measurement of frailty and comorbidity in trials and practice.[24] In the UK, the publication of the NCEI/POI joint report highlighted above[20] has been part of a concerted recent effort to redress the balance in favour of the older cancer patient, culminating in the launch of an 'Action for the Elderly in Cancer' initiative as the main priority of the NCEI at the Britain Against Cancer Conference in London (2014). Although geriatric oncology is beginning to become established as a specialty in North America and Europe, this specialist approach is not yet widely available in the UK.

In older cancer patients, the identification of frailty may be especially important to help guide appropriate, shared decision making, irrespective of what treatment is being considered. Frailty is common in older cancer patients and is independently associated with an increased risk of adverse outcomes, including cancer-related mortality, postoperative complications and poor tolerance of chemotherapy. It has also been identified as a better discriminator of those at risk of adverse outcomes in the surgical and community settings. There are available tools to assess frailty in older patients and inform decisions on therapy, but they are not routinely used in oncology. There is no consensus as to which assessment method should be used to identify frailty in older cancer patients, and a variety of methods have been used in the small number of published trials to date.[26]

In order to make progress, we need a patient-centred, multidisciplinary approach to the care of every older cancer patient. This should not be based solely on chronological age but should also include assessment of frailty, comorbidity and patient choice. Where appropriate, we should develop new treatment approaches that are well tolerated in older people and maximize clinical research activity in older cancer patients. These may include methods to stratify trial participants on the basis of frailty and to maximize the transferability of evidence from trials in younger patients to older populations, for example by appropriate baseline assessment to allow regression-based adjustment; and running parallel observational 'current practice' studies alongside trials. In the absence of evidence from randomized controlled trials, evidence-based medicine has not become routine or possible for many older cancer patients. In some settings, alternatives to randomized trials may become essential. There is a need for the development and application of geriatric decision-making tools and their recognition and routine use in oncology, and to ensure that the principle of early diagnosis (underpinning more effective and less aggressive therapy) is applied in older patients as well as in their younger counterparts.

The provision of individualized treatment to older cancer patients may require upfront expenditure but is likely to provide benefits in terms of improved quality of life and survival, fewer treatment complications and use of resources, and could also help to maintain independence. In order to achieve this, the integration of health and social care services for older cancer patients will be vital. In addition to tailored treatment programmes, we must also consider individual patient preferences and priorities regarding treatment acceptability and tolerability. These are often different in older cancer patients compared with their younger counterparts.

The approaches that are developed towards managing cancer in older people will have a profound impact on future cancer policy and outcomes. While cancer survivorship is increasing overall, with the most recent figures indicating 11.7 million cancer survivors in the USA and nearly 14 million in Europe, the percentage is lower in older people compared with the overall population. Thus, cancer survivorship may plateau, or even decline, unless we develop better approaches for the management of older cancer patients.

References

1 Lawler M, Selby P, Aapro M, *et al.* Ageism in cancer care; we need to change our mindset. *BMJ* 2014; 348: g1614.

2 Lichtman SM, Hurria A, Jacobsen PB. Geriatric oncology: an overview. *J Clin Oncol* 2014; 32: 2521–2.

3 *Global AgeWatch Index. Insight report.* London: HelpAge International, 2014. Available from: www.helpage.org/global-agewatch (accessed 8 April 2015).

4 Turner NJ, Haward RA, Mulley GP, *et al.* Cancer in old age – is it inadequately investigated and treated? *BMJ* 1999; 319: 309–12.

5 United States Census Bureau (2014). *2014 National population projections.* Available from: www.census.gov/population/projections/data/national/2014.html (accessed 9 November 2013).

6 European Commission, Economic Policy Committee. *The 2009 ageing report: economic and budgetary projections for the EU-27 member states (2008–2060).* Luxembourg: Office for Official Publications of the European Communities, 2009.

7 Mistry M, Parkin D, Ahmad A, *et al.* Cancer incidence in the United Kingdom: projections to the year 2030. *Br J Cancer* 2011; 105: 1795–803.

8 Coleman MP, Forman D, Bryant H, *et al.* Cancer survival in Australia, Canada, Denmark, Norway, Sweden, and the UK, 1995–2007 (the International Cancer Benchmarking Partnership): an analysis of population-based cancer registry data. *Lancet* 2011; 377: 127–38.

9 Quaglia A, Tavilla A, Shack L, *et al.* The cancer survival gap between elderly and middle-aged patients in Europe is widening. *Eur J Cancer* 2009; 45: 1006–16.

10 De Angelis R, Sant M, Coleman MP, *et al.* Cancer survival in Europe 1999–2007 by country and age: results of EUROCARE-5 – a population-based study. *Lancet Oncol* 2014; 15: 23–34.

11 Hall P, Handforth C, Spencer K, *et al.* Age as an independent predictor of chemotherapy treatment decisions in 20 common cancers. *J Clin Oncol* 2014; 32 (5 suppl): abstract 9550.

12 Collado M, Blasco MA, Serrano M. Cellular senescence in cancer and aging. *Cell* 2007; 130: 223–33.

13 Finkel T, Serrano M, Blasco MA. The common biology of cancer and ageing. *Nature* 2007; 448: 767–74.

14 Falandry C, Bonnefoy M, Freyer G, Gilson E. Biology of cancer and aging: a complex association with cellular senescence. *J Clin Oncol* 2014; 32: 2604–10.

15 Fung C, Dale W, Mohile SG. Prostate cancer in the elderly patient. *J Clin Oncol* 2014; 32: 2523–30.

16 McCleary NJ, Dotan E, Browner I. Refining the chemotherapy approach for older patients with colon cancer. *J Clin Oncol* 2014; 32: 2570–80.

17 Aapro M, Wildiers H. Triple-negative breast cancer in the older population. *Ann Oncol* 2012; 23 (suppl 6): vi52–5.

18 Tew WP, Muss HB, Kimmick GG, *et al.* Breast and ovarian cancer in the older woman. *J Clin Oncol* 2014; 32: 2553–61.

19 Hershman DL, Shao T, Kushi LH, *et al.* Early discontinuation and non-adherence to adjuvant hormonal therapy are associated with increased mortality in women with breast cancer. *Breast Cancer Res Treat* 2011; 126: 529–37.

20 Department of Health. *The impact of patient age on decision making in oncology.* London: Department of Health, 2012.

21 NHS England. *Are older people receiving cancer drugs? An analysis of patterns in cancer drug delivery according to the age of patient.* Available from: www.england.nhs.uk/wp-content/uploads/2013/12/old-people-rec-cancer-drugs.pdf (accessed 8 June 2015).

22 Smith GL, Smith BD. Radiation treatment in older patients: a framework for clinical decision making. *J Clin Oncol* 2014; 32: 2669–78.

23 Korc-Grodzicki B, Downey RJ, Shahrokni A, *et al.* Surgical considerations in older adults with cancer. *J Clin Oncol* 2014; 32: 2647–53.

24 Wildiers H, Mauer M, Pallis A, *et al.* End points and trial design in geriatric oncology research: a joint European Organisation for Research and Treatment of Cancer–Alliance for Clinical Trials in Oncology–International Society of Geriatric Oncology position article. *J Clin Oncol* 2013; 31: 3711–18.

25 Hurria A, Dale W, Mooney M, *et al.* Designing therapeutic clinical trials for older and frail adults with cancer: U13 conference recommendations. *J Clin Oncol* 2014; 32: 2587–94.

26 Handforth C, Clegg A, Young C, *et al.* The prevalence and outcomes of frailty in older cancer patients: a systematic review. *Ann Oncol* 2015; 26: 1091–101.

02 Clinical Epidemiology and Patterns of Care for Cancer in Older Patients

Rebecca J. Birch, Katie L. Spencer, Eva J.A. Morris

Background

Cancer is predominantly a disease of older people. With an ageing population, this poses a major challenge to healthcare systems. In 1985, around 15% of the UK population was over the age of 65, but by 2010 this proportion had increased, by an additional 1.7 million people, to 17% of the population.[1] This trend is set to continue, and it is projected that by 2035 more than 23% of the population will be over 65.[1]

Cancer incidence is highest in older people, with 63% of all cancers diagnosed in those aged 65 or over.[2] Figure 2.1 shows the increasing incidence of cancer in individuals aged 65 and over between 1971 and 2009. It is anticipated that there will continue to be large increases in the number of older people diagnosed with cancer over the forthcoming decades.[2] By 2040, it is estimated that almost a quarter of people over the age of 65 will have experienced the disease (amounting to 4.1 million people).[3] As such, ensuring that high-quality services are available to care for this rapidly growing population is a major challenge for healthcare providers.

The scale of the challenge is compounded when it is considered alongside current concerns that those diagnosed in older age groups are experiencing inequalities and inequities in both their care and prognosis.[4-6] These anxieties have been heightened by international comparisons repeatedly showing that the 5 year cancer survival rates attained in the UK lag behind those of many economically comparable countries, due to poorer outcomes for older patients.[7-11] There is also a growing body of evidence suggesting that older patients are undertreated and do not have access to the best care.[7] Improving outcomes for older patients has, therefore, become a priority; but, before steps can be taken to reduce the deficits, it is important to understand how they have arisen. The available evidence suggests that a number of factors, across the entire care pathway, may be responsible.

Diagnosis and presentation

First, there appear to be differences in relation to diagnosis and presentation.[6,12] The best outcomes for solid tumours are achieved when individuals are diagnosed with early-stage disease.[13] It is unfortunate, therefore, that it appears that a greater proportion of older patients present with advanced disease compared with younger patients.[14,15]

A greater proportion of older patients also present as emergencies.[16] A national population-based study of all cancer patients over a 5 year period in England identified that 15% of those under the age of 50 had presented as an emergency, which rose to 43% in those over 85.[16] A recent systematic review confirmed this effect for lung and colorectal cancer.[12] Emergency presentation is known to be associated with a more advanced stage of cancer;[16] however, even after adjustment for this, there remain poorer outcomes[17] and lower rates of treatment with curative intent.[18]

Colorectal, lung and prostate cancer

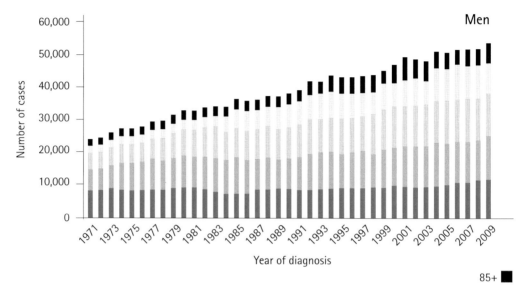

Colorectal, lung and breast cancer

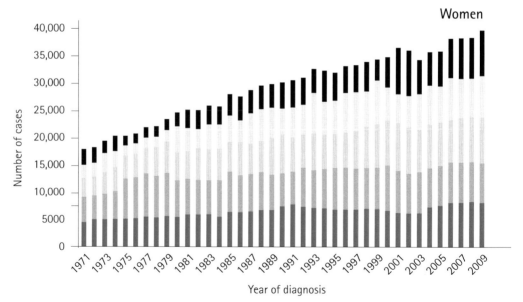

Figure 2.1 Registrations in England, between 1971 and 2009, of newly diagnosed colorectal, lung and prostate cancers in men, and of newly diagnosed colorectal, lung and breast cancers in women (adapted from Sinha et al.[56]).

Reasons behind these differing diagnostic pathways in older people are not fully understood but may include lack of awareness of cancer symptoms, differing symptomatology, lack of social support and variation in help-seeking behaviour.

Management

After diagnosis, age-related differences persist in the management of cancer. Surgery is the main curative treatment option for the majority of individuals with solid tumours, but it appears that surgical intervention rates are significantly reduced in older people.[6,19-21] Similarly, age-related inequalities are apparent in the use of both chemotherapy[5,6,22] and radiotherapy.[6] This variation in practice has caused significant concern and led some to argue that older people are facing discrimination and being denied access to potentially curative treatment.[4] However, this variation in treatment may be clinically appropriate.[23-26] Two of the most important confounding factors may be the presence of comorbid disease and frailty, both of which are known to increase with age (Figure 2.2).[27-32] Both can reduce physiological reserve, increasing the complexity of cancer management and potentially making individuals unsuitable for treatment. Studies have suggested that, whilst some older patients may not be fit enough for standard treatment, they may benefit from adapted treatment regimens.[33-36] Quantifying the impact of these factors is vitally important to assess whether true inequities exist, but it is also extremely difficult with the population-based data currently available.

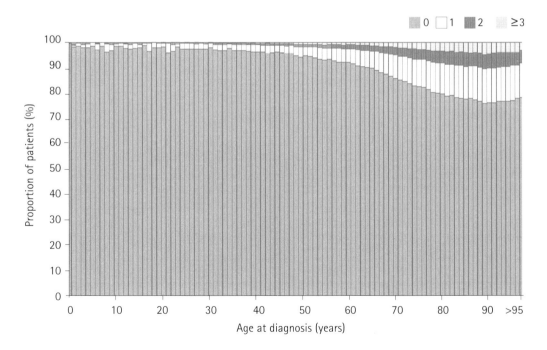

Figure 2.2 Charlson Comorbidity Index scores of patients diagnosed with cancer in England between 2006 and 2010 (all cancers excluding non-melanoma skin cancer). Diagnostic data for comorbidities provided by inpatient Hospital Episode Statistics records, matched at a patient level to cancer registration records and supplied by the National Cancer Registration Service (www.ncr.nhs.uk).

Comorbidity and frailty

Objective tools to measure burden of comorbidity are available. The Charlson Comorbidity Index[37] and Elixhauser Comorbidity Measure[38] have been used to quantify levels of comorbidity using routinely available data. They tend, however, to capture only the more severe illnesses and, consequently, only provide a relatively crude indicator of the extent of any concomitant illness.[39,40] Epidemiological studies using these indices tend to suggest, therefore, that comorbidity does not explain all the age-related variation in care observed.[41] More rigorous population-based comorbidity data are required to determine whether this variation is inequitable.

The situation is similar with respect to frailty. To date, no national epidemiological analyses have been able to assess the contribution of frailty to age-related variation in care and outcome. A number of frailty indices exist,[42] but none are available that enable the extent of the condition to be quantified via routine data at a population level. Higher resolution prospective studies have assessed comorbidity and functional status in greater depth; however, despite this, variation in treatment with chronological age persists.[43] Frailty is such an important factor to consider in analyses that further evidence quantifying its presence across the population is urgently needed.

Outcomes

Survival

Age-related differences in management pathways exist in parallel with significant age-related differences in outcome. The best indicator of the effectiveness of a cancer care system is the survival of the individuals it treats. Unfortunately, when comparing survival rates across age groups, both within the UK[44] and internationally,[8,11,45–47] significant differences are observed. In England, after adjusting for deaths due to other causes, the lowest overall 5 year cancer survival rate is observed in those over the age of 80.[48] Again, many factors may contribute to these outcome differences, including underlying differences in tumour biology and patient behaviour, lower active treatment rates and differing levels of comorbidity and frailty. To determine the true extent of any age-related inequalities or inequities it is important to gain a better understanding of how these factors interact with age.

Patient experience and quality of life

Whilst there are undoubtedly lower treatment rates in older people, NHS England's National Cancer Patient Experience Survey suggests that older patients actually report, overall, a more positive experience of their care compared with younger patients.[49] These annual patient experience surveys have indicated that older age groups were more likely to feel they had been treated with dignity and respect and felt their views were taken into consideration when making treatment decisions.[49] By no means were all the aspects of care included in the survey found to be better in the older age groups: for example, the proportion of older people who felt they had adequate information about side effects was lower than for younger ages, but generally the older English cancer population report a good patient experience.

Another area of cancer care where there are fewer obvious inequalities with respect to older people is around the health-related quality of life of survivors. Large surveys using population-based sampling approaches suggest that older people actually report better health-related quality of life than those in the youngest age groups.[50,51] Again, understanding exactly what is driving these differences is complex, as many of the factors strongly predictive of a worse health-related quality of life are correlated with increasing age. Further evidence is again, therefore, required to fully understand the relationship and ensure that the needs of the growing population of older cancer survivors are met.

Clinical trials

The best medical evidence via which to determine this, and, hence, generate the gold standard treatment pathways for older patients, would be derived from randomized controlled trials. Unfortunately, however, older people are often underrepresented in such studies and, as a result, the current evidence base to inform optimal cancer management in older people is somewhat limited.[27,52,53] Furthermore, the individuals entered into such studies, particularly those who are older, may not be entirely representative of the population at large, as trials tend to recruit younger, more affluent people with better prognosis disease and low levels of comorbidity and frailty.[54] So, again, extrapolating the findings of these studies to inform the optimal management of the older population may be misleading. Assessment of treatment benefit in older people tends, therefore, to rely on data gathered from observational studies. However, the analysis of such observational data to generate robust conclusions is methodologically difficult. Failure to consider or make adjustment for confounding variables can lead to biased results. A recent systematic review determined that such methodological mistakes were common.[55]

Conclusion

 It is clear that major differences exist, at a population level, in both cancer management and outcomes in older people. The currently available epidemiological evidence would strongly suggest that care is inequitable, but, in the absence of stronger data on many of the poor prognostic factors (such as stage, emergency presentation, comorbidity and frailty) correlated with age, it is difficult to draw firm conclusions. Further evidence is, therefore, urgently needed. It must be borne in mind, however, that epidemiology is the study of disease in a population and not individuals. Every person is different and healthcare providers must seek to ensure that they do not make assumptions about any individual's ability to withstand treatment or their personal preferences simply based on chronological age. In this way true inequities in care can be eliminated.

References

1 Office for National Statistics (2012). *Population ageing in the United Kingdom, its constituent countries and the European Union*. Available from: www.ons.gov.uk/ons/dcp171776_258607. pdf (accessed 22 June 2015).

2 Mistry M, Parkin DM, Ahmad AS, Sasieni P. Cancer incidence in the United Kingdom: projections to the year 2030. *Br J Cancer* 2011; 105: 1795–803.

3 Maddams J, Utley M, Moller H. Projections of cancer prevalence in the United Kingdom 2010–2040. *Br J Cancer* 2015; 107: 1195–202.

4 Macmillan Cancer Support. *The age old excuse: the under treatment of older cancer patients*. London: Macmillan Cancer Support, 2015.

5 Haematological Malignancy Research Network. *Patient's age and treatment for haematological malignancy: a report from the Haematologixal Malignancy Research Network (HMRN)*. York: Haematological Malignancy Research Network, 2014.

6   National Cancer Intelligence Network. *Older people and cancer*. London: Public Health England, 2015.

7   Allemani C, Weir HK, Carreira H, *et al*. Global surveillance of cancer survival 1995–2009: analysis of individual data for 25,676,997 patients from 279 population-based registries in 67 countries (CONCORD-2). *Lancet* 2014; 385: 977–1010.

8   Coleman MP, Forman D, Bryant H, *et al*. Cancer survival in Australia, Canada, Denmark, Norway, Sweden and the UK, 1995–2007 (the International Cancer Benchmarking Partnership): an analysis of population-based cancer registry data. *Lancet* 2011; 377: 127–38.

9   Holmberg L, Sandin F, Bray F, *et al*. National comparisons of lung cancer survival in England, Norway and Sweden 2001–2004: differences occur early in follow-up. *Thorax* 2010; 65: 436–41.

10 Moller H, Sandin F, Bray F, *et al*. Breast cancer survival in England, Norway and Sweden: a population-based comparison. *Int J Cancer* 2010; 127: 2638.

11 Morris EJ, Sandin F, Lambert PC, *et al*. A population-based comparison of the survival of patients with colorectal cancer in England, Norway and Sweden between 1996 and 2004. *Gut* 2011; 60: 1087–93.

12 Mitchell ED, Pickwell-Smith B, Macleod U. Risk factors for emergency presentation with lung and colorectal cancers: a systematic review. *BMJ Open* 2015; 5: e006965.

13 National Cancer Intelligence Network. *Cancer survival in England by stage*. London: Public Health England, 2014.

14 Lyratzopoulos G, Abel GA, Brown CH, *et al*. Socio-demographic inequalities in stage of cancer diagnosis: evidence from patients with female breast, lung, colon, rectal, prostate, renal, bladder, melanoma, ovarian and endometrial cancer. *Ann Oncol* 2013; 24: 843–50.

15 Lyratzopoulos G, Greenberg DC, Rubin GP, *et al*. Advanced stage diagnosis of cancer: who is at greater risk? *Exp Rev Anticancer Ther* 2012; 12: 993.

16 Elliss-Brookes L, McPhail S, Ives A, *et al*. Routes to diagnosis for cancer: determining the patient journey using multiple routine data sets. *Br J Cancer* 2012; 107: 1220–6.

17 McPhail S, Elliss-Brookes L, Shelton J, *et al*. Emergency presentation of cancer and short-term mortality. *Br J Cancer* 2013; 109: 2027–34.

18 Palser TR, Cromwell DA, Hardwick RH, *et al*. Impact of route to diagnosis on treatment intent and 1-year survival in patients diagnosed with oesophagogastric cancer in England: a prospective cohort study. *BMJ Open* 2013; 3: e002129.

19 Colorectal Cancer Collaborative Group. Surgery for colorectal cancer in elderly patients: a systematic review. *Lancet* 2000; 356: 968–74.

20 Louwman WJ, Vulto JCM, Verhoeven RHA, *et al*. Clinical epidemiology of breast cancer in the elderly. *Eur J Cancer* 2007; 43: 2242–52.

21 Simmonds PD, Best L, George S, *et al*. Surgery for colorectal cancer in elderly patients: a systematic review. *Lancet* 2000; 356: 968–74.

22 NHS England (2013). *Are older people receiving cancer drugs? An analysis of patterns in cancer drug delivery according to the age of patient*. Available from: www.england.nhs.uk/wp-content/uploads/2013/12/old-people-rec-cancer-drugs.pdf (accessed 30 March 2015).

23 Puts MTE, Tapscott B, Fitch M, *et al.* A systematic review of factors influencing older adults' decision to accept or decline cancer treatment. *Cancer Treat Rev* 2015; 41: 197–215.

24 Fentiman IS, Tirelli U, Monfardini S, *et al.* Cancer in the elderly: why so badly treated? *Lancet* 1990; 335: 1020–2.

25 Fentiman IS. Are the elderly receiving appropriate treatment for cancer? *Ann Oncol* 1996; 7: 657–8.

26 National Cancer Equality Initiative, Pharmaceutical Oncology Initiative (2012). *The impact of patient age on clinical decision-making in oncology.* Available from: file:///C:/Users/user/Downloads/NCAT_DH_ImpactAgeOnco_FINAL.pdf (accessed 21 June 2015).

27 Townsley CA, Selby R, Siu LL. Systematic review of barriers to the recruitment of older patients with cancer on to clinical trials. *J Clin Oncol* 2005; 23: 3112–24.

28 Extermann M. Measurement and impact of comorbidity in older cancer patients. *Crit Rev Oncol Hematol* 2000; 35: 181–200.

29 Audisio RA, Bozzetti F, Gennari R, *et al.* The surgical management of elderly cancer patients: recommendations of the SIOG surgical task force. *Eur J Cancer* 2004; 40: 926–38.

30 Janssen-Heijnen ML, Maas HA, Houterman S, *et al.* Comorbidity in older surgical cancer patients: influence on patient care and outcome. *Eur J Cancer* 2007; 43: 2179–93.

31 Yancik R, Ganz PA, Varricchio CG, Conley B. Perspectives on comorbidity and cancer in older patients: approaches to expand the knowledge base. *J Clin Oncol* 2001; 19: 1147–51.

32 Handforth C, Clegg A, Young C, *et al.* The prevalence and outcomes of frailty in older cancer patients: a systematic review. *Ann Oncol* 2015; 26: 1091–101.

33 Kim JH. Chemotherapy for colorectal cancer in the elderly. *World J Gastroenterol* 2015; 21: 5158.

34 Lichtman SM, Wildiers H, Launay-Vacher V, *et al.* International Society of Geriatric Oncology (SIOG) recommendations for the adjustment of dosing in elderly cancer patients with renal insufficiency. *Eur J Cancer* 2007; 43: 14–34.

35 Extermann M, Chen H, Cantor AB, *et al.* Predictors of tolerance to chemotherapy in older cancer patients: a prospective pilot study. *Eur J Cancer* 2002; 38: 1466–73.

36 Kasenda B, Ferreri AJ, Marturano E, *et al.* First-line treatment and outcome of elderly patients with primary central nervous system lymphoma (PCNSL) – a systematic review and individual patient data meta-analysis. *Ann Oncol* 2015; 26: 1305–13.

37 Charlson ME, Pompei P, Ales KL, MacKenzie CR. A new method of classifying prognostic comorbidity in longitudinal studies: development and validation. *J Chronic Dis* 1987; 40: 373–83.

38 Elixhauser A, Steiner C, Harris RD, Coffey RM. Comorbidity measures for use with administrative data. *Med Care* 1998; 36: 8–27.

39 de Groot V, Beckerman H, Lankhorst GJ, Bouter LM. How to measure comorbidity: a critical review of available methods. *J Clin Epidemiol* 2003; 56: 221–9.

40 Humphries KH, Rankin JM, Carere RG, *et al.* Co-morbidity data in outcomes research. Are clinical data derived from administrative databases a reliable alternative to chart review? *J Clin Epidemiol* 2000; 53: 343–9.

41 Lavelle K, Downing A, Thomas J, *et al.* Are lower rates of surgery amongst older women with breast cancer in the UK explained by comorbidity? *Br J Cancer* 2012; 107: 1175–80.

42 Bouillon K, Kivimaki M, Hamer M, *et al.* Measures of frailty in population-based studies: an overview. *BMC Geriatr* 2013; 13: 64.

43 Lavelle K, Sowerbutts AM, Bundred N, *et al.* Is lack of surgery for older breast cancer patients in the UK explained by patient choice or poor health? A prospective cohort study. *Br J Cancer* 2014; 110: 573–83.

44 Office for National Statistics (2014). *Cancer survival in England: adults diagnosed 2008 to 2012, followed up to 2013*. Available from: www.ons.gov.uk/ons/rel/cancer-unit/cancer-survival-in-england--adults-diagnosed/2008-to-2012--followed-up-to-2013/stb-cancer-survival.html (accessed 21 June 2015).

45 Maringe C, Walters S, Rachet B, *et al.* Stage at diagnosis and colorectal cancer survival in six high-income countries: a population-based study of patients diagnosed during 2000–2007. *Acta Oncol* 2013; 52: 919–32.

46 Walters S, Maringe C, Butler J, *et al.* Breast cancer survival and stage at diagnosis in Australia, Canada, Denmark, Norway, Sweden and the UK, 2000–2007: a population-based study. *Br J Cancer* 2013; 108: 1195–208.

47 De Angelis R, Sant M, Coleman MP, *et al.* Cancer survival in Europe 1999–2007 by country and age: results of EUROCARE-5 – a population-based study. *Lancet Oncol* 2014; 15: 23–34.

48 Vercelli M, Capocaccia R, Quaglia A, *et al.* Relative survival in elderly European cancer patients: evidence for health care inequalities. *Crit Rev Oncol Hematol* 2000; 35: 161–79.

49 Quality Health. *2010 national cancer patient experience survey.* London: Quality Health, 2010.

50 Downing A, Morris EJ, Richards M, *et al.* Health-related quality of life after colorectal cancer in England: a patient-reported outcomes study of individuals 12 to 36 months after diagnosis. *J Clin Oncol* 2015; 33: 616–24.

51 Glaser A, Fraser L, Corner J, *et al.* Patient-reported outcomes of cancer survivors in England 1–5 years after diagnosis: a cross-sectional survey. *BMJ Open* 2013; 3: e002317.

52 Aapro MS, Köhne CH, Cohen HJ, Extermann M. Never too old? Age should not be a barrier to enrollment in cancer clinical trials. *Oncologist* 2005; 10: 198–204.

53 Murthy VH, Krumholz HM, Gross CP. Participation in cancer clinical trials: race-, sex-, and age-based disparities. *JAMA* 2004; 291: 2720–6.

54 Morris EJA, Jordan C, Thomas JD, *et al.* Comparison of treatment and outcome information between a clinical trial and the National Cancer Data Repository. *Br J Surg* 2011; 98: 299–307.

55 de Glas NA, Kiderlen M, de Craen AJM, *et al.* Assessing treatment effects in older breast cancer patients: systematic review of observational research methods. *Cancer Treat Rev* 2015; 41: 254–61.

56 Sinha R, Coyle C, Stokoe J, Ring A. New registrations of prostate, breast, colorectal and lung cancer in patients aged 65 and over in England, 1971–2009. Presented at: 12th conference of the International Society of Geriatric Oncology, Manchester, UK, 25–27 October 2012.

03 Improving Care for Older Cancer Patients in the NHS

Sean Duffy, Mike Birtwistle

NHS cancer services are improving. We are diagnosing more patients before their cancer has spread and providing more effective treatments delivered by expert teams. The experience reported by patients is increasingly positive and we know more about how to support people in living well after a diagnosis of cancer. There is much reason for encouragement and it is right that we celebrate the progress that has been made. Yet there is no room for complacency. Our outcomes are still not as good as in some national comparator countries, and the needs of cancer patients are changing. Worryingly, our outcomes appear to be poorer in the demographic group in which cancer will increase the most: older people. Cancer is predominantly a disease of older age and our population is ageing. More people will be diagnosed with cancer and their needs will be more complex.

Nearly two-thirds of cancer diagnoses occur in the over-65s and one-third in people aged 75 and over. In 2012, over 102,000 people over the age of 75 were diagnosed with cancer. Nearly 32,000 of them were over the age of 85.[1] By 2020 there will be nearly two million people aged 65 and over alive following a diagnosis of cancer. The growing impact of cancer in older people is reflected in the demand for cancer services. More than a quarter of all admitted episodes for cancer in England occur in the over-75s.[2] In the past decade, the increase in admissions in this group has far outstripped the increase observed for cancer patients of all ages.

Today's cancer services, however, were largely designed in the 1990s, a time when the average age of cancer patients was significantly younger. We are now faced with a choice: we can seek to perfect the existing model of cancer care or we can redesign cancer services to better meet the needs of older people. We firmly believe that we must take the latter approach, both so that we may achieve the best outcomes and make the best use of the resources available to us.

The needs of older people are not uniform, just as they are not for any group in society. The nature of malignancy, socioeconomic status, sex and ethnicity all play a role in shaping people's needs and outcomes. Equally, the needs of active older people in otherwise good health will be very different from those of people living with frailty and other health conditions. Yet there is evidence to suggest that older people appear to experience poorer outcomes. Older people are more likely to be diagnosed with cancer following an emergency admission, which diminishes their chances of long-term survival. They also experience poorer survival after diagnosis with a cancer that has already spread. Seeking to make earlier diagnosis in older people should be a major priority. We need to increase awareness of signs and symptoms of cancer, but we also need to increase motivation to seek help. Fear of cancer and the consequences of treatment may inhibit some people from seeking help. For older people, perhaps scarred by memories of old-fashioned cancer treatment received by friends or loved ones, this may be particularly potent. We need to better understand the factors that can lead to late diagnosis in older people.

We know that older patients are also less likely to receive active cancer treatment, be it surgery, radiotherapy or cancer drugs. In some cases, there will be good reasons for this. Frailty and other issues can reduce a person's ability to tolerate treatment and can result in an unacceptable impact on quality of life. Older people may also opt not to receive treatment. Yet we know that treatment plays a vital role in improving outcomes. It is implausible that the reduction in treatment rates can be explained by patient comorbidities or patient preference alone, and factors that depend on professional attitudes are likely to play a part.

The social context for older people is relevant to the cancer care they might receive. Half of all people aged 75 and over live alone, and one in 10 people have less than monthly contact with friends, family and neighbours. Isolation can be particularly difficult when a person is receiving ongoing treatment.[3] Furthermore, one in five people aged 75 and over state they find it very difficult to get to their local hospital.[4] Caring responsibilities can also reduce the probability of people accepting treatment: over half a million people aged 65 and over have caring responsibilities that take up at least 20 h per week.[5] It is necessary to assess whether a patient is physically and mentally able to tolerate treatment and whether a patient has the right social and care support in place to help him or her recover.

Overall, older people report a positive experience of cancer treatment and care. NHS services should be congratulated on their continued efforts to improve patient experience. In particular, older patients are more likely to report confidence in doctors and nurses and feel that they were treated with dignity and respect. Patient experience surveys nonetheless also identify areas for improvement. In particular, older people are less likely to have access to a clinical nurse specialist or report being given information on side effects of treatment. These issues are particularly concerning given that older people are more likely to have other health issues which will impact on their quality of life during and after treatment and which may necessitate enhanced support.

For older people with cancer who are near the end of their life, there are substantial variations in the length of time they spend in hospital, suggesting that some areas of the country are better than others in supporting people in the community. There is substantial scope to improve both the quality and efficiency of care in this respect.

Older people are less likely to have the chance to participate in cancer research, meaning that opportunities to develop the evidence base on how best to treat older people are missed. This not only potentially hinders their care but also compromises our ability to do the very best for future patients. As clinicians we should lament the absence of evidence on treatment in older people without doing everything we can to address it, including seeking to involve a greater number of older people in clinical trials and studies.

One estimate suggests that, if the UK matched US levels of survival for the over-75s, then 14,000 lives could be saved.[6] Yet the outcomes we seek for older people should go beyond survival. Ensuring we treat older people safely and that we do all we can to protect their quality of life and help them recover from treatment as quickly and fully as possible are also important, as is doing what we can to ensure a positive experience of cancer care. There is also a strong economic argument for improving the way in which we support older people affected by cancer. There is nothing as inefficient as a treatment that is ineffective, so we must do more to ensure that the treatment we do provide delivers the outcomes that matter most to older people. Effective, tailored treatment can prevent recurrences or further spread of cancer and can also help to maintain a person's independence. Treatment for earlier stage cancer is less expensive than treatment for advanced disease.[7] We must therefore do more to ensure that older people are diagnosed before their cancer has spread.

Age alone should never be a barrier to treatment, but asserting this is easier than removing the barriers that do exist. These barriers are not about funding or access to services: that would be illegal. They are, unfortunately, far more problematic to address than that. Any clinical decision will be influenced by a range of factors in a clinician's life: his or her own attitudes, training, the service context, as well as previous experiences. On each of these issues, there is more that we can do to help our clinicians.

We should therefore do more to help clinicians assess a person's suitability for treatment, take steps to address factors that might limit the effectiveness of a treatment and, where necessary, tailor treatment options to suit a person's circumstances. Support needs to start with training, but we also need to support the existing workforce in managing older people more effectively. Furthermore, we must join up the medical aspects of care with the wider social factors that will impact on a person's cancer journey. To ignore either is to risk failing our patients when they need us the most. Of course, not all of these factors are in the direct control of cancer clinicians, but we need to look beyond the immediate issues we confront in our clinics and consider the whole picture.

References

1   National Cancer Intelligence Network. *Cancer and equality groups: key metrics – 2014 report.* London: Public Health England, 2014. Available from: www.ncin.org.uk/ view?rid=2697 (accessed 6 June 2015).

2   Health and Social Care Information Centre (2013). *Hospital episode statistics, inpatient statistics by primary diagnosis, 2012/13.* Available from: www.hscic.gov.uk/ catalogue/ PUB12566/hosp-epis-stat-admi-diag-2012-13-tab.xlsx (accessed 6 June 2015).

3   Office for National Statistics (2012). *General lifestyle survey overview* (Table 3.3). Available from: www.ons.gov.uk/ons/rel/ghs/general-lifestyle-survey/2010/general-lifestyle-survey-overview-report-2010.pdf (accessed 6 June 2015).

4   Department for Communities and Local Government (2008). *Housing in England 2006/07: a report based on the 2006/07 survey of English housing* (Table 7.6). Available from: http:// webarchive.nationalarchives.gov.uk/20121108165934/http://www.communities.gov.uk/ publications/corporate/statistics/housingengland2006-07 (accessed 6 June 2015).

5   Office for National Statistics, Department of Work and Pensions (2012). *Family resources survey, United Kingdom 2010/11.* Available from: www.gov.uk/government/ uploads/ system/ uploads/attachment_data/file/222839/ frs_2010_11_report.pdf (accessed 6 June 2015).

6   Moller H, Flatt G, Moran A. Higher cancer mortality rates in the elderly in the UK. *Cancer Epidemiol* 2011; 35: 407–12.

7   Incisive Health (2014) *Saving lives, averting costs. An analysis of the financial implications of achieving earlier diagnosis of colorectal, lung and ovarian cancer.* Available from: www.incisivehealth.com/uploads/Saving lives averting costs.pdf (accessed 6 June 2015).

04 Strategies to Improve Outcomes for Older Cancer Patients: Learning from the Improving Cancer Treatment Assessment and Support for Older People Project

Jane Maher

Introduction

Cancer is primarily a disease of older age.[1] There are now more than 130,000 people living with cancer in the UK who have survived at least 10 years after being diagnosed at age 65 or over, including 8000 diagnosed with cancer at 80 years or over.[2] Six in 10 new cases each year in the UK occur in those aged 65 or over,[3] and 13% of the total UK population aged 65 or over have been diagnosed with cancer at some point in their life.[4] However, the relative 5 year survival of this group in the UK is 14% lower than the European average.[5]

While UK patients appear to present with cancer at a later stage than in comparable countries, there are concerns that they do not access effective cancer treatments to the same extent as comparable younger patients. A survey of 101 UK oncologists found that while 81% would prescribe chemotherapy for a high-risk breast cancer patient aged 68, only 47% would recommend the same treatment for an otherwise identical patient aged 73.[6] There are a range of possible explanations for this, including: inappropriate assessment of fitness for treatment; lack of support for older people before, during and after treatment; and inadequate training of clinical and non-clinical staff in relation to issues more common in older people, such as falls, incontinence, multi-drug use, and sensory and cognitive impairment.

Older people with cancer increasingly have more than one other comorbidity: one US study reported an average of three comorbidities in cancer survivors aged 70 years and above,[7] and one in three older people have existing problems with medication prior to cancer treatment.[8] Antihypertensive medication, in particular, is frequently associated with dizziness, falls and renal impairment. Over 70% of those over 70 have a hearing impairment,[9] which may be confused with cognitive impairment, complicating communication about treatment choices. Older patients living alone are less likely to accept cancer treatment,[10] and people who have more fragile social support networks are not as likely to make favourable treatment decisions.[11] One in five of those aged over 75 state it is difficult to get to their local hospital,[12] and lack of transportation affects acceptance of treatment. In 2011, 14% of older people living in households in England and Wales provided unpaid care: the largest increase in proportion was for those aged 65 and over, who provided ≥50 h/week of unpaid care.[13] Ahead of all other types of care, grandparents were the main child care arrangement for 35% of families where the mother was working or studying when the child was 9 months old.[14] Older people may defer management of their own health issues because of such responsibilities.

Of course, overtreatment can be as inappropriate as undertreatment. As well as a lack of older people in cancer treatment clinical trials, there is a dearth of routinely collected data about life quality in the months and years following treatment. While treatment may initially be tolerated in the majority of cases, small changes in cognitive function, continence and mobility may significantly affect longer term quality of life. Persistent treatment-related symptoms such as fatigue are particularly tough for older people with some physical limitations[15] and can be unexpectedly difficult to manage, even for the previously fit, who report losing confidence in their physical and mental abilities. Lack of such data can make informed decision making a challenge.

Oncologists and cancer surgeons have highlighted that they need more support to both recognize and manage medical issues specific to older people in general: in a survey of 98 UK oncology trainees, 60% reported that they had never received any training in the particular needs of older people with cancer.[16]

What could make a difference?

Elderly care specialists are experienced in co-managing multiple health conditions and polypharmacy, as well as engaging and mobilizing a range of community-based health and social services to provide practical support, but they are rarely involved in decision making related to cancer treatment.

An evidence-based assessment approach such as Comprehensive Geriatric Assessment (CGA) can help ensure more people are assessed for treatment based on their general fitness, not their chronological age,[1] but CGA is not used routinely in oncology multidisciplinary team (MDT) assessments.

The voluntary sector in the UK plays an important role in the management of older people, providing direct services such as assessment of practical needs, financial advice, befriending, transport, assistance with household tasks and correspondence, signposting and coordinating care, but their role in supporting cancer patients during and after treatment is currently limited in that many clinicians do not routinely tell their patients about these services.

There are, however, a number of drivers for change. The provisions contained within the Equality Act 2010,[17] which prohibits age discrimination, were extended to public services in 2012 to ensure that there is no discrimination in the delivery of health services to older people with cancer.

A series of cancer experience surveys have demonstrated that older people are less likely to be offered the name of a clinical nurse specialist, provided with understandable written information about side effects, or directed to sources of financial help or support for self-help.[18]

Clinicians have reported that they do not have enough information to assess older patients in order to make informed decisions about cancer treatment options. Issues such as lack of practical and social support at home, and management of comorbidities and multiple medications, can be barriers to receiving the most effective cancer treatment.

The value of comprehensive assessment, including: medical assessment (problems from the patient's perspective: comorbidity, medication, nutrition); functioning (activities of daily living); psychological (mood and cognition); social (informal care resources, financial); and environmental (home safety, telehealth, transport), has been demonstrated in a Cochrane systematic review of a CGA approach.[19] Data from this review suggested a reduction in early re-hospitalization as a result of CGA,[20] with a higher likelihood of being both alive and living at home a year after treatment if CGA were used in hospital.[19] CGA can benefit older people at any point in their cancer journey, including into survivorship beyond treatment completion when they may be struggling with the chronic consequences of cancer and cancer treatment.

Improving Cancer Treatment Assessment and Support for Older People Project

In 2010, the Improving Cancer Treatment Assessment and Support for Older People Project was set up in partnership between the Department of Health and the charities Macmillan Cancer Support and Age UK. Its findings were reported in 2012.[21] The aims of the project were to 'improve cancer outcomes by increasing access to appropriate cancer treatment for people aged 70 and over' by:

- Testing new methods of clinical assessment based around CGA as the gold standard.
- Coordinating and delivering packages of practical support during treatment.
- Testing ways to ensure that staff receive appropriate support and training.

In addition, since 2012, Macmillan Cancer Support has been running a programme bringing specialists and primary care teams together to consider the 'top tips' that would help oncologists provide better care for their older cancer patients.

New ways to assess older patients were tested by 14 trusts involving 700 patients. Five cancer networks throughout England were chosen take part in the pilot: Mersey and Cheshire, Thames Valley, North East London, South East London, and Sussex.

Assessment

Pilot sites used a CGA approach to patient assessment. CGA is regularly used in geriatric medicine but is new to cancer care in this country. The International Society of Geriatric Oncology recommends the use of CGA prior to medical or surgical intervention in older cancer patients.[22]

A variety of approaches were tested by the five cancer networks to assess patients, involving a range of tools, staff and settings, including:

- Self-completed screening assessment to identify patients requiring a full CGA.
- Deployment of cancer clinical nurse specialists to undertake assessment.
- Elderly care specialists leading the assessment of older cancer patients.
- Testing the feasibility of undertaking assessment in primary care.
- A variety of settings for assessment: home, outpatient clinics, inpatient wards, via telephone and in general practice.

Strong relationships were also formed between the pilot sites and charities such as Age UK and the British Red Cross. These organizations were able to assess practical support needs and provide support services such as financial advice, befriending, transportation, help with household tasks and completion of forms.[21]

While it proved feasible for a range of different staff in different settings to perform CGAs, there was a risk that it would simply be a paper exercise unless it were incorporated into decision making by MDTs and linked to services that could manage other health conditions, as well as to those that could provide practical support. In practice, care of the elderly teams were best placed to do this, although with appropriate systems in place it would be possible for a range of staff to be involved.

Communication and documentation

The project highlighted the need for better communication.[21] Key areas for improvement were identified as:

- Information provided on referral from primary care regarding comorbidity, sensory disability and medication.
- Comprehensiveness of information recorded in the patient notes.
- Feedback of assessment findings to MDT meetings and cancer clinicians.
- Communication between clinicians and patients.
- Ongoing communications between cancer services, elderly care services and primary care.
- Social care and voluntary sector services throughout care and at end of life.

There was evidence of duplication and a need for information-sharing agreements with the voluntary sector so that patients did not have to continually retell their story. Some findings revealed limited feedback of assessments to MDTs to inform clinical decision making, or evidence of modification of management communication between acute sector and voluntary sector services. To avoid assessment being simply a paper exercise, the pilots highlighted the need for integrated systems to link assessment to services to meet the needs identified, such as adjustment of medication, management of non-cancer-related health conditions, and practical support during and after treatment. Documentation and influential communication appeared to be most effective when care of the elderly and primary care professionals were engaged.

Practical support

Service level agreements were established with voluntary sector organizations, i.e. Age UK, British Red Cross and Macmillan Cancer Support, and 300/700 patients assessed were referred to the voluntary sector for practical support. One network produced a directory of services with access to services facilitated by a specialist nurse. Clinical staff were unsure how to make referrals to important services such as falls prevention, pet care or help with household tasks. One network successfully tested a single point of referral via the voluntary sector: Age UK coordinated access to six other voluntary organizations. A key learning point was that availability of services alone was not enough to ensure that patients accessed them. Patients expressed reluctance to take up services, as 'someone else needs them more than me', and staff unfamiliarity affected how these services were presented. For example, where cancer specialist nurses performed the assessment, there was a lower than expected referral to the voluntary sector (other than transportation), reflecting unfamiliarity with the value of these services; however, when elderly care specialists performed the assessment, uptake was higher. Nevertheless, when other specialties carried out assessment, there were case studies demonstrating improved care: for example, where therapeutic radiographers conducted an assessment, those with sensory impairment, dementia, mental health issues and learning disabilities were better managed.

Involvement of elderly care specialists

Two out of the five networks employed older care specialists, and these networks appeared to be more effective in assessing and meeting the needs of elderly cancer patients than networks that did not employ elderly care specialists. Without these specialists, assessments were less likely to influence treatment recommendations: for example, recommendations in relation to morbidity management were less likely to be acted upon. The following were particularly valued by oncologists: support in relation to decision making for the frail; support in the management of those with additional needs such as dementia and sensory impairment; better communication with multiple staff outside the immediate cancer MDT; and enhancement of the skills of the cancer workforce. Nevertheless, therapeutic radiographers proved able to perform assessments in relation to reasonable adjustment of treatment, and cancer pharmacists proved able to assess and adjust polypharmacy.

What should age-friendly services look like?

As a result of the project some clear recommendations could be made:

- Elderly care specialists are part of the cancer care team.

- Ensure appropriate and timely assessment before, during and after cancer treatment linked to decision making in relation to treatment, management of other health conditions and practical support during and after cancer treatment.

- Ensure effective management and coordination of multiple medications and other health conditions, with reasonable adjustment of cancer management in patients with problems uncovered by CGA.

- Establish services and referral pathways to address needs: in particular, links with specialist services such as falls prevention, continence and dementia.

- Establish effective coordination systems to enable coordinated, practical support services, e.g. financial advice, befriending, gardening, household tasks, form filling and transport.

- Ensure that clinical and non-clinical staff have the time and resources to enable them to have the support and training to manage the needs of the older cancer patient before, during and after cancer treatment.

There is now a clear mandate to make changes to improve access to cancer treatment for older patients.

References

1 Maher J. Silver survivors: how do we know if people are 'too old' for cancer treatment? *Future Oncol* 2014; 10: 1811–13.

2 Macmillan Cancer Support. *The Macmillan–NCIN work plan: the UK cancer prevalence project.* Available from: www.ncin.org.uk/about_ncin/segmentation (accessed 15 September 2014).

3 Cancer Research UK. *Cancer incidence by age.* Available from: www.cancerresearchuk.org/cancer-info/cancerstats/incidence/age/#Cancer (accessed 15 September 2014).

4 Maddams J, Utley M, Møller H. Projections of cancer prevalence in the United Kingdom, 2010–2040. *Br J Cancer* 2012; 107: 1195–202.

5   *EUROCARE-5 survival analysis 2000–2007.* Available from: https://w3.iss.it/ site/EU5Results/ Default.aspx (accessed 15 September 2014).

6   Ring A. The influences of age and co-morbidities on treatment decisions for patients with HER2-positive early breast cancer. *Crit Rev Oncol Hematol* 2010; 76: 127–32.

7   Extermann M, Overcash J, Lyman GH, *et al.* Comorbidity and functional status are independent in older cancer patients. *J Clin Oncol* 1998; 16: 1582–7.

8   Lees J, Chan A. Polypharmacy in elderly patients with cancer: clinical implications and management. *Lancet Oncol* 2011; 13: 1249–57.

9   Action on Hearing Loss (2011). *Facts and figures on hearing loss and tinnitus.* Available from: www.actiononhearingloss.org.uk/~/media/Files/Factsheets/Deaf%20awareness/ pdf/Facts%20and%20figures%20on%20deafness%20and%20tinnitus%20July%202011.ashx (accessed 20 April 2015).

10 Cavalli-Björkman N, Qvortrup C, Sebjörnson S, *et al.* Lower treatment intensity and poorer survival in metastatic colorectal cancer patients who live alone. *Br J Cancer* 2012; 107: 189–94.

11 Mor V, Allen S, Malin M. The psychosocial impact of cancer on older versus younger patients and their families. *Cancer* 1994; 74 (suppl 7): 2118–27.

12 Department for Communities and Local Government (2008). *Housing in England 2006/07.* Available from: http://webarchive.nationalarchives.gov.uk/20121108165934/http://www. communities.gov.uk/documents/corporate/pdf/971061.pdf (accessed 20 April 2015).

13 Office for National Statistics (2013). *What does the 2011 census tell us about older people?* Available from: www.ons.gov.uk/ons/dcp171776_325486.pdf (accessed 20 April 2015).

14 Statham J (2011). *Grandparents providing child care. Briefing paper.* Available from: www.gov.uk/government/uploads/system/uploads/attachment_data/file/181364/CWRC-00083-2011.pdf (accessed 20 April 2015).

15 Karakoç T, Yurtsever S. Relationship between social support and fatigue in geriatric patients receiving outpatient chemotherapy. *Eur J Oncol Nurs* 2010; 14: 61–7.

16 Kalsi T, Payne S, Brodie H, *et al.* Are the UK oncology trainees adequately informed about the needs of older people with cancer? *Br J Cancer* 2013; 1018: 1936–41.

17 Government Equalities Office (2015). *Equality Act 2010: guidance.* Available from: www.gov.uk/equality-act-2010-guidance (accessed 15 April 2015).

18 Department of Health (2012). *Cancer experience survey 2011/12.* National report. Available from: www.gov.uk/government/uploads/system/uploads/attachment_data/file/212860/ Cancer-Patient-Experience-Survey-National-Report-2011-12.pdf (accessed 15 April 2015).

19 Ellis G, Whitehead MA, O'Neill D, *et al.* Comprehensive geriatric assessment for older adults admitted to hospital. *Cochrane Database Syst Rev* 2011; 7: CD006211.

20 Stuck A, Iliffe E. Comprehensive geriatric assessment for older adults. *BMJ* 2011; 343; d6799.

21 Macmillan Cancer Support, Department of Health, Age UK (2012). *Cancer services coming of age: learning from the Improving Cancer Treatment Assessment and Support for Older People Project.* Available from: www.gov.uk/government/uploads/system/ uploads/attachment_data/ file/213205/DH_Macmillan_Age-UK_Report_Final.pdf (accessed 20 April 2015).

22 Extermann M, Aapro M, Bernabel R, *et al.*; Task Force on CGA of the International Society of Geriatric Oncology. Use of comprehensive geriatric assessment in older cancer patients: recommendations from the task force on CGA of the International Society of Geriatric Oncology (SIOG). *Crit Rev Oncol Hematol* 2005; 55: 241–52.

05 A European Perspective on Cancer Care in Older People

Gilbert Zulian, Hans Wildiers, Etienne Brain

Introduction

Recently, health authorities and politicians have begun to recognize the healthcare impact of an ageing population, with its profound consequences for health and for the quality, cost and outcome of healthcare services. It has now become an urgent matter to address the needs of older cancer patients in Europe. In cancer medicine, the situation was anticipated over 25 years ago. Yancik and colleagues[1] showed how ageing and cancer incidence were linked, because time is required to allow cancer to develop. They broadly predicted today's situation in Europe. However, limited attention was paid to the subject of cancer and ageing. Cancer specialists continued to concentrate more specifically on developing local and systemic therapies, whereas geriatricians emphasized the global care and functional capacity of the older patient. To remedy this situation, individuals and organizations in Europe and internationally have set out to bring the different specialities together, to establish programmes of research, and to disseminate their findings and educate healthcare professionals of all disciplines, as well as healthcare services managers and political leaders.

In this chapter, we summarize the work of three organizations that are having a positive impact, and describe the notable efforts of one country as an example.

The International Society of Geriatric Oncology (SIOG)

At the beginning of the 1990s, after a conference held in Italy, a group of medical oncologists gathered in Paris to plan regular meetings on the subject of cancers occurring in older people. For strategic reasons linked to the development of the US Senior Adult Cancer Program, the first scientific meeting on geriatric oncology was organized in the USA.[2] Other meetings have followed every year on alternate sides of the Atlantic and have emphasized the need to properly assess not only the cancer but also the broad clinical, functions and holistic impact of the disease on the patient. Multidimensional geriatric assessment, evaluating the function and functional reserves of an individual, became the cornerstone of geriatric oncology.

In 2000, the International Society of Geriatric Oncology (SIOG) was founded under Swiss law (www.siog.org). Since then, every effort has been made to bring together people and specialities that focus on caring for an ageing population and are concerned about cancer incidence, diagnosis and management, and all aspects of cancer care. Health professionals attending SIOG annual meetings can thus teach and learn about all aspects of the problems and challenges encountered by older patients confronted with cancer, including physical, psychological, social and spiritual domains. As a scientific body, SIOG's current strategy includes supporting research, but without a direct sponsorship role, promoting education, promoting career development and expanding internationally. This is embodied in the SIOG 10 priorities initiative.[3]

Besides its annual meeting, SIOG has produced numerous clinical guidelines on the most pertinent subjects of cancer care in older people, which have been published in peer-reviewed journals including its own official publication, the *Journal of Geriatric Oncology*. In addition, most common geriatric screening and assessment tools are available on the SIOG website to help health professionals capture the full range of problems older patients may have, such as functional dependence, comorbidity, polypharmacy, malnutrition, cognitive dysfunction and depression. To detect hidden problems otherwise not identifiable, SIOG recommends using a valid screening tool and, if the screen is positive, to complete the procedure with a geriatric assessment carried out by a trained professional. Taken together, these scientific initiatives can make a great difference in the management of cancer in older people, with the objective of providing not only adequate care but also care adapted to the individual needs and potential of the patient.

A significant contribution of SIOG is the achievement of the French programme on geriatric oncology, termed *oncogériatrie*, led by the Institut National du Cancer (National Institute of Cancer).[4] Twenty-four coordination units and four outposts have been established throughout France and its overseas territories (Figure 5.1). They provide standard basic cancer care offered by the regional health agency and adapt the treatment to the needs of older patients through a mandatory joint oncologist–geriatrician decision process. Depending on local availability and staffing, the programme is led by a geriatrician or a cancer specialist, working together, with help from specialized nurses, to carry out geriatric assessment before deciding which treatment should be offered to the patient. They promote access to care for all older cancer patients, contribute to the development of research in the field, and provide teaching to health professionals and information to the public.

The Belgian National Cancer Plan also emphasizes geriatric oncology.

The European Society for Medical Oncology (ESMO)

While the American Society of Clinical Oncology developed a geriatric track for its annual meeting, in Europe the European Society for Medical Oncology (ESMO) developed a programme to highlight the challenges of cancer in older people. The *Annals of Oncology* (the official ESMO journal) developed a geriatric oncology section. In addition, sponsored sessions, joint sessions and mutual recognition of educational sessions have slowly demonstrated how pertinent professional connections are between ESMO and SIOG. The most important achievement of the close collaboration between ESMO and SIOG is probably the *ESMO handbook of cancer in the senior patient*,[5] first published in 2010 and about to issue its second edition. ESMO has also appointed a faculty group to promote multidisciplinary care for older patients and to help with education of present and future medical oncologists.[6] Such initiatives are likely to help the coming generation of medical oncologists to better understand the complexities of ageing and to better integrate their knowledge of tumours in the management of cancers in older people. Geriatrics input can now be found in almost every ESMO tumour group, with an emphasis on assessment. Geriatric oncology is considered to influence all medical oncology. This is an ongoing process that requires patience, persuasion, education and scientific evidence.

The European Organisation for Research and Treatment of Cancer (EORTC)

The European Organisation for Research and Treatment of Cancer (EORTC) established the Elderly Task Force (ETF) to develop, conduct, coordinate and stimulate research in older patients with cancer across different countries. Towards this goal, the ETF has established close interactions with disease-oriented EORTC groups, and it reviews every new protocol for elderly-

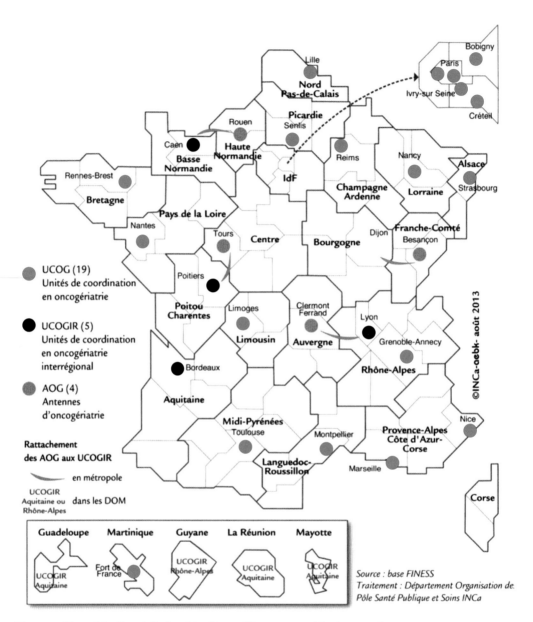

Figure 5.1 Map of the French National Institute of Cancer *oncogériatrie* network.

specific questions within EORTC's protocol review process, aiming to reduce 'ageism' within study protocols. The ETF focuses on three aspects:

1. Specific methodology for clinical trials in the older population.[7]

2. The creation of a common language for describing heterogeneity between older individuals, using the EORTC minimal dataset for geriatric assessment in older cancer patients, including the G8 Geriatric Screening Tool.[8]

3. The performance of clinical trials in the older population.

The ETF has managed to initiate three clinical trials devoted to older cancer patients, one in metastatic breast cancer (EORTC 75111-10114), one in metastatic colorectal cancer (EORTC 40085-75083, now closed), and one prospective cohort study on cancer in nursing homes (EORTC-1221), with integration of geriatric assessment and translational research on biomarkers of ageing. In addition, from 2014 onwards, the G8 Geriatric Screening Tool has been integrated at baseline in all patients aged 70 or older included in any EORTC trial. This tool considers the synergistic effects of a timely diagnosis with an objective assessment of the individual's functional reserves before embarking on treatment. This is expected to result in a marked improvement in the general care of older cancer patients and will be the subject of further research.

The work done by SIOG, ESMO and EORTC in Europe is providing new scientific information about the problems of cancer care in an older population of patients and their comorbidities. This demands the sharing of skills and expertise to bring together the fast-moving world of oncology, with a traditional emphasis on biomedicine and geriatrics in order to obtain a holistic portrait of the patient through Comprehensive Geriatric Assessment. Studies of ageing and cancer provide us with an opportunity to understand the functioning of those who live longer than expected, and to learn from them medically and socially. Health professionals must work to improve the care of older patients with cancer: an immense challenge to our medical skill and humanity.

References

1 Yancik R, Kessler L, Yates JW. The elderly population. Opportunities for cancer prevention and detection. *Cancer* 1988; 62 (8 suppl): 1823–8.

2 Balducci L, Beghe C, Parker M, Chausmer A. Prognostic evaluation in geriatric oncology: problems and perspectives. *Arch Gerontol Geriatr* 1991; 13: 31–41.

3 International Society of Geriatric Oncology. *SIOG 10 priorities.* Available from: www.siog.org/index.php?option=com_content&view=article&id=218&Itemid=135 (accessed 12 February 2015).

4 Institut National du Cancer. *Oncogériatrie.* Available from: www.e-cancer.fr/en/soins/prises-en-charge-specifiques/oncogeriatrie (accessed 18 February 2015).

5 Schrijvers D, Aapro M, Zakotnik B, *et al. ESMO handbook of cancer in the senior patient.* London: Informa Healthcare, 2010.

6 European Society for Medical Oncology. *ESMO faculty.* Available from: www.esmo.org/About-Us/ESMO-Faculty (accessed 12 February 2015).

7 Wildiers H, Mauer M, Pallis A, *et al.* End points and trial design in geriatric oncology research: a joint European Organisation for Research and Treatment of Cancer–Alliance for Clinical Trials in Oncology–International Society of Geriatric Oncology position article. *J Clin Oncol* 2013; 31: 3711–18.

8 Pallis AG, Ring A, Fortpied C, *et al.* EORTC workshop on clinical trial methodology in older individuals with a diagnosis of solid tumors. *Ann Oncol* 2011; 22: 1922–6.

06 Clinical Trials in Older Patients with Cancer

Khurum Khan, Matthew Seymour, Alistair Ring, Peter Johnson

Introduction

Clinical trials are conducted in patients with cancer in order to determine the optimal treatment for a patient population. This might include evaluation of a new therapeutic agent, best use of an existing drug or intervention, assessment of safety, or identification of which patients are most likely to benefit from treatment.[1] The information gained from such studies may be submitted to regulatory authorities and inform best practice guidelines, and will often be required to make decisions on whether an intervention may be funded by those commissioning healthcare. However, a unifying feature of these applications of clinical trial results is that the evidence base is established in a population that is representative of the population we are planning to treat. Unfortunately, this is not necessarily the case when considering the care of older patients with cancer.[2]

At present, more than 160,000 people aged 70 and over are diagnosed with cancer every year in the UK, representing 50% of all cancer diagnoses.[3] With the ageing of the population, both the proportion of cancers diagnosed in older patients and the absolute number of cancer diagnoses in this patient group are likely to rise, such that by 2030 it is anticipated that 70% of cancers will occur in people aged over 65,[4] with very similar projections for the USA.[5] Therefore, attending to the needs of the increasingly large population of older patients with cancer must become a priority for those involved in cancer care, and this should include recruitment to clinical trials in order to inform best care.

Are older patients with cancer represented in clinical trials?

Several studies have shown that recruitment of older patients to clinical trials is not in proportion to the age distribution of the cancer population.[6,7] A 2004 analysis reported on the recruitment of older patients to registration trials of new drugs or new indications approved by the US Food and Drug Administration between 1995 and 2002.[7] The proportion of the trial populations aged >65, >70 and >75 years were 36%, 20% and 9%, compared with 60%, 46% and 31%, respectively, in the US cancer population. Statistically significant underrepresentation of the older patient was noted for all cancer treatments except for breast cancer hormonal therapies.[7] Similar observations can be made regarding trials on the Cancer Research UK portfolio (Figures 6.1–6.3), providing further evidence that older patients are underrepresented in clinical trials.

Why are older patients underrepresented in clinical trials?

It is conceivable that the underrepresentation of older patients in clinical trials reflects the lower rates of treatment in older patients in general, rather than a particular feature of clinical trials. In 2011, a report from the UK National Cancer Intelligence Network described a significant reduction in the proportion of patients receiving a major resection for cancer with increasing age.[8] Furthermore, in 2013, NHS England reported a significant reduction in the likelihood of patients

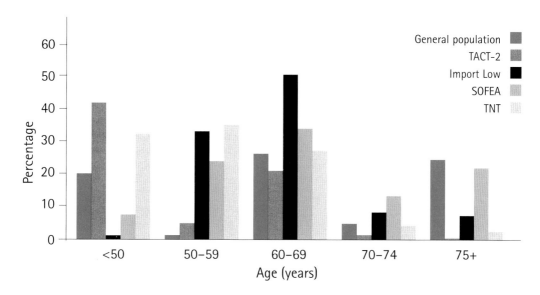

Figure 6.1 Breast cancer studies: comparing trial populations with a general population undergoing cancer therapy. TACT-2, adjuvant chemotherapy: 2 vs 3 weekly epirubicin + CMF (cyclophosphamide, methotrexate and 5-FU) or capecitabine;[30] Import Low (ClinicalTrial.gov registration no. NCT00814567), different ways of giving radiotherapy for low-risk early-stage breast cancer; SOFEA, fulvestrant +/– anastrozole vs exemestane in postmenopausal women with metastatic breast cancer;[31] TNT (ClinicalTrial.gov registration no. NCT00532727), chemotherapy for advanced triple negative breast cancer.

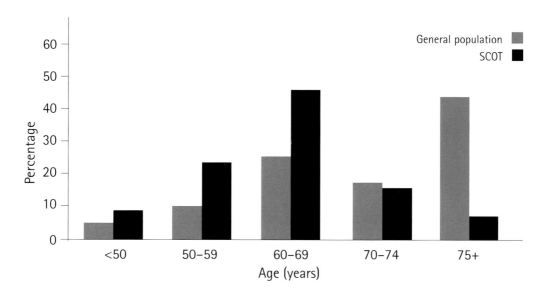

Figure 6.2 Colorectal cancer study: comparing a trial population with a general population undergoing cancer therapy. SCOT (ClinicalTrial.gov registration no. ISRCTN59757862), short course (12 vs 24 weeks) adjuvant chemotherapy after surgery for bowel cancer.

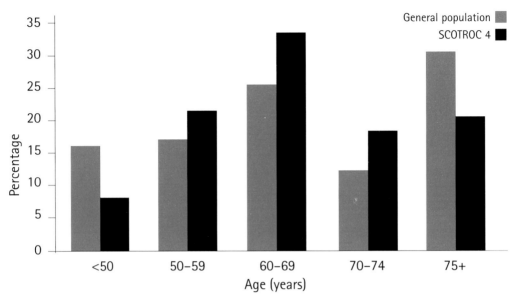

Figure 6.3 Ovarian cancer study: comparing a trial population with a general population undergoing cancer therapy. SCOTROC 4 (ClinicalTrial.gov registration no. NCT00098878), a prospective, multicentre, randomized trial of carboplatin flat dosing vs intrapatient dose escalation in first-line chemotherapy of ovarian, Fallopian tube and primary peritoneal cancers.

aged 65 or over receiving chemotherapy.[9] Whilst many clinicians may have understandable concerns about fitness for cancer therapies in older patients, due to their comorbidities, polypharmacy or biological decline of organ function with age, it is clear that selected older patients can benefit from such interventions.[10–14] As a result, any analysis of the inclusion of older patients in clinical trials (and interventions to address this) needs to take into account the background lower rates of treatment in this patient group in normal clinical care.

There may also be specific features of clinical trial protocols that contribute to underrepresentation. Historically, a number of pivotal clinical trials restricted the inclusion criteria of the patients to those below the age of 75.[15–17] In contemporary trials, upper age limits for trial enrolment are less commonly seen, but older patients may be excluded by default on the basis of comorbidities that are protocol exclusions. An analysis of 59,300 patients enrolled in National Cancer Institute trials found that protocol restrictions based on organ-specific abnormalities and functional status limitations were associated with low rates of inclusion of older patients in clinical trials.[18] The study estimated that relaxation of exclusions based on organ-specific abnormalities alone or functional status could increase enrolment of patients aged 65 and over from 32% to 47% and 60%, respectively.[18] It is, of course, important to acknowledge that some comorbidities may be specifically excluded in the protocol for safety reasons. However, even when controlling for comorbidity and physical functioning it appears that older patients are less likely to be offered entry to clinical trials.[19] Even if an older patient is offered entry to a clinical trial, he or she may choose not to participate because of the requirement for more frequent hospital visits or travel to a more distant cancer centre, or because they are reluctant to accept treatments with potentially greater side effects.[20] Trial involvement may be further limited in older patients with impaired cognition, in whom it may be challenging to gain reliable informed consent. Intriguingly, it is also apparent that there may be an interaction between older age, disease burden, comorbidities and cognitive impairment.[21] In itself this may influence both the treatment approach and potential clinical trial participation. The inevitable corollary of these factors is that older patients who do enter clinical trials represent a selected subset of older patients who may have low burdens of comorbidity, who are well-supported socially and who are highly motivated. As such they may not necessarily be representative of older patients seen routinely in the clinic by most practising clinicians. Caution should therefore be exercised in generalizing the information gained from older patients in such trials into clinical practice.

Can the recruitment of older patients to clinical trials be improved?

The European Organisation for Research and Treatment of Cancer (EORTC) established an Elderly Task Force, with the aim of improving access to clinical trials and research in order to deliver high-quality evidence-based care for the older population with cancer. A joint position paper between the EORTC, the Alliance for Clinical Trials in Oncology and the International Society of Geriatric Oncology specifies a roadmap for research and clinical trials in older people.[22,23] This guidance suggests an absolute requirement for clinical trials to be without an upper age limit, and it also recommends the need for standardized approaches to the measurement of frailty and comorbidity in clinical trials and practice.[22] This second recommendation should receive high priority: much of the geriatric oncology literature calls for the incorporation of objective assessments (of factors such as comorbidities, functional status, nutrition, cognition and social support) into management decisions.[24] In principle, clinical cancer trials offer the ideal opportunity to validate such tools against relevant outcomes, such as toxicity, and to examine in a multivariate analysis whether such individual factors maintain their significance as important factors predictive of outcomes. A further potential key question for clinical trials in older patients will be the definition of the development of key endpoints, in particular with respect to toxicity. Whilst grade 3 and 4 toxicities are routinely reported in clinical trials, lower grade toxicities may determine treatment modifications/discontinuation, particularly in older patients.[25] The incorporation of objective assessments of health and relevant endpoints into clinical trials of interventions pertinent to older patients can lead to practice-influencing clinical trials, as illustrated by the Fluorouracil, Oxaliplatin, Irinotecan: Use and Sequencing (FOCUS)2 trial.[26] This was a UK phase III randomized trial in which older and frail patients with inoperable colorectal cancer were randomized 1:1:1:1 to receive treatment with infusional fluorouracil (5-FU)/levofolinic acid or capecitabine, or either fluoropyrimidine schedule with the addition of oxaliplatin, all at 80% of the standard drug doses. The study succeeded in randomizing 459 patients, and furthermore explored the use of a novel composite endpoint (overall treatment utility) which included objective measures of response and toxicity, as well as clinician and patient perceptions of treatment benefit.[26] This study, along with a few notable others,[27,28] is an excellent example of how well-designed trials asking questions sensitive to the needs of older patients with cancer can be successfully conducted and inform future practice.

Unfortunately, randomized controlled trials in the older population have not always been successful. The Endocrine +/− Surgical Therapy for Elderly Women with Mammary Cancer (ESTEeM), Adjuvant Cytotoxic Chemotherapy in Older Women (ACTION) and Chemotherapy Adjuvant Studies for Women at Advanced Age (CASA) were trials that were designed to compare surgery and primary endocrine therapy (ESTEeM) and to investigate the role of chemotherapy (ACTION and CASA) in older women with breast cancer.[29] All three trials closed early due to poor recruitment, demonstrating the challenges associated with non-blinded studies that have major differences between the allocated groups. Nonetheless, the questions being addressed by these studies are fundamental to the effective management of older patients with cancer, and, as such, alternative approaches to randomized trials may need to be considered. These might include the establishment of prospective hypothesis-driven cohort studies, incorporating objective health assessments and novel endpoints but not involving randomization. A secondary advantage of such studies might be that relatively permissive inclusion criteria may also minimize the selection bias associated with some randomized trials. However, it is uncertain whether the evidence acquired from such studies would be sufficient to inform and change clinical practice. These challenges notwithstanding, clinical trials within this population do provide an opportunity to investigate low toxicity interventions and pilot novel trial designs in a group of patients where they are most relevant (Table 6.1).

Table 6.1 Emerging opportunities and challenges in cancer trials in older patients.	
Trial design	Flexibility: cohort studies and patient preference studies in addition to randomized trials
	Entry criteria permitting comorbidities
	Incorporation of geriatric assessments to define and stratify study population
	Manageable investigation schedules
	Age-appropriate consent processes
Interventions	Surgical prehabilitation to reduce postoperative complications
	Minimally invasive surgery
	Modern radiotherapy techniques with reduced toxicity and increased convenience: intraoperative therapy, brachytherapy and hypofractionation
	Antibody-drug conjugates and targeted therapy to reduce systemic exposure
Endpoints	Pharmacokinetics and biomarkers of ageing
	Measurements of low-grade toxicities and their impact on quality of life
	Impact of treatment on functional independence

Conclusion

Cancer is a disease associated with ageing, and although the majority of cancer diagnoses are made in those aged over 65 years this population is underrepresented in clinical trials. There are many reasons for this underrepresentation; however, the end result is a lack of robust evidence to underpin many management decisions made during the care of older people with cancer. Nonetheless, it is possible to design high-quality clinical trials which can successfully recruit older patients and provide the necessary evidence base for clinical decision making. These require careful framing of the research question and collaborative working, drawing on the expertise of the geriatrics community, and working with patients to design trials that will be acceptable to potential participants.

References

1 McAlearney AS, Song PH, Reiter KL. Why providers participate in clinical trials: considering the National Cancer Institute's Community Clinical Oncology Program. *Contemp Clin Trials* 2012; 33: 1143–9.

2 Scher KS, Hurria A. Under-representation of older adults in cancer registration trials: known problem, little progress. *J Clin Oncol* 2012; 30: 2036–8.

3 Cancer Research UK. *Cancer incidence by age.* Available from: http://info.cancerresearchuk.org/cancerstats/incidence/age/ (accessed 29 January 2015).

4 Mistry M, Parkin D, Ahmad A, *et al.* Cancer incidence in the United Kingdom: projections to the year 2030. *Br J Cancer* 2011; 105: 1795–803.

5 Edwards BK, Howe HL, Ries LA, *et al.* Annual report to the nation on the status of cancer, 1973–1999, featuring implications of age and aging on U.S. cancer burden. *Cancer* 2002; 94: 2766–92.

6 Hutchins LF, Unger JM, Crowley JJ, *et al.* Underrepresentation of patients 65 years of age or older in cancer-treatment trials. *N Engl J Med* 1999; 341: 2061–7.

7 Talarico L, Chen G, Pazdur R. Enrollment of elderly patients in clinical trials for cancer drug registration: a 7-year experience by the US Food and Drug Administration. *J Clin Oncol* 2004; 22: 4626–31.

8 National Cancer Intelligence Network (2011). *Major surgical resections, England, 2004–2006.* Available from: file:///C:/Users/user/Downloads/NCIN_Major_surgical_resections_report_web_v2.pdf (accessed 8 June 2015).

9 NHS England (2013). *Are older people receiving cancer drugs? An analysis of patterns in cancer drug delivery according to the age of patient.* Available from: www.england.nhs.uk/wp-content/uploads/2013/12/old-people-rec-cancer-drugs.pdf (accessed 8 June 2015).

10 Frasci G, Lorusso V, Panza N, *et al.* Gemcitabine plus vinorelbine versus vinorelbine alone in elderly patients with advanced non-small-cell lung cancer. *J Clin Oncol* 2000; 18: 2529–36.

11 Zietman AL, Bae K, Slater JD, *et al.* Randomized trial comparing conventional-dose with high-dose conformal radiation therapy in early-stage adenocarcinoma of the prostate: long-term results from Proton Radiation Oncology Group/American College of Radiology 95-09. *J Clin Oncol* 2010; 28: 1106–11.

12 D'Amico AV, Chen MH, Renshaw AA, *et al.* Androgen suppression and radiation vs radiation alone for prostate cancer: a randomized trial. *JAMA* 2008; 299: 289–95.

13 Muss HB, Woolf S, Berry D, *et al.* Adjuvant chemotherapy in older and younger women with lymph node-positive breast cancer. *JAMA* 2005; 293: 1073–81.

14 Clarke M, Collins R, Darby S, *et al.* Effects of radiotherapy and of differences in the extent of surgery for early breast cancer on local recurrence and 15-year survival: an overview of the randomised trials. *Lancet* 2005; 366: 2087–106.

15 Douillard JY, Cunningham D, Roth AD, *et al.* Irinotecan combined with fluorouracil compared with fluorouracil alone as first-line treatment for metastatic colorectal cancer: a multicentre randomised trial. *Lancet* 2000; 355: 1041–7.

16 de Gramont A, Figer A, Seymour M, *et al.* Leucovorin and fluorouracil with or without oxaliplatin as first-line treatment in advanced colorectal cancer. *J Clin Oncol* 2000; 18: 2938–47.

17 Tournigand C, Andre T, Achille E, *et al.* FOLFIRI followed by FOLFOX6 or the reverse sequence in advanced colorectal cancer: a randomized GERCOR study. *J Clin Oncol* 2004; 22: 229–37.

18 Lewis JH, Kilgore ML, Goldman DP, *et al.* Participation of patients aged 65 years of age or older in cancer clinical trials. *J Clin Oncol* 2003; 21: 1383–9.

19 Kemeny MM, Peterson BL, Kornblith AB, *et al.* Barriers to clinical trial participation by older women with breast cancer. *J Clin Oncol* 2013; 21: 2268–75.

20 Basche M, Baron AE, Eckhardt SG, *et al.* Barriers to enrollment of elderly adults in early phase clinical trials. *J Oncol Pract* 2008; 4: 162–8.

21 Mandelblatt J, Jaconsen P, Ahles T. Cognitive effects of cancer systemic therapy: implications for the care of older patients and survivors. *J Clin Oncol* 2014; 32: 2617–26.

22 Wildiers H, Mauer M, Pallis A, *et al.* End points and trial design in geriatric oncology research: a joint European Organisation for Research and Treatment of Cancer–Alliance for Clinical Trials in Oncology–International Society of Geriatric Oncology position article. *J Clin Oncol* 2013; 31: 3711–18.

23 Hurria A, Dale W, Mooney M, *et al.* Designing therapeutic clinical trials for older and frail adults with cancer: U13 conference recommendations. *J Clin Oncol* 2014; 32: 2587–94.

24 Pallis AG, Ring A, Fortpied C, *et al.* EORTC workshop on clinical trial methodology in older individuals with a diagnosis of solid tumors. *Ann Oncol* 2011; 22: 1922–6.

25 Kalsi T, Babic-Illman G, Fields P, *et al.* The impact of low-grade toxicity in older people with cancer undergoing chemotherapy. *Br J Cancer* 2014; 111: 2224–8.

26 Seymour MT, Thompson LC, Wasan HS, *et al.* Chemotherapy options in elderly and frail patients with metastatic colorectal cancer (MRC FOCUS2): an open-label, randomised factorial trial. *Lancet* 2011; 377: 1749–59.

27 Aparicio T, Jouve JL, Teillet L, *et al.* Geriatric factors predict chemotherapy feasibility: ancillary results of FFCD 2001–02 phase III study in first-line chemotherapy for metastatic colorectal cancer in elderly patients. *J Clin Oncol* 2013; 31: 1464–70.

28 Kunkler IH, Williams LJ, Jack WJ, *et al.* Breast-conserving surgery with or without irradiation in women aged 65 years or older with early breast cancer (PRIME II): a randomised controlled trial. *Lancet Oncol* 2015; 16: 266–73.

29 Ring A, Reed M, Leonard RCF, *et al.* The treatment of early breast cancer in women over the age of 70. *Br J Cancer* 2011; 105: 189–93.

30 Bliss J, Canney P, Velikova G, *et al.* TACT2 Randomised Adjuvant Trial in Early Breast Cancer (EBC): tolerability and toxicity of standard 3 weekly epirubicin (E) versus accelerated epirubicin (aE) followed by capecitabine (X) or CMF in 129 UK hospitals (CRUK/05/019). *Cancer Res* 2010; 70 (24 suppl): 5–10-07.

31 Johnston SR, Kilburn LS, Ellis P, *et al.* Fulvestrant plus anastrozole or placebo versus exemestane alone after progression on non-steroidal aromatase inhibitors in postmenopausal patients with hormone-receptor-positive locally advanced or metastatic breast cancer (SoFEA): a composite, multicentre, phase 3 randomised trial. *Lancet Oncol* 2013; 14: 989–98.

07 Comprehensive Geriatric Assessment and Available Tools

Danielle Harari, Tania Kalsi

What is Comprehensive Geriatric Assessment?

UK national policy now advocates comprehensive assessments for older people at the time of cancer treatment decision making.[1] Comprehensive Geriatric Assessment (CGA) is a 'multidimensional interdisciplinary diagnostic process focused on determining a frail older person's medical, psychological and functional capability in order to develop a coordinated and integrated plan for treatment and long-term follow-up'.[2] CGA involves a review of comorbidities, geriatric syndromes (e.g. frailty, falls, incontinence), mental health, functional difficulties and social circumstances. Although the term CGA implies it is an assessment, it is in fact a four-part clinical process (Figure 7.1).

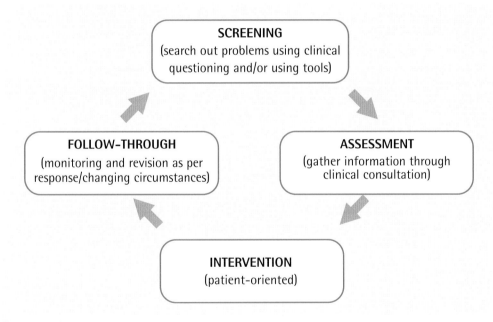

Figure 7.1 CGA process.

It is essential to ask about the patient's own goals for the treatment experience (e.g. 'to go to my granddaughter's wedding in a month'). Randomized controlled trials, meta-analyses and a 2011 Cochrane review[3] have shown that CGA reduces mortality and institutionalization. Studies of geriatrician-delivered CGA in orthopaedics and surgery have shown reduced length of stay, mortality and postoperative complications.[4,5] Based on such evidence, the International Society of Geriatric Oncology (SIOG) recommends CGA in cancer patients over the age of 70 years.[6,7]

Studies in cancer patients have demonstrated that the four-stage CGA process influences oncological treatment decision making,[8,9] impacts clinical care by resulting in a number of intervention plans,[8,9] increases postoperative survival,[10] and, for geriatrician-led CGA, improves chemotherapy tolerance.[11] Studies of one-stage CGA (i.e. screening alone without follow-through) have identified that patient factors such as function, nutrition, comorbidity and falls are associated with lower survival, postoperative complications and chemotherapy toxicity.[12–14] Caution should be applied to interpreting these factors as definitive predictors of poor outcome in cancer treatment, however, because these studies crucially lack the key element of intervention and clinical optimization that may impact the associations (e.g. diabetes care, dietary supplementation, referring to falls strength and balance programmes).

What does CGA include and how can we apply this to cancer care?

CGA covers multiple domains that ideally are all screened for but that can also be sub-selected to best assess particular patient needs (e.g. bladder and bowel function for those undergoing pelvic irradiation). Relevant domains can also be added, so for cancer patients this would include cancer-related symptoms and how these impact independent functioning and quality of life, e.g. European Organisation for Research and Treatment of Cancer Quality of Life Questionnaire (EORTC QLQ-C30), potential risks of treatment toxicity and optimization to reduce those risks, and preoperative assessment for those undergoing surgery, e.g. American Society of Anesthesiologists (ASA) score. Table 7.1 summarizes these domains with clinical scenarios illustrating referral pathways and optimization if abnormalities are detected through screening. Patients with single-organ comorbidities can be appropriately referred for specialist review (e.g. cardiology or GP). More frequently, however, several domains require management and in such cases a geriatrician review may usefully avoid multiple referrals.

Oncologists increasingly need to consider how they can integrate the broader approach of CGA into routine oncology practice. CGA screening can feasibly be delivered in the oncology clinic,[15] but full CGA can take an hour in complex patients. CGA needs identified through screening may require a second visit, which can be co-managed by geriatrics specialists, or indeed by oncologists (doctors or advanced nurse practitioners) trained and supported in CGA delivery by geriatricians. Table 7.2 gives an example of CGA screening-based guidance, co-developed by geriatricians, surgeons, anaesthetists and pre-assessment nurses, to indicate when preoperative clinics should refer older people undergoing elective (including cancer) surgery to geriatricians for more in-depth CGA.[16] Although there are currently few formal shared care arrangements between oncology and geriatrics in UK hospitals, there are existing frameworks for cross-specialty advice and review whereby such clinically pragmatic referral pathways can potentially be agreed upon.

What CGA screening tools should I use in the oncology clinic?

CGA screening should be used to identify those needing more in-depth CGA and not as a scoring tool to decide who is fit or not fit for cancer treatment. CGA screening tools also lack in-depth diagnostic ability, making follow-on clinical assessment for those with needs imperative. This is also pertinent to performance status (PS), commonly used in oncological care. PS 2 in an older person may cause concern for that person's ability to tolerate full curative treatment, while in fact the reduced mobility and fatigue may be due to pain from arthritis.

When choosing CGA screening tools, providers should aim for the most comprehensive and relevant assessment within whatever practical limitations the application may have. Self-reported

Table 7.1 Specific domains included in CGA with exemplar real-life clinical cases showing referral pathways and benefits of optimization.

CGA domain	Example clinical scenario
Comorbidity	75-year-old woman with ovarian cancer assessed for paclitaxel and carboplatin
	CGA screening in oncology clinic identified poor diabetes control
	Referred to diabetic team: diabetic medications adjusted; pre-emptive plan made for when given dexamethasone; re-reviewed through treatment for further adjustments
	Improved diabetic control through treatment and improved QOL (less hyperglycaemic nocturia, resulting in less sleep disturbance)
Medications (polypharmacy)	78-year-old man with bladder cancer assessed for gemcitabine and cisplatin
	Renal impairment (eGFR 48 ml/min) and pre-syncope identified on CGA screening
	Referred to geriatrician: postural BP drop identified; NSAIDs, bendroflumethiazide and furosemide discontinued
	Pre-syncope symptoms and eGFR improved to 62 ml/min, enabling cautious platinum-based chemotherapy
Cognition and delirium risk	72-year-old patient assessed for palliative capecitabine
	Cognitive impairment identified on CGA screening
	Referred to geriatrician: mild dementia with executive function difficulties identified; mental capacity assessed and found to have capacity for chemotherapy decision making
	Chemotherapy delivered with appointment diary and text alerts; transport arranged; family-administered capecitabine; supportive medications in blister packs by community pharmacist; nurse specialist provided extra telephone check-ups
Mood and anxiety	Fit 85-year-old man with potentially curative colorectal cancer refusing surgery
	CGA screening identified low mood
	Referred to GP: identified that the patient's daughter had recently died (she had supported him with shopping and transport to hospital and bingo) and he was now socially isolated and worried about coping after surgery
	Bereavement counselling arranged; antidepressants started; Age UK arranged for shopping, be-a-friend volunteer visits and transport to bingo; hospital transport arranged for hospital appointments; patient referred to social services for re-enablement support at home after surgery
	Agreed to proceed to surgery
Continence (urine and faecal)	81-year-old woman with bladder cancer assessed for radiotherapy
	CGA screening identified urinary incontinence
	Referred to continence clinic (available in hospital or community): started pelvic floor and bladder retraining exercises; tolterodine prescribed for mixed urge and stress incontinence
	Symptoms improving and agreed to radiotherapy; urge symptoms worsened through treatment: reassessed and tolterodine increased with sufficient improvement to complete treatment
Falls	87-year-old patient with locally advanced pancreatic cancer; palliative chemotherapy discontinued in other centre due to falls
	Referral to falls clinic identified multifactorial causes: bradycardia secondary to amiodarone; reduced strength and balance; peripheral neuropathy related to diabetes and vitamin B_{12} deficiency; bifocal glasses with no optician visit for 5 years

	Amiodarone stopped; pulse improved; vitamin B_{12} replaced; physiotherapy started; occupational therapy home visit identified trip hazards and equipment needs; optician arranged for visual assessment and single focal lens
	Fewer falls and improved QOL
Osteoporosis and bone health	84-year-old man with prostate cancer on goserelin
	CGA screening in clinic identified Colles' fracture 4 years earlier
	Referred to osteoporosis clinic: other osteoporosis risk factors identified (smoking, BMI 21 kg/m²); FRAX score indicated high risk for fracture, so started on alendronate without DEXA
Nutrition	73-year-old man with oesophageal cancer planned for neoadjuvant EOX
	CGA screening identified poor nutrition
	Referred to dietitian before treatment: dentures lost in hospital; wife recently ill so no longer able to do cooking
	Nutritional needs identified; dietary and supplement plan made including arranging meals-on-wheels for both him and his wife; urgent replacement dentures facilitated
Sensory (vision, hearing)	70-year-old patient with NSCLC planned for vinorelbine and cisplatin
	Potential hearing impairment identified on CGA screening
	Referred to audiology: significant wax identified and removed; subsequent hearing assessment revealed no significant hearing impairment
	Went on to treatment as planned
Sleep	81-year-old patient being considered for palliative chemotherapy, with significant baseline fatigue and multiple comorbidities
	CGA screening questionnaire identified poor sleep
	Referral to geriatrician identified causes of sleep disturbance: 7× nocturia due to untreated BPH; sleeping on sofa as toilet downstairs and painful osteoarthritis made stairs difficult at night
	BPH treated; bedside urine bottles and stair rail provided by occupational therapy; analgesia optimized for osteoarthritis
	Sleep and fatigue improved, resulting in improved QOL; received dose-reduced palliative chemotherapy
Pain	76-year-old man with prostate cancer on active surveillance
	CGA screening identified significant pain
	Referral to GP found pain was related to undiagnosed osteoarthritis: paracetamol and codeine phosphate started with laxative cover; NSAIDs stopped, as on aspirin
	QOL functional improvement with pain relief
Tissue viability	87-year-old nursing home patient with a large rectal tumour, for de-functioning colostomy
	CGA screening on the ward identified a high Waterlow score (i.e. risk of pressure sores): urgent pressure-relieving mattress requested on ward
	Referred on day of admission to occupational therapy and district nurses for pressure-relieving mattress and cushion to be provided in care home on discharge
	As identified and requested early, hospital-acquired pressure sores were prevented and early discharge expedited

Mobility including exercise tolerance	78-year-old woman, considered for palliative chemotherapy, PS 2
	CGA screening identified mobility difficulties
	Referral to geriatrician identified poor mobility related to painful osteoarthritis and undiagnosed early Parkinson's disease: regular analgesia and Parkinson's medications commenced; no physiotherapy required
	Improved mobility and PS; chemotherapy given; domperidone given instead of metoclopramide supportive medication to avoid worsening of Parkinson's symptoms
Function (basic ADL and instrumental ADL)	85-year-old man on palliative chemotherapy; grade 3 nausea and grade 2 fatigue with cycle 2; keen to continue as wants to make Christmas
	CGA screening identified functional difficulties
	Referral to geriatrician identified that the patient was confused about supportive medications and was unable to use telephone due to hearing, so was unable to call acute oncology when in difficulty; felt too tired to get the bus to the hospital/GP and did not want to bother ambulance; unable to get into bath due to fatigue: audiology referral; telephone for hearing-impaired arranged; supportive medications arranged into blister pack; hospital transport arranged; extra nurse specialist phone calls; occupational therapy provided bath board and grab rails
	Continued to cycle 2 on 20% dose reduction, later re-escalated to full dose as coping well with the additional support
Social circumstances	71-year-old woman seen at routine follow-up 2 years after surgically treated breast cancer
	CGA screening identified difficulties at home
	Referred to social worker, who put a package of care into place and organized day centre visits, improving her QOL
QOL	88-year-old patient with locally advanced lung cancer, receiving palliative care alone
	Repeat CGA screening noted a decline in a number of QOL measures (social activities, pain, nausea, mood, fatigue)
	Referred to geriatrician and palliative care: pain and nausea treated; additional social support provided through social services, Macmillan and Age UK; reversible contributors to fatigue (untreated hypothyroidism, anaemia) treated

ADL, activities of daily living; BPH, benign prostatic hypertrophy; eGFR, estimated glomerular filtration rate; EOX, epirubicin, oxaliplatin and capecitabine; FRAX, Fracture Risk Assessment Tool (www.shef.ac.uk/FRAX/tool.aspx); NSAIDs, non-steroidal anti-inflammatory drugs; NSCLC, non-small-cell lung carcinoma; QOL, quality of life.

CGA questionnaires have the advantage of being easier to adapt to the specific needs of a patient group and are less time-consuming for the clinician.[15] The CGA-GOLD questionnaire is an example of a self-completed screening questionnaire evaluated in a UK cancer centre.[11] Patients can complete the questionnaire by post or in the waiting room prior to clinical review, so the responses can be looked at by oncologists in clinic to: (1) identify fit patients who have no coexisting problems; (2) review patients with needs and decide on immediate treatment (e.g. antihypertensives) and/or ongoing referrals to optimize them for cancer treatment; and (3) broaden patient–oncologist communication.

Clinician-completed screening has the advantage of incorporating CGA as part of the clinical assessment and can be undertaken by providers of any discipline or specialty trained in its use. Oncologists can choose combinations of individual domain tools pertinent to their clinical practice, with some being more comprehensive than others (Table 7.3).

Table 7.2 Referral guidance for geriatric liaison for older people undergoing elective surgery being screened in pre-assessment clinic by surgical or anaesthetic staff (from Harari et al.[9]).

- Cardiovascular: uncontrolled hypertension (BP above 160/90 mmHg), recent history of myocardial infarction, unstable angina, current treatment for heart failure
- Poorly controlled diabetes
- Previous stroke
- Currently taking warfarin
- Chronic lung disease, which you consider may put your patient at risk
- Poor nutritional status (BMI <20 kg/m^2, or weight loss of 5 kg or more over past 6 months)
- Two or more falls from standing height in the past year
- Significant memory problems or history of confusion or known dementia
- Needs personal help with getting to the toilet, moving from bed to chair, standing up, dressing, walking
- Likely to need a complex discharge package

Table 7.3 CGA domains and commonly available screening and assessment tools.

CGA domain	Tool (n)	Potential relevance
Comorbidities	Adult Comorbidity Evaluation-27 (ACE-27) (n=27)	Comprehensive: includes assessment of disease severity and uses clinical data which are mainly available in routine care, so can guide comorbidity optimization; score is less clinically helpful than using individual domain content, as based on score of worst single disease decompensation, and difficult to interpret for those with mild decompensations of multiple diseases; copyrighted
	Cumulative Illness Rating Scale–Geriatrics (CIRS-G) (n=14)	Comprehensive and takes into account disease severity; validated for use in older people; manual is needed to score correctly
	Charlson Comorbidity Index (n=17)	Simplistic; easy to complete with routine clinical information; does not take into account disease severity, so insufficient detail for optimization
Medications (polypharmacy)	Screening Tool in Older Persons for Potentially Inappropriate Prescriptions and Screening Tool to Alert Doctors to the Right Treatment (STOPP/START) (n=114; 80 STOPP, 34 START medications)	Lists medications that should be avoided or used with caution in older people with comorbidities and the potential for interaction and side effects; can improve appropriate prescribing
	Beers Criteria	Similar to above; US criteria
	≥4 scheduled medications	Simple screening for polypharmacy, alerting need for medication review
Cognition	Abbreviated Mental Test Score (AMTS) (n=10)	Quick; does not need experience to use; well established as screening tool in different settings; useful for delirium (where status is fluctuating)
	Short Portable Mental Status Questionnaire (SPMSQ) (n=10)	Quick; easy to use as above as screening tool

	Clock-drawing test (draw a clock and put in hands reading 10 past 11) Mini-Cog (*n*=3)	Can pick up subtle problems with executive cognitive function (e.g. minute hand pointing to 10 rather than 2), so may be used where above screening tools have picked up a deficit; combines clock-drawing test with recall of three words, so additional screen for short-term memory loss
	Mini-Mental State Examination (*n*=30)	More comprehensive (10 min); has been widely used; copyrighted
	Montreal Cognitive Assessment (*n*=30)	Comprehensive (10 min), so useful when short screening is positive; informs clinician as patient completes it on areas of cognitive difficulty
Mood	Single question 'Are you depressed?'	Validated to have high sensitivity and specificity and positive predictive value for screening in palliative care patients[19]
	Geriatric Depression Scale (GDS-4 and GDS-15)	Quick, with simple yes/no answers; four-item scale can be used for screening; 15-item scale has higher positive and negative predictive value (against DSM IV definition), so can be used if patient screens positive with single question or GDS-4
	Hospital Anxiety and Depression Scale (HADS) (*n*=14)	As above; more detailed and assesses anxiety as well as depression
Basic function	Barthel Index (*n*=10)	Quick and reasonably comprehensive screen for basic function (e.g. walking, stairs, transfers, washing, toilet use, etc.); may not identify milder functional impairment
	Nottingham Extended Activities of Daily Living (NEADL)	Can be used by postal questionnaire or by phone
	Katz Index of Independence in Activities of Daily Living (*n*=6)	Quick, but less detailed; does not assess mobility beyond transfers
Advanced function	Lawton–Brody Instrumental Activities of Daily Living (IADL) (*n*=8)	More sensitive, detecting milder functional deficits which could benefit from support (e.g. cooking, cleaning, telephone use)
Mobility	Timed Up and Go (TUG) test	Time in seconds to walk 3 m and back from seated position; quick; indicates mobility or balance problems requiring further assessment with >20 s as cut-off
	Falls Risk Assessment Tool (FRAT)	Can use first question of part 1 'Have you fallen in the past 12 months?' and proceed to rest of assessment if yes
Nutrition	Malnutrition Universal Screening Tool (MUST) (*n*=3)	Recent weight loss and reduced appetite; BMI measure; note of recent acute illness
	Mini-Nutritional Assessment Short Form (*n*=6)	As above; plus mobility and cognition/mood question
QOL	European Organisation for Research and Treatment of Cancer Quality-of-Life Questionnaire (EORTC QLQ-C30) (*n*=20); also has geriatric version	Covers a wide number of issues (mobility, mood, pain, diarrhoea, fatigue) and impact on social functioning; can be self-completed; issues are in relation to the past 7 days; can be used throughout cancer treatment to assess wider impact on well-being

n, number of items; QOL, quality of life.

Table 7.4 Abbreviated screening tools (adapted from Decoster et al.[20]).

Abbreviated tool	CGA domain included	Number of items/ questions	Sensitivity for detecting need for in-depth assessment (%)	Specificity for detecting need for in-depth assessment (%)
SIOG Geriatric Screening Tool (G8)[21]	Nutrition Mobility Cognition Mood Medication General health	8	65–92	3–75
Vulnerable Elders Survey-13 (VES-13)[22]	Function Mobility	13	39–88	62–100
Abbreviated Comprehensive Geriatric Assessment (aCGA)[23]	Function Cognition Depression	15	51	97
Groningen Frailty Indicator (GFI)[24]	Vision Hearing Mobility Nutrition Cognition Comorbidity Psychosocial Physical fitness	15	39–66	86–87
Edmonton Frailty Scale[25]	Cognition Health status Functional dependence Social support Medication Nutrition Mood Urinary incontinence Functional performance	11		

Brief CGA and frailty tools have been applied in oncology (e.g. G8 and VES-13) (Table 7.4) but require particular caution as some lack the breadth of self-completed questionnaires and detail of multiple individual tools and so may over- or underestimate clinical problems.[16] As with other screening instruments, they cannot define who is 'too frail' for cancer treatment but can identify who requires further optimization and support. The Edmonton Frailty Scale[17] (clinician-completed) has been applied less in the cancer setting, but it combines several tests, includes the largest number of CGA domains from the abbreviated tools and is the screening tool recommended by the British Geriatrics Society in the elective surgical setting.[18]

Conclusion and learning points

- CGA is an evidence-based clinical process: screening, assessment, and, importantly, intervention and follow-through.
- CGA screening in the oncology clinic is feasible and useful to identify unmet needs requiring further assessment and management plans to optimize patients for cancer treatment. This may include referral to appropriate specialists.
- CGA screening and frailty tools are not treatment decision-making tools.

References

1 Macmillan Cancer Support, Department of Health, Age UK (2012). *Cancer services coming of age: learning from the Improving Cancer Treatment Assessment and Support for Older People Project.* Available from: www.macmillan.org.uk/Documents/AboutUs/Health_professionals/OlderPeoplesProject/CancerServicesComingofAge.pdf (accessed 23 June 2015).

2 Rubenstein LZ, Stuck AE, Siu AL, Wieland D. Impacts of geriatric evaluation and management programs on defined outcomes: overview of the evidence. *J Am Geriatr Soc* 1991; 39 (9 part 2): 17–18S.

3 Ellis G, Whitehead MA, O'Neill D, *et al.* Comprehensive geriatric assessment for older adults admitted to hospital. *Cochrane Database Syst Rev* 2011; 7: CD006211.

4 Harari D, Hopper A, Dhesi J, *et al.* Proactive care of older people undergoing surgery ('POPS'): designing, embedding, evaluating and funding a comprehensive geriatric assessment service for older elective surgical patients. *Age Ageing* 2007; 36: 190–6.

5 Vidan M, Serra JA, Moreno C, *et al.* Efficacy of a comprehensive geriatric intervention in older patients hospitalized for hip fracture: a randomized, controlled trial. *J Am Geriatr Soc* 2005; 53: 1476–82.

6 Extermann M, Aapro M, Bernabel R, *et al.*; Task Force on CGA of the International Society of Geriatric Oncology. Use of comprehensive geriatric assessment in older cancer patients: recommendations from the task force on CGA of the International Society of Geriatric Oncology (SIOG). *Crit Rev Oncol Hematol* 2005; 55: 241–52.

7 Wildiers H, Heeren P, Puts M, *et al.* International Society of Geriatric Oncology consensus on geriatric assessment in older patients with cancer. *J Clin Oncol* 2014; 28: 8347.

8 Caillet P, Canoui-Poitrine F, Vouriot J, *et al.* Comprehensive geriatric assessment in the decision-making process in elderly patients with cancer: ELCAPA study. *J Clin Oncol* 2011; 29: 3636–42.

9 Chaibi P, Magne N, Breton S, *et al.* Influence of geriatric consultation with comprehensive geriatric assessment on final therapeutic decision in elderly cancer patients. *Crit Rev Oncol Hematol* 2011; 79: 302–7.

10 McCorkle R, Strumpf NE, Nuamah IF, *et al.* A specialized home care intervention improves survival among older post-surgical cancer patients. *J Am Geriatr Soc* 2000; 48: 1707–13.

11 Kalsi T, Babic-Illman G, Ross PJ, *et al.* The impact of comprehensive geriatric assessment interventions on tolerance to chemotherapy in older people. *Br J Cancer* 2015; 112: 1435–44.

12 Extermann M, Boler I, Reich RR, *et al.* Predicting the risk of chemotherapy toxicity in older patients: the Chemotherapy Risk Assessment Scale for High-Age Patients (CRASH) score. *Cancer* 2011; 118: 3377–86.

13 Hurria A, Togawa K, Mohile SG, *et al.* Predicting chemotherapy toxicity in older adults with cancer: a prospective multicenter study. *J Clin Oncol* 2011; 29: 3457–65.

14 Wildes TM, Ruwe AP, Fournier C, *et al.* Geriatric assessment is associated with completion of chemotherapy, toxicity and survival in older adults with cancer. *J Geriatr Oncol* 2013; 4: 227–34.

15 Hurria A, Lichtman SM, Gardes J, *et al.* Identifying vulnerable older adults with cancer: integrating geriatric assessment into oncology practice. *J Am Geriatr Soc* 2007; 55: 1604–8.

16 Hamaker ME, Jonker JM, de Rooij SE, *et al.* Frailty screening methods for predicting outcome of a comprehensive geriatric assessment in elderly patients with cancer: a systematic review. *Lancet Oncol* 2012; 13: e437–44.

17 Dasgupta M, Rolfson DB, Stolee P, *et al.* Frailty is associated with postoperative complications in older adults with medical problems. *Arch Gerontol Geriatr* 2009; 48: 78–83.

18 British Geriatrics Society (2014). *Fit for frailty. Consensus for best practice guidance for the care of older people living with frailty in community and outpatient settings.* Available from: www.bgs.org.uk/campaigns/fff/fff_full.pdf (accessed 19 April 2015).

19 Lloyd-Williams M, Spiller J. Which depression screening tools should be used in palliative care? *Palliat Med* 2003; 17: 40–3.

20 Decoster L, Van Puyvelde K, Mohile S, *et al.* Screening tools for multidimensional health problems warranting a geriatric assessment in older cancer patients: an update on SIOG recommendations. *Ann Oncol* 2015; 26: 288–300.

21 Bellera CA, Rainfray M, Mathoulin-Pélissier S, *et al.* Screening older cancer patients: first evaluation of the G-8 geriatric screening tool. *Ann Oncol* 2012; 23: 2166–72.

22 Luciani A, Ascione G, Bertuzzi C, *et al.* Detecting disabilities in older patients with cancer: comparison between comprehensive geriatric assessment and vulnerable elders survey–13. *J Clin Oncol* 2010; 28: 2046–50.

23 Overcash JA, Beckstead J, Extermann M, Cobb S. The abbreviated comprehensive geriatric assessment (aCGA): a retrospective analysis. *Crit Rev Oncol Hematol* 2005; 54: 129–36.

24 Steverink N, Slaets JPJ, Schuurmans H, van Lis M. Measuring frailty: development and testing of the Groningen Frailty Indicator (GFI). *Gerontologist* 2001; 41 (special issue 1): 236–7.

25 Rolfson DB, Majumdar SR, Taher A, Tsuyuki RT. Development and validation of a new instrument for frailty. *Clin Invest Med* 2000; 23: 336.

26 Johnson C, Fitzsimmons D, Gilbert J, *et al.*; EORTC Quality of Life Group. Development of the European Organisation for Research and Treatment of Cancer quality of life questionnaire module for older people with cancer: The EORTC QLQ-ELD15. *Eur J Cancer* 2010; 46: 2242–52.

Further reading

• Owusu C, Berger NA. Comprehensive geriatric assessment in the older cancer patient: coming of age in clinical cancer care. *Clin Pract* 2014; 11: 749–62.

• Sattar S, Alibhai MH, Wildiers H, Puts MTE. How to implement a geriatric assessment in your clinical practice. *Oncologist* 2014; 19: 1056–68.

• Chow WB, Rosenthal RA, Merkow RP, *et al.* Optimal preoperative assessment of the geriatric surgical patient: a best practices guideline. *J Am Coll Surg* 2012; 215: 453–66.

08 Special Issues Concerning Radiotherapy in Older Cancer Patients

Allan Price

Introduction

In 2011, among the three commonest cancers for which radiotherapy is the standard treatment, 22,000 women over the age of 65 were diagnosed with breast cancer, 32,000 men and women over 65 with lung cancer, and 31,000 men with prostate cancer.[1] Delaney and coworkers[2] estimated the ideal use of radiotherapy in these populations as 83%, 76% and 60%, respectively, amounting to 61,000 individuals for these three cancers alone. Other sites for which over half of patients were expected to receive radiotherapy included rectum, head and neck, oesophagus, stomach, pancreas, lymphoma, bladder and CNS. There is therefore a large pool of older patients for whom radiotherapy is likely to represent a component of their treatment pathway.

A number of studies have suggested lower rates of use of radiotherapy in older patients than would be expected, particularly when compared with younger populations.[3-5] Even the use of palliative radiotherapy has been reported to be 25–44% lower in those aged over 80 years.[5] This may relate to perceived benefit from and tolerance of radiotherapy. A Dutch study[6] examined health-related quality of life after radiotherapy in patients over 80 years old. Quality of life was maintained until the end of radiotherapy. Six months after the completion of radiotherapy it had, however, deteriorated in general and in elderly-specific areas, indicating potentially limited benefit and also the need to develop specific supportive interventions for this age group.[6]

In older patients, the delivery of radiotherapy may be further complicated by the need to integrate chemotherapy with radiotherapy for locally advanced cancers for many tumour sites. De Ruysscher and coworkers[7] looked at the eligibility for concomitant chemotherapy of 711 patients with stage III non-small-cell lung carcinoma (NSCLC) diagnosed between 2002 and 2005. One or more severe comorbidities were considered to exclude patients from this treatment. Approximately a quarter were over 75 years old and all of this age group had at least one major comorbidity. A similar number were aged between 70 and 74 years, of whom over half had at least one comorbidity.

This chapter describes examples of a number of possible solutions to these problems, including attempting to identify those at greatest risk of harm, avoiding radiotherapy where possible, modifying treatment and ameliorating side effects.[7]

Can we identify older people who are at increased risk of harm from radiotherapy?

Many instruments have been developed to identify patients with frailty. A systematic review of the literature from 2010 to 2012[8] identified 33 studies published in English and one in French that applied geriatric assessment tools to older people with newly diagnosed cancer. Treatment decisions were changed in a quarter of individuals so assessed. Performance status (PS) and reduced independence in activities of daily living (ADL) were associated with increased mortality. A range of different tools were used but none were clearly better than any of the others.

None of these studies specifically addressed patients receiving radiotherapy. The same authors reported a prospective study of 112 patients with newly diagnosed cancer, of whom seven received radiotherapy alone and 33 radiotherapy with another treatment modality.[9] Low grip strength was associated with increased toxicity, while reduced PS and ADL disability predicted increased mortality. Ulger and coworkers[10] reported treatment-related toxicities in 30 patients who underwent Comprehensive Geriatric Assessment (CGA) before commencing radical radiotherapy. None of the toxicities were dose limiting. Only hand strength showed a trend towards an association with radiation-induced toxicity. Kenis and colleagues[11] reported 1967 patients in 10 hospitals screened initially with the G8 tool and then with CGA. Seventy-one percent of initial G8 screens warranted the more detailed assessment. Half of patients had a previously unidentified problem and a quarter required geriatric intervention before treatment.[11]

In summary, despite much work in this area on assessing patients with cancer in general, little work has been done on geriatrics assessment tools and radiotherapy specifically, and there is no foreseeable prospect of these being used routinely in patients about to receive radiotherapy, to identify those at greater risk for whom special measures might be taken.

Are there patient groups in whom radiotherapy can be avoided?

While there is no evidence that cancer is less aggressive in older people, there are some low-risk situations where the reduced time at risk because of competing causes of mortality may reduce the likely benefit of radiotherapy. Thus, the International Society of Geriatric Oncology guideline on management of prostate cancer[12] recommends that patients at low risk (T1–T2a, Gleason score ≤6, prostate-specific antigen <10 g/l) should only receive radiotherapy if life expectancy is greater than 20 years. However, a comparative effectiveness study in older men with locally advanced prostate cancer using the Surveillance, Epidemiology, and End Results database[13] found that, in those aged 75–85 years, the addition of radiotherapy to androgen deprivation significantly reduced mortality. Kunkler and colleagues[14] randomized 1326 women over age 65 with low-grade, oestrogen receptor-positive, node-negative breast cancer to hormones alone after lumpectomy or to hormones and radiotherapy. Survival at 5 years was 94% in both groups. Local recurrence was 1% with and 4% without radiotherapy, suggesting radiotherapy could safely be omitted in this group.

This indicates that, depending on the tumour type, risks of recurrence (based on tumour biology) and risks from competing causes of mortality, individualizing the use or omission of radiotherapy should be discussed with older patients, emphasizing where the risk from cancer might be low, the time at which risk is reduced and the time at which risk of harm is increased.

Can changes be made safely in radiotherapy delivery?

Radiotherapy doses and fractionation schedules have been developed over many decades. Improvements in technology and greater understanding of the radiobiology of cancers and normal tissues have allowed better selection of fractionation schemes for individual patients which are equally applicable to younger and older patients. Reduced numbers of fractions, minimizing hospital attendances and avoiding admission if possible, is a key aim in older patients. In patients with stage I NSCLC, the introduction of stereotactic ablative radiotherapy using 3–5 fractions rather than 20–36 fractions, which appears to improve local control without increasing toxicity, meets this aim.[15] In women with breast cancer, the FAST-Forward trial is looking at whether radical treatment can be delivered in five rather than 15 fractions.[16] In men with localized prostate cancer, the Conventional or Hypofractionated High-Dose Intensity

Modulated Radiotherapy for Prostate Cancer (CHHiP) trial compared 37, 20 and 19 fractions of radiotherapy.[17] No difference in toxicity between 37 and 20 fractions was seen, but morbidity was reduced in patients with 19 fractions.

Erridge and Rampling[18] have reviewed the evidence for radiotherapy in older patients with glioblastoma. A randomized trial comparing surgery plus postoperative radiotherapy with radiotherapy alone in 81 patients over 70 years old reported a 12 week increase in median survival (from 17 to 29 weeks) after 50.4 Gy in 28 fractions over 5.5 weeks.[19] Various studies have been conducted to reduce numbers of fractions, and, hence, treatment intensity and toxicity. A study comparing 40 Gy in 15 fractions with 60 Gy in 30 fractions in 100 patients over 60 years found no difference in survival.[20] A further trial reported that temozolomide alone and 34 Gy in 10 fractions over 2 weeks each gave better survival compared with conventional radiotherapy.[21] The results of an intergroup study of over 500 patients comparing 40 Gy in 15 fractions with or without temozolomide, but with no chemotherapy-alone arm, will be reported shortly.

Ortholan and colleagues[22] reviewed the management of oral cancer in those over 80 years old. While, even within this age group, age under or over 84 years old was a prognostic factor, age-adapted treatments using hypofractionated or split-course regimens did not seem to compromise survival. In line with this, a meta-analysis of accelerated and hyperfractionated regimens did not show survival benefit in those over 70 years old, as it had in those who were younger, suggesting that improvements in local control were balanced by increases in toxicity.[23]

Chakraborty and colleagues[24] compared patients under and over 65 years old treated for cervical cancer with volumetric modulated-arc therapy. One out of 43 younger patients and eight out of 23 older patients did not receive chemotherapy. In seven patients (median age 75 years, interquartile range 74–78 years), old age was the only reason given. No differences were seen in chemotherapy interruptions or cessation, treatment toxicity, local control or survival between the two groups.

In summary, in a number of settings it may be possible to improve the use of radiotherapy in older people with the greater precision of modern radiotherapy using stereotactic ablative radiotherapy or volumetric modulated-arc therapy. Hypofractionated regimens to reduce time away from home also seem to have potential in this age group. It is unclear why the supposed disadvantages of increased late toxicity with this strategy have not been more prominent.

Can the toxicities of radiotherapy be ameliorated?

Following on from a randomized trial carried out by the European Organisation for Research and Treatment of Cancer,[25] patients with stage III NSCLC have been treated at the Netherlands Cancer Institute with 66 Gy in 24 fractions over 4.5 weeks and concomitant daily cisplatin.[26] The addition of a pre-hydration regimen of 1 l saline with each cisplatin dose reduced the median decrease in glomerular filtration rate from 24% to 8%, the grade 2 or greater oesophageal toxicity from 62% to 34%, and the discontinuation of cisplatin from 19% to 2%. Such approaches could benefit many patients, but older patients who are at particular risk of nephrotoxicity might be the group with the most to gain.

Conclusion

Radiotherapy is a frequently used and critical component of cancer treatments in older people, who may be more susceptible to its side effects. While many tools are available to identify patients at risk, they have not been widely researched in the context of radiotherapy. Patient groups can be identified in whom radiotherapy might not be necessary. When it is necessary, hypofractionation may be a way of making radiotherapy more tolerable and easier to complete, but caution must be applied that elderly-specific regimens not represent a compromise in some aspect of treatment outcomes; what is best and safest for younger patients is also likely to be so for older patients. Smith and Smith[27] have made recommendations for how radiotherapy should be approached in older patients. Our understanding of what older people want from radiotherapy, what they can tolerate and can benefit from, and whether modified treatments are justified requires specific studies of all these issues.

References

1   Cancer Research UK. *Statistics by cancer type*. Available from: www.cancerresearchuk.org/health-professional/cancer-statistics/statistics-by-cancer-type (accessed 8 June 2015).

2   Delaney G, Jacob S, Featherstone C, Barton M. The role of radiotherapy in cancer treatment: estimating optimal utilization from a review of evidence-based clinical guidelines. *Cancer* 2005; 104: 1129–37.

3   Joerger M, Thürlimann B, Savidan A, *et al*. Treatment of breast cancer in the elderly: a prospective, population-based Swiss study. *J Geriatr Oncol* 2013; 4: 39–47.

4   Landrum MB, Keating NL, Lamont EB, *et al*. Reasons for underuse of recommended therapies for colorectal and lung cancer in the Veterans Health Administration. *Cancer* 2012; 118: 3345–55.

5   Wong J, Xu B, Yeung HN, Roeland EJ, *et al*. Age disparity in palliative radiation therapy among patients with advanced cancer. *Int J Radiat Oncol Biol Phys* 2014; 90: 224–30.

6   Kaufmann A, Schmidt H, Ostheimer C, *et al*. Quality of life in very elderly radiotherapy patients: a prospective pilot study using the EORTC QLQ-ELD14 module. *Support Care Cancer* 2015; 23: 1883–92.

7   De Ruysscher D, Botterweck A, Dirx M, *et al*. Eligibility for concurrent chemotherapy and radiotherapy of locally advanced lung cancer patients: a prospective, population-based study. *Ann Oncol* 2009; 20: 98–102.

8   Puts MT, Santos B, Hardt J, *et al*. An update on a systematic review of the use of geriatric assessment for older adults in oncology. *Ann Oncol* 2014; 25: 307–15.

9   Puts MT, Monette J, Girre V, *et al*. Are frailty markers useful for predicting treatment toxicity and mortality in older newly diagnosed cancer patients? Results from a prospective pilot study. *Crit Rev Oncol Hematol* 2011; 78: 138–49.

10   Ulger S, Kizilarslanoglu MC, Kilic MK, *et al*. Estimating radiation therapy toxicity and tolerability with comprehensive assessment parameters in geriatric cancer patients. *Asian Pac J Cancer Prev* 2015; 16: 1965–9.

11   Kenis C, Bron D, Libert Y, *et al*. Relevance of a systematic geriatric screening and assessment in older patients with cancer: results of a prospective multicentric study. *Ann Oncol* 2013; 24: 1306–12.

12   Droz JP, Aapro M, Balducci L, *et al*. Management of prostate cancer in older patients: updated recommendations of a working group of the International Society of Geriatric Oncology. *Lancet Oncol* 2014; 15: e404–14.

13   Bekelman JE, Mitra N, Handorf EA, *et al*. Effectiveness of androgen-deprivation therapy and radiotherapy for older men with locally advanced prostate cancer. *J Clin Oncol* 2015; 33: 716–22.

14 Kunkler IH, Williams LJ, Jack WJ, *et al.*; PRIME II Investigators. Breast-conserving surgery
    with or without irradiation in women aged 65 years or older with early breast cancer (PRIME
    II): a randomised controlled trial. *Lancet Oncol* 2015; 16: 266–73.

15 Cannon NA, Iyengar P, Choy H, *et al.* Stereotactic ablative body radiation therapy for
    tumors in the lung in octogenarians: a retrospective single institution study. *BMC Cancer*
    2014; 14: 971.

16 Institute of Cancer Research. *FAST-Forward. Randomised clinical trial testing a 1 week course
    of curative whole breast radiotherapy against a standard 3 week schedule in terms of local cancer
    control and late adverse effects in patients with early breast cancer.* Available from: www.icr.ac.uk/
    our-research/our-research-centres/clinical-trials-and-statistics-unit/clinical-
    trials/fast_forward_page (accessed 8 June 2015).

17 Dearnaley D, Syndikus I, Sumo G, *et al.* Conventional versus hypofractionated high-dose
    intensity-modulated radiotherapy for prostate cancer: preliminary safety results from the
    CHHiP randomised controlled trial. *Lancet Oncol* 2012; 13: 43–54.

18 Erridge SC, Rampling R. Management of central nervous system tumours in the elderly. *Clin
    Oncol (R Coll Radiol)* 2014; 26: 431–7.

19 Keime-Guibert F, Chinot O, Taillandier L, *et al.* Radiotherapy for glioblastoma in the elderly.
    N Engl J Med 2007; 356: 1527–35.

20 Roa W, Brasher P, Bauman G, *et al.* Abbreviated course of radiation therapy in older patients
    with glioblastoma multiforme: a prospective randomized clinical trial. *J Clin Oncol* 2004; 22:
    1583–8.

21 Malmstrom A, Gronberg BH, Marosi C, *et al.* Temozolomide versus standard 6-week
    radiotherapy versus hypofractionated radiotherapy in patients older than 60 years with
    glioblastoma: the Nordic randomised, phase 3 trial. *Lancet Oncol* 2012; 13: 916–26.

22 Ortholan C, Lusinchi A, Italiano A, *et al.* Oral cavity squamous cell carcinoma in 260 patients
    aged 80 years or more. *Radiother Oncol* 2009; 93: 516–23.

23 Bourhis J, Overgaard J, Audry H, *et al.*; Meta-analysis of Radiotherapy in Carcinomas of Head
    and Neck (MARCH) Collaborative Group. Hyperfractionated or accelerated radiotherapy in
    head and neck cancer: a meta-analysis. *Lancet* 2006; 368: 843–54.

24 Chakraborty S, Geetha M, Dessai S, *et al.* How well do elderly patients with cervical cancer
    tolerate definitive radiochemotherapy using RapidArc? Results from an institutional audit
    comparing elderly versus younger patients. *Ecancermedicalscience* 2014; 8: 484.

25 Belderbos J, Uitterhoeve L, van Zandwijk N, *et al.* Randomised trial of sequential versus
    concurrent chemoradiotherapy in patients with inoperable non-small-cell lung cancer
    (EORTC 08972-22973). *Eur J Cancer* 2007; 43: 114–21.

26 Uyterlinde W, Chen C, Nijkamp J, *et al.* Treatment adherence in concurrent chemoradiation
    in patients with locally advanced non-small cell lung carcinoma: results of daily intravenous
    prehydration. *Radiother Oncol* 2014; 110: 488–92.

27 Smith GL, Smith BD. Radiation treatment in older patients: a framework for clinical decision
    making. *J Clin Oncol* 2014; 32: 2669–78.

09 Special Issues Concerning Systemic Anticancer Therapy in Older Cancer Patients

Satish Kumar

Introduction

People over the age of 65 are the fastest growing segment of the UK population. By 2034, their number is projected to rise by 50%,[1] when the over-65s will make up more than 20% of the population. This changing demographic has resulted in a >50% cancer incidence in the 50–74 age group; a third of all new cancer diagnoses are in the >75 age group.[2] Three-quarters of all cancer deaths occur in the >65 age group and a half of all cancer deaths occur in the >70 age group. While the cancer burden is highest in the older age group, the evidence for systemic anticancer therapy (SACT) comes largely from retrospective and subgroup analyses of prospective clinical trials, and caution should be exercised in extrapolating results to the general older population. The data, however, suggest that SACT can be safe and effective for these patients, although there is a tendency to greater treatment-related morbidity. This chapter will consider the important aspects of SACT prescribing and the clinical data underpinning its use in older people.

General aspects of SACT in older patients

As with all patients, treatment decisions in older patients require expert knowledge of altered drug pharmacology and biology (which is well characterized in breast cancer, for example), the type of therapy (cytotoxic, small molecules, immunotherapy), the expected benefits and the intent of treatment (curative adjuvant therapy or palliative). It is important to individualize therapy, particularly in older patients. Optimal therapy requires characterization of the functional reserve of an individual patient, both physical and mental, assessment of the extent and severity of comorbidity, identification of malnutrition (low albumin, anaemia) and the degree of social support. Treatment decisions have to be made in the context of life expectancy. The expansion of the therapeutic armamentarium with targeted small molecules, monoclonal antibodies and immunotherapy is likely to expand the number of patients it will be possible to treat who would not otherwise have been suitable for traditional cytotoxic therapy. The newer agents, however, have specific toxicities that may make older patients more susceptible to them.

Altered pharmacokinetics

The physiological and pathological decline in hepatic and renal function together with reduced bone marrow reserve associated with ageing are key contributors to the altered pharmacokinetic and pharmacodynamic characteristics of many cancer drugs. This, along with the potential for drug interactions due to the polypharmacy associated with older patients, and factors such as germline mutations in drug-metabolizing enzymes and altered pharmacogenomics, can complicate dosing issues especially for cytotoxic agents with narrow therapeutic ratios. Table 9.1 highlights important age-related physiological changes and their consequences for chemotherapy prescribing. Most pharmacokinetic studies are small and include few older patients. On the whole, most studies show that significant pharmacokinetic changes are based on hepatic and renal function and not on age. Not surprisingly, myelosupression from cytotoxic therapy is more common in older patients. Table 9.2 shows the safety aspects of specific drugs in older patients.

Evidence for SACT in older patients

Prostate cancer

Prostate cancer is primarily a disease of older men, and many clinical trials of systemic therapy have a high proportion of those above the age of 65 or 70. Subgroup analyses of trials of docetaxel,[4] cabazitaxel, abiraterone and enzalutamide have shown that survival improvements accrue to these patients to a similar degree to those in younger patients but with greater toxicity. Docetaxel, however, was not shown to be feasible in frail older patients above the age of 75.[5]

Hormonal therapy remains the standard initial medical therapy, although it carries risks of fractures, metabolic syndrome, cardiac side effects and depression. The majority of patients, however, tolerate it well. Greater attention needs to be paid to long-term complications of such therapy, particularly with regard to bone health and cardiovascular risks especially in those with pre-existing comorbidity. Consideration should be given to calcium and vitamin D supplementation, especially in those with suspected dietary deficiencies, as well as advice on lifestyle modification to include weight-bearing exercise, smoking cessation and control of alcohol consumption. Abiraterone and enzalutamide are good options in treating castration-resistant patients not deemed suitable for docetaxel chemotherapy.

Breast cancer

Hormone therapy use in older women with breast cancer is generally safe and should be offered to all patients irrespective of age, provided it is medically feasible to do so. On the basis of data from the Early Breast Cancer Trialists' Collaborative Group (EBCTCG), adjuvant aromatase

Table 9.1 General dosing considerations in SACT prescribing (adapted from Repetto[3]).

Physiological change	Pharmacokinetic implication
Decreased gastrointestinal motility, decreased splanchnic blood flow, decreased secretion of digestive enzymes, mucosal atrophy	Reduced drug absorption
Malnutrition and low albumin	Increased concentration of protein-bound drugs
Decreased hepatic blood flow, mass and cytochrome P450 function (more important when combined with pharmacogenomic alterations)	Altered drug metabolism
Reduced glomerular filtration rate	Altered pharmacokinetic of renally excreted drugs: capecitabine, carboplatin, methotrexate, cisplatin
Polypharmacy	Drug interactions, increased toxicity or reduced effectiveness
Increased body fat and reduction in lean body mass	Altered drug distribution
Greater anaemia, low albumin	Increased levels of circulating drugs
Reduced stem cell mass/bone marrow reserve	Slower recovery of blood and mucosal cells, i.e. prolonged neutropenia

inhibitors have proven to be superior to tamoxifen in the 60–69 and >70 years age groups. Tamoxifen, however, is a good alternative if cardiovascular and bone health or tolerability are an issue with aromatase inhibitors. Tamoxifen may be considered for those oestrogen receptor-positive breast tumours that have an excellent prognosis. Extended duration hormonal therapy with aromatase inhibitors beyond 5 years of tamoxifen or switch after 2–3 years of tamoxifen should be considered in selected patients with high-risk features such as node-positive or high-grade tumours. DEXA scans with supplemental vitamin D and calcium are important in following up these patients.

Chemotherapy for older patients requires a balanced approach, bearing in mind the biology of breast cancer in older patients (more indolent histology, greater hormone receptor positivity, lower human epidermal growth factor receptor 2 [HER2] positivity); the known cardiac and haematological toxicities of anthracyclines and taxanes, respectively; the life expectancy of a

Table 9.2 Safety aspects of selected SACT in older patients.

Systemic agent	Risk of treatment
Doxorubicin, epirubicin, trastuzumab, 5-FU	Greater risk of congestive heart failure and left ventricular dysfunction
Taxanes, oxaliplatin	Paclitaxel: greater drug exposure in older patients; higher risks of neutropenia and neuropathy; weekly paclitaxel is less toxic
Capecitabine, 5-FU	Angina, myocardial infarction, arrhythmia, cardiogenic shock, sudden death; consider starting at reduced dose for reduced creatine clearance; important interaction with warfarin, with exaggerated activity; caution in those on folate supplementation
Carboplatin, cisplatin, methotrexate	Dosing based on creatine clearance; caution with methotrexate in pleural effusion; ascites
Opioids (e.g. codeine)	Great interpatient variability in exposure due to renal dysfunction and pharmacogenomic changes
Sunitinib	Consider first-line dose reduction (no decrease in efficacy); greater fatigue and anorexia in >70 years
Pazopanib	Standard initial doses
Axitinib	Standard dose
Cetuximab	Safe at standard dose
Bevacizumab	Greater drug-induced hypertension in >75 years, greater number of arterial thromboembolic events; screen for vascular risk factors
Gefitinib	Better tolerated than vinorelbine (similar efficacy)
Erlotinib	Greater rash, stomatitis, dehydration, anorexia and fatigue
Pertuzumab, trastuzumab emtansine	No additional cardiac toxicity to trastuzumab, but close cardiac monitoring in older patients recommended
Ipilimumab	Careful patient selection, ideally trial-eligible patients
Vemurafenib, dabrafenib	No dosage alterations first line; hepatic function-dependent

given patient; and the functional status of any given patient. Caution has to be exercised in the use of online programmes such as Adjuvant! Online (www.adjuvantonline.com) for predictive and prognostic purposes, as these models are not well validated in those above age 70 and do not take into account the burden of comorbidity, which is highly variable in this population.

The EBCTCG meta-analysis had too few patients above the age of 70 to enable any conclusions to be drawn about the benefits of adjuvant polychemotherapy. A French study of older breast cancer patients showed that weekly epirubicin with tamoxifen resulted in improved recurrence-free survival but no increase in overall survival (OS) when compared with tamoxifen alone.[6] Oral capecitabine was shown in a Cancer and Leukemia Group B (CALGB) study to be inferior to standard chemotherapy (cyclophosphamide, methotrexate and fluorouracil [5-FU], and cyclophosphamide and doxorubicin).[7] Anthracycline-based adjuvant chemotherapy regimens may be considered for fit, older patients, recognizing greater risk of cardiac toxicity even with normal baseline cardiac function. A Surveillance, Epidemiology, and End Results (SEER) database analysis of more than 40,000 patients showed cardiac failure rates at 10 years of 38%, 33% and 29% in those receiving anthracyclines, non-anthracyclines and no chemotherapy, respectively.[8] Non-anthracycline-containing regimens, namely docetaxel and cyclophosphamide, and oral cyclophosphamide, methotrexate and 5-FU (where both anthracyclines and taxanes are to be avoided), should be considered in less fit patients. In the HER2-positive group, the use of trastuzumab and chemotherapy (such as paclitaxel and carboplatin) is favoured in those with high-risk features, especially in those with hormone receptor-negative disease. It is necessary to proactively assess and manage women with coronary artery disease, hypertension or a subnormal ejection fraction by carrying out a cardiology consultation and instituting medical therapy to optimize cardiac function before embarking on trastuzumab or anthracyclines.

In the metastatic setting, a randomized phase II study in older women comparing weekly paclitaxel and docetaxel showed a greater response rate and progression-free survival (PFS) for paclitaxel: there was more myelosupression and neuropathy with paclitaxel, and more fatigue and oedema with docetaxel.[9] Other drugs with a good safety profile include vinorelbine, liposomal doxorubicin and capecitabine (consider an initially reduced dose and estimate renal function). Anthracyclines can be used cautiously with cardiac monitoring and weekly administration or use of liposomal formulations, as well as dexrazoxane as a cardioprotectant against doxorubicin-mediated cardiomyopathy (when more than 300 mg/m^2 cumulative doses have been used). Trastuzumab use in combination with chemotherapy reduces breast cancer mortality compared with chemotherapy alone in HER2-positive disease.[10] Sequential use of single agents is preferred. The choice of agents depends on the patient's clinical status and on patient tolerability, keeping in mind the schedule and toxicity of specific agents. Supportive therapy with growth factors should be considered when using agents with a greater than 20% chance of myelosupression.

Hormonal therapy in the metastatic setting should be offered as first line in all patients who do not have rapidly progressive visceral disease. Aromatase inhibitors are generally first line; second-line therapy would be fulvestrant or exemestane in combination with an mTOR inhibitor. They may be combined with HER2 inhibitors in those with HER2-positive disease. In people above the age of 85, and with limited life expectancy and comorbidity, primary hormonal therapy alone is a justifiable option.

Ovarian cancer

A retrospective analysis of SACT use in ovarian cancer was carried out in the Elderly Women Ovarian Cancer trial of the French GINECO group. Retrospective analysis of two studies in >70-year-old patients treated with a platinum-based doublet revealed that advanced age, depression at baseline and International Federation of Gynecology and Obstetrics (FIGO) stage IV were predictive for prognosis, and paclitaxel use was an independent predictor for worse survival.[11] Prospective studies are underway to confirm or refute these findings.

The GOG-182 trial showed that age is an important risk factor when considering postoperative chemotherapy. Age was associated with poor performance status (PS), lower chemotherapy completion rates, higher toxicity and an 8 month shorter survival.[12] Fit, older patients can be considered for doublet and triplet (with bevacizumab) therapy based on efficacy data. Patients with poor PS can be considered for single-agent carboplatin, weekly carboplatin/paclitaxel and reduced initial doses. Several single agents such as paclitaxel, gemcitabine, doxorubicin hydrochloride and topotecan have useful activity. Less commonly, cyclophosphamide and etoposide are also used.

Non-small-cell lung cancer

The prospective Elderly Lung Cancer Vinorelbine Italian Study (ELVIS) study of 191 patients above the age of 70 with lung metastases, showed a 7 week improvement in OS and quality of life from vinorelbine but did not reach the accrual target of 350 patients.[13] Docetaxel is at least as effective as vinorelbine and has greater myelotoxicity and superior rates of response and PFS. Subgroup analysis of trial data suggests that: (1) chemotherapy is likely to prolong survival in patients with good PS; (2) there are conflicting data on the efficacy of doublet agents versus single agents – non-cisplatin-containing doublet regimens are equivalent to single agents such as gemcitabine and vinorelbine;[14] (3) doublet regimens including carboplatin and paclitaxel have been shown to be efficacious with acceptable toxicity, even in those with PS 2, and more efficacious than non-platinum single agents such as gemcitabine and vinorelbine.

Adjuvant cisplatin-based chemotherapy has been shown to improve OS in older patients to a similar extent to that of their younger counterparts, but there are more dose reductions and earlier discontinuations, so patient selection and consideration of patient preferences and comorbidities were important in making treatment decisions. Carboplatin can substitute cisplatin with some reduction in efficacy, but lack of prospective data should limit its routine use in the adjuvant setting.

Targeted therapy such as erlotinib and crizotinib can have dramatic effects in older patients and, even in patients with poor PS, has been shown to improve both PFS and OS, though with greater rash, fatigue and dehydration.[15] Single agents in older patients with poor PS can result in a median survival of 18 months, and 1 year survival rates of 63%.

Colorectal cancer

More than 70% of colorectal cancer patients are above the age of 65. In general, 5-FU and capecitabine-based adjuvant chemotherapy benefits older patients to a similar extent to their younger counterparts, though at the cost of cardiotoxicity sustained by a higher proportion of older patients. A pooled analysis of 5-FU and folinic acid in more than 3300 postoperative patients with stage II and III disease, showed a 24% reduction in mortality and a 32% decrease in disease recurrence in all age groups including those over 70:[16] only one study showed a greater risk of grade 3 neutropenia. The evidence for adding oxaliplatin to 5-FU is conflicting, but on the whole it results in little incremental benefit and should be reserved for the fittest stage III and high-risk stage II patients with reasonable life expectancy.

In metastatic disease, the combination of oxaliplatin or irinotecan with 5-FU is efficacious in older patients but may be accompanied by greater myelosupression, nausea, vomiting, neuropathy and diarrhoea; in less fit patients, it is reasonable to reduce the initial dose. In the latter group, oxaliplatin combination regimens may produce greater response rates and a trend to improvement in both PFS and OS;[17] in the case of irinotecan, there may also be a greater predisposition to delayed diarrhoea. Capecitabine combined with oxaliplatin was associated with slightly inferior response rates, similar PFS and a greater risk of grade 3–4 nausea, vomiting, diarrhoea, anorexia and hand-foot syndrome.[17] A pooled analysis of trials showed that combination therapy benefited PS 2 patients as much as PS 1 patients but at the cost of increased nausea and vomiting.[18]

Irinotecan, either single agent or in combination with 5-FU and folinic acid, is generally safe and efficacious in older patients[19] but is less toxic when given with infusional 5-FU and folinic acid rather than in bolus doses. The addition of bevacizumab in triplet therapy has to be tempered with the known increased risk of thromboembolic disease with this agent.

Conclusion

The judicious use of SACT in older patients requires knowledge of altered physiology and resultant altered pharmacology of oncology drugs. This, coupled with incorporation of geriatric assessment, would enable safe and effective prescribing. The challenge is to adapt service provision to manage these complex patients who have greater needs and who are probably not best served in busy oncology clinics. Individualized and biomarker-led therapy can potentially refine patient selection so as to maximize response to therapy and minimize toxicity.

The use of risk prediction tools such as those developed by Extermann *et al.*[20] (Chemotherapy Risk Assessment Scale for High-Age Patients [CRASH]) or by Hurria *et al.*[21] includes both treatment and patient-related factors to predict chemotherapy toxicity. However, these studies are subject to limitations. They do not agree entirely on which patient factors are important. They do not provide a framework for intervention, which is a highly desirable feature of such approaches. Ongoing work will improve the tools to predict toxicity and increase their role and value.

SACT datasets containing both treatment and outcome details should be a priority and are likely to have significant benefits for generating research hypotheses, benchmarking outcomes and enhancing services for the complex and multidisciplinary needs of older patients. The need for education and training in geriatric oncology should be recognized in order to meet the challenges of treating a burgeoning older population in the future.

References

1. Office for National Statistics (2013). *National population projections, 2012-based statistical bulletin.* Available from: www.ons.gov.uk/ons/dcp171778_334975.pdf (accessed 20 March 2015).

2. Cancer Research UK. *Cancer mortality by age.* Available from: www.cancerresearchuk.org/cancer-info/cancerstats/mortality/age (accessed 20 March 2015).

3. Repetto L. Greater risks of chemotherapy toxicity in elderly patients with cancer. *J Support Oncol* 2003; 1 (suppl 2): 18–24.

4. Berthold DR, Pond GR, Soban F, *et al.* Docetaxel plus prednisone or mitoxantrone plus prednisone for advanced prostate cancer: updated survival in the TAX 327 study. *J Clin Oncol* 2008; 26: 242–5.

5. Mourey L, Gravis G, Sevin E, *et al.* Feasibility of docetaxel-prednisone (DP) in frail elderly (age 75 and older) patients with castration-resistant metastatic prostate cancer (CRMPC): GERICO10-GETUG P03 trial led by Unicancer (abstract). Presented at: American Society of Clinical Oncology genitourinary cancer symposium, 2014.

6 Fargeot P, Bonneterre J, Roché H, *et al.* Disease-free survival advantage of weekly epirubicin plus tamoxifen versus tamoxifen alone as adjuvant treatment of operable, node-positive, elderly breast cancer patients: 6-year follow-up results of the French adjuvant study group 08 trial. *J Clin Oncol* 2014; 22: 4622–30.

7 Muss HB, Berry DA, Cirrincione CT, *et al.* Adjuvant chemotherapy in older women with early-stage breast cancer. *N Engl J Med* 2009; 360: 2055–65.

8 Pinder MC, Duan Z, Goodwin JS, *et al.* Congestive heart failure in older women treated with adjuvant anthracycline chemotherapy for breast cancer. *J Clin Oncol* 2007; 25: 3808–15.

9 Beuselinck B, Wildiers H, Wynendaele W, *et al.* Weekly paclitaxel versus weekly docetaxel in elderly or frail patients with metastatic breast carcinoma: a randomized phase-II study of the Belgian Society of Medical Oncology. *Crit Rev Oncol Hematol* 2010; 75: 70–7.

10 Griffiths RI, Lalla D, Herbert RJ, *et al.* Infused therapy and survival in older patients diagnosed with metastatic breast cancer who received trastuzumab. *Cancer Invest* 2011; 29: 573–84.

11 Wright JD, Ananth CV, Tsui J, *et al.* Comparative effectiveness of upfront treatment strategies in elderly women with ovarian cancer. *Cancer* 2014; 120: 1246–54.

12 Tew WP, Java J, Chi D, *et al.* Treatment outcomes for older women with advanced ovarian cancer: results from a phase III clinical trial (GOG182). *J Clin Oncol* 2010; 28 (suppl): abstract 5030.

13 The Elderly Lung Cancer Vinorelbine Italian Study Group. Effects of vinorelbine on quality of life and survival of elderly patients with advanced non-small-cell lung cancer. *J Natl Cancer Inst* 1999; 91: 66–72.

14 Gridelli C, Perrone F, Gallo C, *et al.*; MILES Investigators. Chemotherapy for elderly patients with advanced non-small-cell lung cancer: the Multicenter Italian Lung Cancer in the Elderly Study (MILES) phase III randomized trial. *J Natl Cancer Inst* 2003; 95: 362–72.

15 Inoue A, Kobayashi K, Usui K, *et al.*; North East Japan Gefitinib Study Group. First-line gefitinib for patients with advanced non-small-cell lung cancer harboring epidermal growth factor receptor mutations without indication for chemotherapy. *J Clin Oncol* 2009; 27: 1394–400.

16 Sargent DJ, Goldberg RM, Jacobson SD, *et al.* A pooled analysis of adjuvant chemotherapy for resected colon cancer in elderly patients. *N Engl J Med* 2001; 345: 1091–7.

17 Seymour MT, Thompson LC, Wasan HS, *et al.*; FOCUS2 Investigators, National Cancer Research Institute Colorectal Cancer Clinical Studies Group. Chemotherapy options in elderly and frail patients with metastatic colorectal cancer (MRC FOCUS2): an open-label, randomised factorial trial. *Lancet* 2011; 377: 1749–59.

18 Folprecht G, Rougier P, Saltz L, *et al.* Irinotecan in first line therapy of elderly and non-elderly patients with metastatic colorectal cancer: meta-analysis of four trials investigating 5-FU and irinotecan. *J Clin Oncol* 2006; 24 (suppl): abstract 3578.

19 Sargent DJ, Köhne CH, Sanoff HK, *et al.* Pooled safety and efficacy analysis examining the effect of performance status on outcomes in nine first-line treatment trials using individual data from patients with metastatic colorectal cancer. *J Clin Oncol* 2009; 27: 1948–55.

20 Extermann M, Boler I, Reich RR, *et al.* Predicting the risk of chemotherapy toxicity in older patients: the Chemotherapy Risk Assessment Scale for High-Age Patients (CRASH) score. *Cancer* 2012; 118: 3377–86.

21 Hurria A, Togawa K, Mohile SG, *et al.* Predicting chemotherapy toxicity in older adults with cancer: a prospective multicenter study. *J Clin Oncol* 2011; 29: 3457–65.

10 Special Issues in the Selection of Older Cancer Patients and Delivery of Their Surgery

Anita Hargreaves, William Cross, Paul Finan, Riccardo Audisio

Background

We live in an ageing population. Life expectancy has doubled over the last century; the number of people aged >65 years has doubled and the number over 85 years has quadrupled.[1] By 2050, those over 65 years of age will account for 20% of the population in the developed world.[2] This epidemiological explosion places a tremendous burden on health resources and provides unique challenges in the area of geriatric oncology. Senescence generates numerous physiological and biological changes that can impact on treatment selection. Patients are presenting who would never have previously been considered for cancer treatment. Are we able to holistically assess them? Can we accurately predict perioperative risk and overall survival (OS) for the different treatment options using assessment tools designed for a younger population? Is their consent supported and informed as it is with their younger counterparts? Do we have a clear understanding of their psycho-oncological and social needs? Is their overall management truly multidisciplinary? In this chapter, we consider the general issues surrounding cancer surgery in older patients and include specific comments on the four commonest cancers: breast, lung, prostate and colorectal.

Modern oncological treatment planning is based on evidence. Unfortunately, there are no national standards of care or evidence-based guidelines for older cancer patients because in this age group they have often been excluded from trials. Following publication of trial results, there has been limited independent validation of cancer treatments for older patients. Older patients are underrepresented in clinical trials[3] and we regularly offer treatment options as the gold standard based on clinical trials undertaken in younger population groups. This includes the use of breast-conserving surgery and radiotherapy instead of mastectomy, based on the results of the Milan trials, which did not recruit any individuals over the age of 70 years. Even some recent trials targeted at this patient group (Endocrine +/− Surgical Therapy for Elderly Women with Mammary Cancer [ESTEeM][4] and Adjuvant Cytotoxic Chemotherapy in Older Women [ACTION][5]) have closed early due to recruitment problems. Methodologically sound investigations do not readily transpose to the geriatric oncology setting, as illustrated in the area of total mesorectal excision for rectal cancer, which has significantly reduced loco-regional recurrence and survival in younger patients but may not do so in older patients.[6] As care providers, we must be cognizant of the limited validity of evidence-based practice in the setting of cancer in the older cancer population.

Surgery remains the most effective cancer ablative therapy. The increase in length of stay, requirements for critical care organ support, complication rates and mortality can preclude oncological benefit. Differences in patient management may be related to the lack of clinical evidence to determine treatment efficacy in older women; patient preferences; surgical preferences; anaesthetic assessment; the influence of family, friends and carers; comorbidities and frailty that contraindicate treatment options; and, unfortunately, innate ageism. Undertreatment may be related to a perceived lack of tolerance for the risks or side effects of therapies. Personalized plans should be multifactorial and include tumour characteristics, pre-existing conditions and comorbidities, and informed preferences.

The International Society of Geriatric Oncology advocates the use of Comprehensive Geriatric Assessment (CGA), as age alone is not a good indicator of a patient's ability to withstand treatment. Formal CGA assesses cognitive function, the ability to perform activities of daily living independently, pre-existing medical conditions and comorbidities, polypharmacy, nutritional status, psychosocial needs and generic syndromes. Frailty assessment is mandatory: it may be present in the absence of comorbidity and is an independent predictor of life expectancy, surgical morbidity and mortality.[7] CGA is time-consuming. Quicker, validated screening tools, such as Preoperative Assessment of Cancer in the Elderly (PACE) and Vulnerable Elders Survey (VES)-13, enable us to identify patients who would benefit from preoperative optimization (correction of anaemia/dehydration/malnutrition) or from referral to a geriatrician and early involvement of occupational therapy and physiotherapy to aid recovery and safe discharge. The identification of impaired cognition, hypoalbuminaemia, recurrent falls, low haematocrit, functional dependence and significant burden of comorbidities is directly related to the length of hospital stay. These factors may account for a 50% increase in the risk of postoperative complications, 6 month mortality and institutionalization.[8–10] One-third of older patients develop a new impairment while hospitalized.

Lung cancer

Lung cancer commonly affects the older patient population. Resection via lobectomy or segmentectomy is the treatment standard for resectable tumours. There is no significant survival advantage for either surgical approach over the other.[11] For those with non-resectable tumours, chemotherapy may be withheld from older patients in UK practice due to perceived lack of tolerance. Despite this perception, however, chemotherapy has been shown to be well tolerated in many patients and has a survival advantage.[12]

Colorectal cancer

Over 50% of colorectal cancers are diagnosed in patients >65 years. The incidence of colorectal cancer increases with age, rising from 415 (male) and 257 (female) cases per 100,000 of the population between 75 and 79 years of age to 518 and 333 per 100,000, respectively, for those aged over 85 years. This presents unique problems in the diagnosis and management of the disease. Recent data from the National Cancer Data Repository reveals, where stage can be determined, that fewer than 50% of cases presenting over the age of 80 years are stage I or II. The significant improvement in stage following the introduction of the national screening programme, with 53% being stage I or II,[13] may have an effect on incidence in due course by detection at an earlier age. Older colorectal cancer patients present more frequently as an emergency, rising from 24% in 70- to 79-year-olds to 43% in patients older than 85 years at presentation.[14] This is reflected in outcomes after surgery, with a three- to fourfold increase in perioperative mortality and a greater chance of death within the first year.[15] Even on diagnosis there is recent evidence that the chances of a patient receiving a major resection fall significantly with age (a National Cancer Intelligence Network report on major resections by age is available from www.ncin.org.uk) and this is confirmed by an absence of staging data in over 40% of patients presenting at 85 years of age and over.

Advances in surgical and perioperative treatment have made colorectal cancer surgery safer. Curative resection is well tolerated, particularly if the patient is suitable for a laparoscopic approach.[16,17] The advantages of laparoscopic surgery may be offset by the duration of surgery and we have yet to see the impact of this on survival. Complications for rectal cancer resection show no significant differences between younger and older patients.[18] Routine preoperative physiological testing (cardiopulmonary exercise testing) allows physiological optimization of the patient and laparoscopic surgery, whilst increasing operative time, and reduces the surgical insult to the patient. All these advances are of value in older patients with increased comorbidity and associated long-term conditions. Surgical treatments, particularly for rectal cancer, often lead to problems with continence, and such surgery may be compounded by pre-existing sphincter injuries. According to the National Bowel Cancer Audit (www.hsic.gov.uk), permanent stoma rates at 18 months in patients with rectal cancer are in the region of 45–50%; impairment of eyesight or reduction in manual dexterity associated with older age may further impair quality of life in stoma patients.

Evidence-based adjuvant therapies have emerged in recent years and have led to improvements in survival for stage III colorectal cancer (adjuvant chemotherapy) or reductions in local recurrence rates in rectal cancer (adjuvant radiotherapy). Again, these treatment options appear to be used less frequently in older patients. Use of adjuvant chemotherapy fell from 80% of stage III cases aged 60–64 years to 20% in similarly staged patients over 75 years of age (R. Birch, personal communication). Chemotherapy in the adjuvant and metastatic setting seems to be well tolerated and there are no statistically significant differences in the side effect profile and toxicities between younger and older patient cohorts.[19–21] When studying radiotherapy treatments in patients with rectal cancer a similar effect was noted: the proportion of patients having some form of radiotherapeutic intervention fell from 60% in those younger than 60 years of age to 30% in those aged over 80 years.

Prostate cancer

Prostate cancer disproportionately affects older men: disease incidence, prevalence and mortality are strongly correlated with increasing age. In the UK, prostate cancer is the most frequently diagnosed solid cancer in men: according to Cancer Research UK statistics (www.cancerresearchuk.org), more than one-third of cases are diagnosed in men aged over 75 years. Although prostate cancer survival has improved dramatically in the last 40 years, with now more than eight in 10 men surviving their disease for at least 10 years, 70% of disease-related deaths occur in men aged 75 years or older.[22] It has been estimated that the incidence of prostate cancer in the UK will continue to increase until at least 2030,[23] further highlighting the significance of this condition for the ageing population and for geriatric oncology.

Prostate cancer is a highly heterogeneous disease that follows a variable course in different patients, irrespective of age. One of the greatest challenges in routine practice is to diagnose and treat clinically significant prostate cancer in a timely manner while limiting overdiagnosis and unnecessary treatment of low-risk disease. Men older than 70 years with low-risk prostate cancer, coexisting medical conditions and a relatively limited life expectancy are at particular risk of overtreatment.[22] By contrast, healthy older men presenting with high-risk localized or locally advanced disease are often denied the opportunity of radical therapy and are therefore disadvantaged. The optimal clinical management of this patient group requires shared decision making with a fully informed patient (and family) and a multidisciplinary approach with a team of clinical specialists from diagnosis to treatment and beyond. Van Poppel[24] reviewed the place of prostatectomy in older patients with prostate cancer. Radical prostatectomy is feasible in men in their 70s and 80s and produces good results in patients who are carefully selected, taking into account their level of comorbidity.[25-31] OS is reported to be 65–83% and cancer-specific survival 94–96%,[24] although studies are often small. Definitions of continence rates vary, but using strict criteria (no continence pads required) continence rates were as high as 92% in some series.[24] Radical prostatectomy is an option for older prostate cancer patients depending on comorbidity, frailty and patient choice, and certainly should not be excluded on the basis of chronological age.

Breast cancer

In breast cancer, observational studies illustrate significant delays in cancer detection, under-staging and inferior survival in older patients. The 2009 NHS breast screening programme report concluded that older patients were less likely to have radiotherapy and chemotherapy.[32] This may be due to the higher proportion of grade 3, node-positive cancers in younger women. Avoidance of radiotherapy in low-risk T1 oestrogen receptor (ER)-positive human epidermal growth factor receptor 2-negative cancers may be based on evidence from the PRIME II[33] and CALGB 9343[34] trials. Patient management continues to be strongly influenced by the Preece *et al.* pilot study,[35] despite a Cochrane review concluding that primary endocrine therapy should only be given if the patient is unfit for surgery because of the development of endocrine resistance. The lack of surgical patients with ER-positive breast cancer lacks equipoise with the surgical management of older patients with ER-negative cancer (the perioperative risk is 2 in 1000 patients). Ideally, there would be an equivalent to the Adjuvant! Online (www.adjuvantonline.com) and Predict (www.predict.nhs.uk) systems used by non-surgical oncologists which would combine oncology data and frailty assessment to aid the treatment planning of older breast cancer patients. It is essential to remember that health-related quality of life is a vital endpoint for older women with breast cancer.

Future developments in cancer surgery for older patients should be driven by closer links with geriatrics colleagues following the success seen in the management of older orthopaedic patients. Observational data from studies like Bridging the Age Gap in Breast Cancer and Adjuvant Chemotherapy in Older Women with Breast Cancer (AChEW); systematic reviews (e.g. Liverpool Reviews and Implementation Group); and collaborations such as the European Registration of Cancer Care will help to improve cancer care for older cancer patients across Europe. Clinical research should focus on complication rates, perioperative and postoperative mortality, long-term outcomes and quality of life. We hope that the interest in this challenging field results in improved quality of care and quality of life, as well as in improved overall life expectancy, for the patients of the future.

References

1 Office for National Statistics (2012). *Population ageing in the United Kingdom, its constituent countries and the European Union.* Available from: www.ons.gov.uk/ons/dcp171776_258607 .pdf (accessed 17 July 2015).

2 World Health Organization (2014). *Facts about ageing.* Available from: www.who.int/ageing/ about/facts/en/ (accessed 17 July 2015).

3 National Cancer Intelligence Network. *Older people and cancer.* London: Public Health England, 2015.

4   Reed MW, Wyld L, Ellis P, *et al.*; ACTION and ESTEeM Trial Management Groups. Breast cancer in older women: trials and tribulations. *Clin Oncol (R Coll Radiol)* 2009; 21: 99–102.

5   Leonard R, Ballinger R, Cameron D, *et al.* Adjuvant Chemotherapy in Older Women (ACTION) study – what did we learn from the pilot phase? *Br J Cancer* 2011; 105: 1260–6.

6   Rutten HJ, den Dulk M, Lemmens VE, *et al.* Controversies of total mesorectal excision for rectal cancer in elderly patients. *Lancet Oncol* 2008; 9: 494–501.

7   Habr-Gama A, Perez RO. Non-operative approaches to rectal cancer: a critical evaluation. *Semin Radiol Oncol* 2011; 21: 234–9.

8   Robinson TN, Eiseman B, Wallace JI, *et al.* Redefining geriatric preoperative assessment using frailty, disability and co-morbidity. *Ann Surg* 2005: 250: 449–55.

9   Robinson TN, Wu DS, Pointer LF, *et al.* Pre-operative cognitive dysfunction is related to adverse postoperative outcomes in the elderly. *J Am Coll Surg* 2012; 215: 12–17.

10   PACE participants, Audisio RA, Pope D, *et al.* Shall we operate? Preoperative assessment in elderly cancer patients (PACE) can help. A SIOG surgical task force prospective study. *Crit Rev Oncol Haematol* 2008; 65: 156–63.

11   Allen MS, Darling GE, Pechet TT, *et al.* Morbidity and mortality of major pulmonary resections in patients with early stage lung cancer: initial results of the randomized, prospective ACOSOG Z0030 trial. *Ann Thorac Surg* 2006; 81: 1013–19.

12   Fisher S, Al-Fayea TM, Winget M, *et al.* Uptake and tolerance of chemotherapy in elderly patients with small cell lung cancer and impact on survival. *J Cancer Epidemiol* 2012; 2012: 708936.

13   Morris EJA, Whitehouse LE, Farrell T, *et al.* A retrospective observational study examining the characteristics and outcomes of tumours diagnosed within and without of the English NHS Bowel Cancer Screening Programme. *Br J Cancer* 2012; 107: 757–64.

14   Elliss-Brookes L, McPhail S, Ives A, *et al.* Routes to diagnosis for cancer – determining the patient journey using multiple routine data sets. *Br J Cancer* 2012; 107: 1220–6.

15   Downing A, Aravani A, Macleod U, *et al.* Early mortality from colorectal cancer in England: a retrospective observational study of the factors associated with death in the first year after diagnosis. *Br J Cancer* 2013; 108: 681–5.

16   National Cancer Institute. *Surveillance, Epidemiology, and End Results Program. SEER stat fact sheets: colon and rectum cancer.* Available from: http://seer.cancer.gov (accessed June 2015).

17   Allardyce RA, Bagshaw PF, Frampton CM, *et al.* Australasian Laparoscopic Colon Cancer Study shows that elderly patients may benefit from lower postoperative complication rates following laparoscopic versus open resection. *Br J Surg* 2010; 97: 86–91.

18   Manceau G, Karoi M, Werne A, *et al.* Comparative outcomes of rectal cancer surgery between elderly and non-elderly patients: a systematic review. *Lancet Oncol* 2005; 13: e2525–36.

19   Köhne CH, Folprecht G, Goldberg RM, *et al.* Chemotherapy in elderly patients with colorectal cancer. *Oncologist* 2008; 13: 390–402.

20   Williams GR, Sanoff HK. Adjuvant chemotherapy in older adults with colon cancer. *Am J Hematol Oncol* 2015; 11: 5–10.

21   Chemotherapy options in elderly patients with metastatic colorectal cancer (MRC FOCUS2): an open-label randomised controlled trial. *Lancet* 2011: 377: 1749–59.

22   Droz J-P, Aapro M, Balducci L, *et al.* Management of prostate cancer in older patients: updated recommendations of a working group of the International Society of Geriatric Oncology. *Lancet Oncol* 2014; 15: e404–14.

23 Mistry M, Parkin DM, Ahmad AS, Sasieni P. Cancer incidence in the United Kingdom: projections to the year 2030. *Br J Cancer* 2011; 105: 1795–803.

24 Van Poppel H. Prostatectomy in elderly prostate cancer patients. In: Droz J-P, Audisio RA, eds. *Management of urological cancers in older people.* London: Springer, 2013; 105–20.

25 Thompson RH, Slezak JM, Webster WS, *et al.* Radical prostatectomy for octogenarians: how old is too old? *Urology* 2006; 68: 1042–5.

26 Richstone L, Bianco FJ, Shah HH, *et al.* Radical prostatectomy in men aged ≥70 years: effect of age on upgrading, upstaging, and the accuracy of a preoperative nomogram. *BJU Int* 2008; 101: 541–6.

27 Barry MJ, Albertsen PC, Bagshaw MA, *et al.* Outcomes for men with clinically nonmetastatic prostate carcinoma managed with radical prostatectomy, external beam radiotherapy, or expectant management: a retrospective analysis. *Cancer* 2001; 91: 2302–14.

28 Pierorazio PM, Humphreys E, Walsh PC, *et al.* Radical prostatectomy in older men: survival outcomes in septuagenarians and octogenarians. *BJU Int* 2010; 106: 791–5.

29 Pfitzenmaier J, Pahernik S, Buse S, *et al.* Survival in prostate cancer patients ≥70 years after radical prostatectomy and comparison to younger patients. *World J Urol* 2009; 27: 637–42.

30 Froehner M, Koch R, Litz RJ, *et al.* Survival analysis in men undergoing radical prostatectomy at an age of 70 years or older. *Urol Oncol* 2010; 28: 628–34.

31 Alibhai SM, Naglie G, Nam R, *et al.* Do older men benefit from curative therapy of localized prostate cancer? *J Clin Oncol* 2003; 21: 3318–27.

32 National Cancer Intelligence Network (2007). *Second all breast cancer report.* Available from: www.ncin.org.uk/search/second+all+breast+cancer+report (accessed 17 July 2015).

33 Kunkler IH, Williams LW, Jack W, *et al.* The PRIME II trial: wide local excision and adjuvant hormonal therapy +/− postoperative whole breast irradiation in women ≥65 years with early breast cancer managed by breast conservation (abstract S2-01). Presented at: San Antonio Breast Cancer Symposium, San Antonio, TX, 11 December 2013.

34 Hughes KS, Schanper LA, Bellon LR, *et al.* Lumpectomy plus tamoxifen with or without irradiation in women age 70 years or older with early breast cancer: long term follow up of CALGB 9343. *J Clin Oncol* 2013; 31: 2382–7.

35 Preece PE, Wood RA, Mackie CR, Cuschieri A. Tamoxifen as initial sole treatment of localised breast cancer in elderly women: a pilot study. *BMJ (Clin Res Ed)* 1982; 284: 869–70.

11 Drug Therapy in Older People: Pharmacology and the Dangers of Polypharmacy

Denis Curtin, Paul Gallagher

Introduction

Prescribing for older patients with cancer is complex and challenging. They are a heterogeneous group, ranging from those who are medically well up until the time of cancer diagnosis to those who have multiple concurrent chronic diseases such as hypertension, coronary artery disease, heart failure, diabetes, chronic kidney disease, falls, stroke disease, depression and dementia. The majority of older patients presenting to oncology services are prescribed medications for treatment of coexisting conditions, in addition to primary and secondary prevention of illness.[1] One British study of 100 older patients with metastatic cancer identified a median of seven prescribed medications (interquartile range 1–17 medications).[1] A Canadian study of 112 older patients with newly diagnosed cancer identified a median of five medications before cancer treatments were initiated.[2]

A new diagnosis of cancer may: (1) change the therapeutic targets for existing conditions, e.g. strict lipid control for prevention of cardiovascular disease may no longer be a priority; (2) result in an altered physiological environment that can affect drug handling and drug response with a requirement for dose adjustment, particularly in the context of organ dysfunction; and (3) contribute to additional drug burden in the form of chemotherapy and supportive drugs to manage cancer symptoms, thus placing older patients at increased risk of additive toxicity, drug interactions and adverse drug events.[3] These negative outcomes increase morbidity and healthcare resource use by requiring additional clinical consultations, laboratory testing and prescriptions to treat new symptoms.[1]

Optimizing drug therapy is an essential part of managing an older patient with cancer. All pharmacological treatments should be goal-directed with realistic regard for expected clinical outcome. Clinicians should be aware of age-related pharmacological changes which influence the appropriateness of drug selection in older patients, as well as the clinical implications of polypharmacy including drug–drug and drug–disease interactions, adverse drug events, prescribing cascades and difficulties with compliance.

Age-related pharmacological changes

Physiological changes associated with ageing can affect drug pharmacokinetics (absorption, distribution, metabolism and excretion) and pharmacodynamics (the effect of drugs on the body).[4] Although normal ageing has little effect on drug absorption, gastric emptying can be increased by prokinetic drugs (e.g. domperidone and erythromycin). Anticholinergic drugs can reduce salivary secretion, thus impeding the rate but not the extent of buccal absorption of drugs such as midazolam or fentanyl.

Systemic bioavailability of most drugs is not affected by normal ageing, other than in those which undergo substantial first-pass hepatic metabolism, e.g. morphine, buprenorphine, midazolam and propranolol. With these drugs, age-related reductions in liver volume and blood flow (up to 30%) can result in significantly higher systemic bioavailability because of reduced first-pass hepatic extraction. Therefore, initial doses of these drugs should be reduced.

Ageing is associated with reduced lean body weight and muscle mass and a relative increase in total body fat, thus increasing the volume of distribution of lipid-soluble drugs, e.g. morphine, benzodiazepines, neuroleptics and amitriptyline. This results in longer elimination half-lives, prolonged drug effect, accumulation with continued use, and greater potential for adverse effects such as sedation and falls. The starting doses of most such drugs should be reduced in older patients, with slow up-titration according to response. The volume of distribution of water-soluble drugs such as lithium, theophylline and gentamicin is reduced, resulting in higher plasma concentrations after initial administration, thereby necessitating lower initial doses.

Many drugs are inactive when bound to circulating plasma proteins and mediate their effects when unbound or free. Though normal ageing does not affect plasma protein concentration, serum albumin levels fall with chronic disease, thereby causing clinically important increases in free drug concentration for compounds that are heavily protein bound, e.g. benzodiazepines, antipsychotics, ibuprofen, warfarin and phenytoin. The volume of distribution of these drugs increases with hypoalbuminaemia, thereby increasing their elimination half-life and potential for toxicity.

Liver enzyme activity is usually preserved in normal ageing. However, prescribers should be aware of potential drug interactions involving inhibition and induction of cytochrome P450 metabolizing enzymes. Enzyme inhibition can lead to a rapid reduction in drug metabolism with resultant toxic accumulation: for example, haloperidol may impede the metabolism of amitriptyline through inhibition of cytochrome P450 2D6, thereby increasing the potential for anticholinergic side effects, orthostatic hypotension and tachyarrhythmias, all of which may contribute to falls. Conversely, drugs such as carbamazepine and phenytoin can induce cytochrome P450 isoenzymes, which accelerate the metabolism and clearance of another drug or unrelated substrate, potentially resulting in treatment failure. Commonly prescribed cytochrome P450 inhibitors, inducers and substrate drugs are presented in Table 11.1.

Renal function declines with age because of reduction in renal size, blood flow and concentrating ability.[5] This is potentiated by conditions such as hypertension and diabetes and is probably the most important age-related pharmacokinetic change. Glomerular filtration rate should be estimated for all older patients at regular intervals and medication doses adjusted accordingly (Table 11.2).

Table 11.1 Inhibitors and inducers of the hepatic cytochrome P450 enzyme system.

Enzyme inhibitor	Enzyme inducer	Substrate drug
Erythromycin, clarithromycin	Carbamazepine	Tyrosine kinase inhibitors
Sulfonamides	Phenytoin	Cyclophosphamide
Ciprofloxacin	Phenobarbital	Etoposide
Fluconazole, miconazole, ketoconazole	Isoniazid	Bicalutamide
Amiodarone	Rifampicin	Taxanes
Diltiazem, verapamil	Ethanol	Aromatase inhibitors
Cimetidine	Primdone	Warfarin
Fluoxetine, paroxetine	St John's Wort	Diazepam
		Opioids

Table 11.2 Drug classes requiring dose adjustment in patients with impaired renal function.

Drug/class	Example
Cardiac drugs	Digoxin, atenolol, sotalol
Lipid-lowering drugs	Rosuvastatin, pravastatin, fibrates
Diuretics	Thiazide diuretics have limited efficacy if creatinine clearance <30 ml/min
	Avoid potassium-sparing diuretics if creatinine clearance <30 ml/min
Hypoglycaemic drugs	Metformin, glibenclamide, glimepiride, gliptins, insulin
Anticoagulants	Apixaban, rivaroxaban, dabigatran, low-molecular-weight heparin
Bone antiresorptive drugs	Avoid bisphosphonates if creatinine clearance <30 ml/min
Analgesic drugs	Opioids (morphine, codeine, pethidine, NSAIDs)
Anticonvulsant drugs	Topiramate, levetiracetam, vigabatrin
Psychotropic drugs	Lithium, gabapentin, amisulpride
Antibiotics	Aminoglycosides, carbapenems, piperacillin/tazobactam, ceftazidime
Antifungals	Fluconazole, sulfamethoxazole
Antivirals	Acyclovir, ganciclovir, famciclovir

NSAIDs, non-steroidal anti-inflammatory drugs.

Table 11.3 Age-related changes in pharmacodynamic response to commonly prescribed drugs.

Drug type	Specific drug	Pharmacodynamic response	Potential clinical consequence
Analgesia	Morphine	↑	Excessive sedation, confusion, constipation, respiratory depression
Anticoagulant	Warfarin	↑	Increased bleeding risk
	Dabigatran in those aged ≥75 years with a body weight <50 kg	↑	
	Apixaban	↑	
Cardiovascular system drugs	Angiotensin receptor blocker	↑	Hypotension
	Diltiazem	↑	
	Enalapril	↑	
	Verapamil	↑	
	Propranolol	↓	
Diuretics	Furosemide	↓	Reduced diuretic effect at standard doses
Psychoactive drugs	Diazepam	↑	Excessive sedation, confusion, postural sway, falls
	Midazolam	↑	
	Temazepam	↑	
	Haloperidol	↑	
	Triazolam	↑	
Others	Levodopa	↑	Dyskinesia, confusion, hallucinations

↑, increased pharmacodynamic response; ↓, reduced pharmacodynamic response.

Ageing is associated with increased pharmacodynamic sensitivity to many drugs. Common examples are presented in Table 11.3. It is usually recommended to start such drugs at the lowest possible dose and to slowly up-titrate according to response.

Polypharmacy: associations and consequences

Polypharmacy refers to the use of several drugs concurrently. Although multiple medications are often clinically justifiable, it is well established that polypharmacy in older patients is associated with inappropriate prescribing (i.e. where the risk of treatment outweighs the potential clinical benefit),[6] adverse drug reactions,[7] and geriatrics syndromes including falls, incontinence, weight loss, and cognitive and functional decline.[8] An adverse drug reaction is an appreciably harmful or unpleasant reaction, resulting from an intervention related to the use of a medicinal product, which predicts hazard from future administration and warrants prevention or specific treatment, alteration of the dosage regimen or withdrawal of the product.[9] Patients taking two concurrent medications have a 13% risk of an adverse drug reaction, which rises to 38% for four medications and 82% for seven or more medications prescribed simultaneously.[7] Adverse consequences of polypharmacy are summarized in Table 11.4.

Table 11.4	Polypharmacy in older patients: clinical associations.	
1.	↑	Risk of adverse drug reactions including drug–drug and drug–disease interactions
2.	↑	Likelihood of inappropriate prescribing including prescription of drugs without clear clinical indication
3.	↑	Likelihood of prescribing cascades, i.e. where a drug is prescribed to treat a symptom attributable to an adverse effect of another drug
4.	↑	Incidence of geriatric syndromes including cognitive and functional decline, weight loss and falls
5.	↑	Risk of non-compliance and poor concordance with medication regimen
6.	↑	Healthcare costs with respect to drug costs and resource use to investigate and manage adverse outcomes

↑, increase.

Chemotherapy regimens typically comprise co-prescription of drugs that are inherently toxic and have narrow therapeutic indices with medications for supportive care including antiemetics, analgesics, corticosteroids and antimicrobials. Such combinations have potential for significant interactions and adverse drug reactions, particularly in the context of co-prescribed non-oncological medications, malnutrition, frailty and organ dysfunction (Tables 11.5 and 11.6). A Canadian study of 405 cancer patients identified at least one moderate or major drug–drug interaction in 109 patients (27%); 87% of interactions involved non-cancer agents such as warfarin, steroids and antiepileptic drugs.[10]

Inappropriate prescribing is highly prevalent in older patients and pertains to overuse (no clinical indication, therapeutic duplication or excessive duration), misuse (risk of drug–drug and drug–disease interactions) and underuse of medication (omission of a clinically indicated drug of therapeutic benefit).[11] Inappropriate prescribing is associated with polypharmacy and it increases the risk of adverse drug events and overuse of healthcare resources.[12] Over 11% of hospital admissions of older patients are related to adverse effects of inappropriately prescribed drugs.[13]

Table 11.5 Clinically significant drug–drug interactions in older patients.

Drug	Drug	Interaction/potential effect	Recommended management
NSAIDs	Antihypertensive agents	NSAIDs antagonize hypotensive effect	Avoid combination
NSAIDs	Methotrexate	Potential for toxic levels of methotrexate	Avoid combination
Aspirin	NSAIDs Oral corticosteroids	↑ Risk of peptic ulceration	Avoid combination or co-prescribe PPI
Warfarin	Capecitabine Etoposide Carboplatin Gemcitabine Gefitinib Paclitaxel Tamoxifen Phenytoin Thyroxine	↑ Anticoagulant effect	Monitor INR closely
Warfarin	Ketoconazole Fluconazole Amiodarone Macrolide antibiotics Ciprofloxacin Metronidazole Sulfonamides	↓ Anticoagulant effect	Monitor INR closely
Digoxin	Diuretics	Diuretic-induced hypokalaemia increases the effect of digoxin (arrhythmic, toxicity)	Monitor for hypokalaemia
Digoxin	Amiodarone Diltiazem Verapamil	↓ Clearance of digoxin ↑ Effect of digoxin (arrhythmia, toxicity)	Avoid combination
TCA	Enzyme inhibitors	↓ Clearance of TCA Arrhythmia, confusion, orthostatic hypotension, falls	Avoid combination or reduce dose of TCA if necessary
Phenytoin Carbamazepine	Sunitinib	↓ Anticancer effect	Avoid combination or consider higher dose of sunitinib with close monitoring
Ondansetron	Cisplatin Cyclophosphamide	↓ Anticancer effect	Avoid combination
Azole antifungals	Tamoxifen Vincristine (itraconazole) Irinotecan Docetaxel Etoposide Paclitaxel Teniposide Cyclophosphamide (itraconazole)	↑ Serum concentration of chemotherapy agent	Avoid combinations if possible

INR, International Normalized Ratio; NSAIDs, non-steroidal anti-inflammatory drugs; PPI, proton pump inhibitor; TCA, tricyclic antidepressant; ↑, increased interaction; ↓, reduced interaction.

Table 11.6 Clinically significant drug–disease interactions in older patients.

Drug	Disease or condition	Drug–disease interaction
Anticholinergics Benzodiazepines Opiates Antipsychotics Vinca alkaloids Taxanes Cisplatin (neurotoxicity)	Falls	↑ Risk of falls, gait instability
Benzodiazepines Anticholinergics Corticosteroids Opiates Hydroxycarbamide Ifosfamide Interferon	Cognitive impairment/dementia	↑ Confusion, delirium
Diuretics Anticholinergics Peripheral vasodilators Nitrates Cisplatin Tricyclic antidepressants	Orthostatic hypotension	Syncope, falls, hip fracture
Corticosteroids	Osteopenia/osteoporosis	Fracture
Anthracyclines Trastuzumab	Cardiac failure	Exacerbation of heart failure
NSAIDs Antithrombotics	Peptic ulcer disease	Haemorrhagic peptic ulcer
NSAIDs Corticosteroids Bevacizumab Sunitinib	Hypertension	↑ BP
NSAIDs Aminoglycosides Cisplatin Carboplatin Carmustine Mitomycin High-dose methotrexate	Renal failure	Acute kidney injury
Metoclopramide Prochlorperazine Antipsychotics	Parkinsonism	Exacerbation of extrapyramidal signs

NSAIDs, non-steroidal anti-inflammatory drugs; ↑, increased interaction; ↓, reduced interaction.

Table 11.7	Key considerations when prescribing for older patients.

1. Use non-pharmacological treatment whenever possible
2. Include the patient (and carer where appropriate) in prescribing decisions
3. Ensure each medication has an appropriate indication and a clear therapeutic goal: this involves careful clinical assessment and appreciation of time to obtain treatment effect and life expectancy; clinical prescribing indicators such as STOPP/START criteria are useful when evaluating prescribing appropriateness
4. Start at the smallest dose and titrate slowly according to response and efficacy
5. Use the simplest dosing regimen (e.g. once a day is preferable to three times a day) and the most appropriate formulation
6. Provide verbal and written instructions on indication, time and route of administration and potential adverse effects of each medication; administer medications via a pre-prepared blister pack if available
7. Maintain an up-to-date list of all medications being taken by the patient, including over-the-counter and complementary/alternative medicines
8. Regularly review prescriptions in the context of coexisting disease states, concurrent medications, functional and cognitive status and therapeutic expectation
9. Be aware that new presenting symptoms may be due to an existing medication, drug–drug interaction or drug–disease interaction (avoid prescribing cascade)
10. When stopping a medication check that it can be stopped abruptly or whether it needs to be tapered, e.g. long-term steroids, benzodiazepines

Polypharmacy: management

Table 11.7 presents key recommendations when prescribing for all older patients. Comprehensive Geriatric Assessment of patients with newly diagnosed cancer involves assessment of prescription and non-prescription medication. Errors in medication histories are common and should be corrected by patient/carer interview, inspection of drug containers or lists, and contact with the community pharmacist or general practitioner.[14] Beers' Criteria[15] and STOPP/START criteria (Screening Tool of Older Persons' Potentially Inappropriate Prescriptions and Screening Tool to Alert Doctors to the Right Treatment)[16] comprise lists of medications that should be avoided or used with caution in older people with common comorbidities or potential for drug–drug and drug–disease interactions. Clinical application of STOPP/START can improve all domains of prescribing appropriateness[17] and reduce the incidence of in-hospital adverse drug reactions.

Ideally, older patients with cancer should be managed by a multidisciplinary team that includes a clinical pharmacist.[18] Medication reconciliation should be performed periodically according to the individual's circumstances. Disease progression should prompt a review of therapeutic goals that may not yield benefits for several years after initiation of treatment, e.g. rigid control of BP, glucose and cholesterol. Functional or cognitive decline and falls often represent adverse drug effects. They should precipitate a medication review and may signal a change in goals of care.

Computerized provider order entry systems require clinicians to directly place orders into an electronic system and ensure standardized and legible orders. Complementary clinical decision support software can check for drug–drug interactions. Uptake of electronic systems has been slow due to resistance to changes in physicians' practice patterns, costs and training time involved, alert fatigue and the absence of evidence that these systems reduce adverse drug reactions.[19] Genomics and proteomics will influence the treatment of older patients with cancer in the future. These emerging techniques will allow targeted antineoplastic treatments based on the patient's phamacogenomic profile and may predict pharmacokinetics, effectiveness and risk of adverse effects of drugs for individual patients.[20]

Conclusion

 Prescribing for older patients with cancer is complex and often challenging, particularly in the context of multiple comorbidities, variable functional and cognitive status, uncertain life expectancy and changes in pharmacokinetics and pharmacodynamics. A multidisciplinary approach with regular reappraisal of the risks and benefits of each medication in light of current status and goals of care is essential.

References

1   Cashman J, Wright J, Ring A. The treatment of comorbidities in older patients with metastatic cancer. *Support Care Cancer* 2010; 18: 651–5.

2   Puts MT, Costa-Lima B, Monette J, *et al.* Medication problems in older, newly diagnosed cancer patients in Canada: how common are they? A prospective pilot study. *Drugs Aging* 2009; 26: 519–36.

3   Scripture CD, Figg WD. Drug interactions in cancer therapy. *Nat Rev Cancer* 2006; 6: 546–58.

4   Mangoni AA, Jackson SHD. Age-related changes in pharmacokinetics and pharmacodynamics: basic principles and practical applications. *Br J Clin Pharmacol* 2004; 57: 6–14.

5   Rowe JW, Andres R, Tobin JD, *et al.* The effect of age on creatinine clearance in men: a cross-sectional and longitudinal study. *J Gerontol* 1976; 31: 155.

6   Gallagher P, Lang PO, Cherubini A, *et al.* Prevalence of potentially inappropriate prescribing in an acutely ill population of older patients admitted to six European hospitals. *Eur J Clin Pharm* 2011; 67: 1175–88.

7   Goldberg RM, Mabee J, Chan L, *et al.* Drug–drug and drug–disease interactions in the ED: analysis of a high-risk population. *Am J Emerg Med* 1996; 14: 447–50.

8   Steinman MA, Hanlon JT. Managing medications in clinically complex elders: 'There's got to be a happy medium.' *JAMA* 2010; 304: 1592–601.

9   Edwards IR, Aronson JK. Adverse drug reactions: definitions, diagnosis, and management. *Lancet* 2000; 356: 1255–9.

10 Riechelmann RP, Tannock IF, Wang L, *et al.* Potential drug interactions and duplicate prescriptions among cancer patients. *J Natl Cancer Inst* 2007; 99: 592–600.

11 Spinewine A, Schmader KE, Barber N, *et al.* Appropriate prescribing in elderly people: how well can it be measured and optimised? *Lancet* 2007; 370: 173–84.

12 Hamilton H, Gallagher P, Ryan C, *et al.* Potentially inappropriate medications defined by STOPP criteria and the risk of adverse drug events in older hospitalized patients. *Arch Intern Med* 2011; 171: 1013–19.

13 Gallagher P, O'Mahony D. STOPP (Screening Tool of Older Persons' potentially inappropriate Prescriptions): application to acutely ill elderly patients and comparison with Beers' criteria. *Age Ageing* 2008; 37: 673–9.

14 Tam VC, Knowles SR, Cornish PL, *et al.* Frequency, type and clinical importance of medication history errors at admission to hospital: a systematic review. *CMAJ* 2005; 173: 510–15.

15 American Geriatrics Society 2012 Beers' Criteria Update Expert Panel. American Geriatrics Society updated Beers' Criteria for potentially inappropriate medication use in older adults. *J Am Geriatr Soc* 2012; 60: 616–31.

16 O'Mahony D, O'Sullivan D, Byrne S, *et al.* STOPP/START criteria for potentially inappropriate prescribing in older people: version 2. *Age Ageing* 2015; 44: 213–18.

17 Gallagher PF, O'Connor MN, O'Mahony D. Prevention of potentially inappropriate prescribing for elderly patients: a randomized controlled trial using STOPP/START criteria. *Clin Pharmacol Ther* 2011; 89: 845–54.

18 Hurria A, Browner IS, Cohen HJ, *et al.* Senior adult oncology. *J Natl Compr Canc Netw* 2012; 10: 162–209.

19 Ranji SR, Rennke S, Wachter RM. Computerised provider order entry combined with clinical decision support systems to improve medication safety: a narrative review. *BMJ Qual Saf* 2014; 23: 773–80.

20 Balducci L, Goetz-Parten D, Steinman MA. Polypharmacy and the management of the older cancer patient. *Ann Oncol* 2013; 24 (suppl 7): vii36–40.

12 Screening for Breast and Prostate Cancer in the Older Population

Jenna Morgan, Freddie Hamdy, Malcolm Reed

Introduction

Screening programmes aim to detect cancer at an early stage when treatment may be more effective and less intense. In the UK, there are well-established programmes in breast and cervical cancer; more recently, programmes have been developed to detect bowel cancer. In some countries, including the UK, these are national programmes with lower and upper age limits which reflect the evidence base for benefits.

Much of the uncertainty around the use of screening tests in older people results from a lack of randomized controlled trials (RCTs) conducted in this population, requiring extrapolation of data on effectiveness from younger patients. Furthermore, most do not account for individual patient characteristics, such as levels of comorbidity, frailty or functional status, which may alter the likelihood of benefit or harm from screening. Additionally, ageing results in a shorter life expectancy; thus, older patients are more likely to die with their cancer rather than from it.

This chapter summarizes the current situation for breast cancer screening, which has been established in the UK since 1988, and prostate cancer screening, which is not yet the subject of a national screening programme. These two subjects provide useful insights into the advantages and disadvantages of cancer screening programmes in the older population.

Recent developments

Screening for breast cancer

The Forrest report published in 1986[1] led to the establishment of the NHS national breast cancer screening programme in 1988. This report was based on a number of international RCTs and it recommended screening by x-ray mammography on a 3 yearly basis between the ages of 50 and 65 years. However, subsequent long-term follow-up and observational studies raised concerns relating to the risks and benefits of breast cancer screening, leading to claims that there was no reliable evidence that mammographic screening decreases breast cancer mortality and that such screening programmes could not be justified.[2] Over the following decade there was increasing debate surrounding breast cancer screening and in 2012 an independent review chaired by Sir Michael Marmot was commissioned in the UK to focus on the beneficial effect of breast cancer screening on mortality and also the risk of overdiagnosis and other harms.[3] The review concluded that screening results in a 20% reduction in breast cancer mortality amongst women invited to the breast cancer screening programme but that there is considerable uncertainty around this estimate (Figure 12.1). This benefit equates to approximately one breast cancer death prevented for every 180 women who attend breast cancer screening within the 50–70 year age group, i.e. the prevention of approximately 1300 breast cancer deaths each year. The review also concluded that overdiagnosis – the detection of cancers which might never have become symptomatic – does occur and represents approximately 20% of cancers detected in women invited for screening. There are thus three cases of overdiagnosis and treatment for every

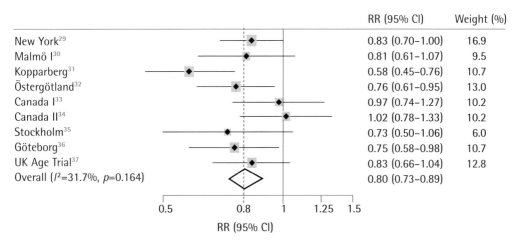

	RR (95% CI)	Weight (%)
New York[29]	0.83 (0.70–1.00)	16.9
Malmö I[30]	0.81 (0.61–1.07)	9.5
Kopparberg[31]	0.58 (0.45–0.76)	10.7
Östergötland[32]	0.76 (0.61–0.95)	13.0
Canada I[33]	0.97 (0.74–1.27)	10.2
Canada II[34]	1.02 (0.78–1.33)	10.2
Stockholm[35]	0.73 (0.50–1.06)	6.0
Göteborg[36]	0.75 (0.58–0.98)	10.7
UK Age Trial[37]	0.83 (0.66–1.04)	12.8
Overall (I^2=31.7%, p=0.164)	0.80 (0.73–0.89)	

Figure 12.1 Meta-analysis of breast cancer mortality after 13 years' follow-up in breast cancer screening trials (adapted from Marmot et al.[3]).

individual death from breast cancer prevented (Table 12.1). This represents a 1% chance of overdiagnosis amongst women invited to attend for breast cancer screening.

A large proportion of overdiagnosis is the result of the detection of preinvasive ductal carcinoma *in situ* (DCIS), which is associated with microcalcification and is detectable on mammography. The incidence of DCIS prior to breast cancer screening was approximately 1–2% of all breast cancers, rising to approximately 20% within screening programmes. Whilst removal of areas of DCIS can prevent cancer, many cases of DCIS might never progress to invasive cancer, the treatment of which typically involves surgery and radiotherapy and may have psychological consequences. A subsequent review by the Swiss government covering the same evidence base concluded that no further extension of breast cancer screening should be undertaken and that the government should consider discontinuing the programme.[4]

The Marmot review[3] also made a number of recommendations for ongoing research particularly to investigate the potential benefits of breast cancer screening in women over the age of 70 and evaluate the optimal treatment of screen-detected DCIS. Only one of the RCTs of breast cancer screening in the Marmot review included women aged over 70 years, despite the fact that over a

Table 12.1 Estimates of overdiagnosis of breast cancer in RCTs without systematic end-of-trial screening of the control group, according to four calculation methods (adapted from Marmot et al.[3]).

RCT	A	B	C	D
Malmö I[30] (age 55–69 years), % (n)	11.7 (82/698)	10.5 (82/780)	18.7 (82/438)	29.1 (82/282)
Canada I[33] (age 40–49 years), % (n)	14.1 (82/581)	12.4 (82/663)	22.7 (82/361)	29.4 (82/279)
Canada II[34] (age 50–59 years), % (n)	10.7 (67/626)	9.7 (67/693)	16.0 (67/420)	19.8 (67/338)

Numbers of excess cancers are expressed as a percentage of different denominators.
A, excess cancers as a proportion of cancers diagnosed over whole follow-up period in unscreened women.
B, excess cancers as a proportion of cancers diagnosed over whole follow-up period in women invited for screening.
C, excess cancers as a proportion of cancers diagnosed during screening period in women invited for screening.
D, excess cancers as a proportion of cancers detected by screening in women invited for screening.

third of newly diagnosed breast cancers occur in women in this age group and that the incidence of breast cancer continues to increase with age (the NHS breast cancer screening programme is open to older women, but this is at the request of the individual rather than by invitation).

In 2007, the UK government recommended the extension of the NHS breast cancer screening programme from 47 to 73 years of age. However, in view of the lack of capacity in the programme to deliver age extension, a pilot study evaluating cluster randomization was undertaken. The pilot study showed that this was feasible and it was subsequently developed into a national trial (the Age Trial) embedded within the NHS breast cancer screening programme.[5] This is effectively two separate trials, one addressing the earlier commencement of breast cancer screening and the other addressing the extension of screening to age 73. This trial is currently one of the largest RCTs in the world, having recruited over 2 million women. The outcome, however, is not expected for approximately 10 years and currently the decision whether or not to undergo continued breast cancer screening beyond the age of 73 is a matter of individual choice based on the potential benefits and harms. These are summarized in a revised information leaflet, *NHS breast screening. Helping you decide.*[6] This leaflet, along with other cancer screening information leaflets, was developed in 2013 by an independent team of experts at King's Health Partners.[7] Individual women seeking advice from their medical practitioner on whether or not to attend for breast cancer screening should be aware that the life expectancy of a healthy 70 year old with good prognosis breast cancer is approximately 15 years, but it may be severely curtailed by any significant, associated comorbidity. A diagnosis of breast cancer after age 80 is less likely to be the subsequent cause of death than other associated diseases; however, apart from those with a very poor prognosis, it remains a significant risk to well-being and survival. Whilst the use of cytotoxic chemotherapy in older patients is much less frequent due to associated toxicity and reduced efficacy of other treatments including surgery, radiotherapy and endocrine therapy, all are associated with side effects. In the most frail older patients, surgery and radiotherapy may be avoided in those with oestrogen receptor positivity. All these factors should be taken into consideration when discussing breast cancer screening in older women.

There is no clear evidence base on which to form an appropriate response to a request from an older woman for advice on whether or not to undergo breast cancer screening. As the Age Trial results will not be available for at least 10 years, a pragmatic approach is required. If the woman has a life expectancy of approximately 10 or more years, it is probable that detection of a malignant lesion may be of benefit in terms of survival and less complex treatment. A woman with a predicted life expectancy of 5 years or less, however, may be unlikely to benefit in terms of survival. At present this remains a matter of individual choice and the NHS breast cancer screening programme will accept self-referral by women of any age who are able to attend and undergo the investigation.

Screening for prostate cancer

Screening for prostate cancer remains one of the most controversial public health issues. At present, prostate cancer screening continues to fall short of the WHO criteria described by Wilson and Jungner.[8] Whilst this ubiquitous malignancy is indeed an important health problem and the most common malignancy in men, its natural history is not yet well understood. The majority of prostate cancer cases detectable through prostate-specific antigen (PSA)-based screening are at low or intermediate risk of progression. Most of these screen-detected cases may never become lethal during an individual's lifetime. However, there is compelling evidence from the European Randomized Study of Screening for Prostate Cancer (ERSPC) that PSA-based screening for prostate cancer can yield a significant survival benefit, as well as a reduction in the burden of metastatic disease, albeit at the cost of exposing unacceptably large numbers of men to radical treatment for each life saved.[9,10] Prostate cancer is a heterogeneous malignancy, with much genomic diversity, and it is becoming increasingly apparent that our definition of 'significant' versus 'insignificant' prostate cancer is inadequate.[11-13] Effective treatments to cure clinically localized prostate cancer, including different forms of radiotherapy and minimally invasive surgery such as robot-assisted laparoscopic radical prostatectomy, are widely available and have excellent outcomes. Paradoxically, many of these patients do not require treatment, as their disease is unlikely to cause harm in the long term, and they are best managed by active surveillance or monitoring with delayed intervention if necessary. However, follow-up protocols are imperfect, and some of these patients can progress whilst monitored. In the UK, the Prostate Testing for Cancer and Treatment (ProtecT) trial is the world's largest RCT comparing the three major treatment options in screen-detected prostate cancer: surgery, radiotherapy and active monitoring. It is due to report its findings in 2016.[14] The Cluster Randomised Trial of PSA Testing for Prostate Cancer (CAP), within which ProtecT is embedded, is a UK-wide primary care-based RCT investigating the clinical and cost-effectiveness of PSA testing of men aged 50–69 years.[15] Over 415,000 men from 573 primary care practices across the UK have been recruited, making CAP the largest study of PSA-based prostate cancer screening to date, and the results will provide a future contribution to the current evidence base.

Multiple genome-wide association studies have reported 77 single nucleotide polymorphisms (SNPs) associated with prostate cancer. Further studies are required to identify whether targeted screening could be performed based on the genetic information obtained from these SNPs. In addition to the familial risk in first-degree relatives of men with prostate cancer, rare and highly penetrant germline mutations are linked to genetic predisposition, such as *HOXB13,* and *BRCA2* in families with a high incidence of breast and ovarian cancer.[16]

The diagnosis of prostate cancer is obtained by measurement of serum PSA levels, followed by transrectal ultrasound-guided biopsy, which in itself can carry morbidity and complications.[17] There is increasing enthusiasm for the use of pre-biopsy multiparametric magnetic resonance imaging (mpMRI) in order to identify or exclude 'significant' lesions[18] and facilitate MRI-transrectal ultrasound fusion biopsies.[19] At present, the use of pre-biopsy mpMRI is not widespread in most countries but is likely to evolve following completion of ongoing clinical trials. Protocols incorporating imaging into screening programmes will need to be evaluated prospectively.

The fact that the ERSPC has clearly demonstrated that prostate cancer screening can reduce the future development of advanced metastatic disease may be used as a powerful argument for the introduction of screening. However, it is likely that the screening process could be further refined through the risk stratification of men at the introduction of the screening process, taking into consideration factors such as family history, race, life expectancy and baseline PSA level,[20,21] with the subsequent screening protocol modified for individuals based on these risk factors. The frequency with which men may need to be screened may also be influenced by their initial PSA test result within a screening programme protocol.[22,23] Other developments in the contemporary prostate cancer diagnosis pathway, such as the use of additional kallikrein markers, targeted screening and the introduction of mpMRI, may improve the performance of a screening protocol such that the benefits could be increased and the risks reduced.[24] These and other future developments are likely to influence the ratio of risks to benefits in favour of the introduction of screening in due course. In the meantime, men who request PSA testing should only receive the test after careful professional counselling about the potential benefits and harms caused by screening for prostate cancer.

In general clinical practice, PSA levels are frequently checked in older men (e.g. for lower urinary tract symptoms), and interpretation of raised levels can be complex: 8% of men aged ≥65 will have a PSA >4.0 ng/ml, increasing with age to 28% in black men aged ≥85.[25] In addition, 25% of men with benign prostatic hypertrophy (BPH) will have a PSA >4 ng/ml, with histological BPH occurring in nearly 80% by the age of 80.[26] Clinical factors (more prevalent in older men) that add to this overlap of cancer, age and BPH in raising PSA levels include active urinary tract infection, prostatitis and recent catheterization. All need consideration in order to avoid unnecessary biopsies. Digital rectal examination (DRE) will evidently inform this decision by demonstrating abnormalities consistent with cancer or BPH, but a normal DRE does not exclude cancer. Cancer detection rates in patients with normal DRE in one study were 8.6%, 13.4%, 21.8%, 41.7% and 85.2% in patients with PSA <4, 4–10, 10.1–20, 20.1–50 and >50 ng ml, respectively.[27] With respect to lower urinary tract symptoms in the context of elevated PSA, prostate cancer is associated with less severe symptoms (e.g. as measured according to the International Prostate Symptom Score), but not enough to have prognostic validity.[28]

Conclusion

Currently there is little hard evidence to support the population-wide cancer screening of older people; however, ongoing research in this area may shed more light on this issue. Older individuals who request cancer screening should be counselled transparently on the relative benefits and harms in relation to their individual circumstances in order to make a personalized choice.

References

1   Forrest APM. *Breast cancer screening. Report to the health ministers of England, Wales, Scotland and Northern Ireland.* London: HMSO, 1986.

2   Gøtzsche PC, Nielson M. Screening for breast cancer with mammography. *Cochrane Database Syst Rev* 2001; 1: CD001877.

3   Marmot MG, Altman DG, Cameron DA, *et al.*; Independent UK Panel on Breast Cancer Screening. The benefits and harms of breast cancer screening: an independent review. *Lancet* 2012; 380: 1778–86.

4   Swiss Medical Board (2013). *Systematisches Mammographie-Screening.* Available from: www.medical-board.ch/fileadmin/docs/public/mb/Fachberichte/2013-12-15_Bericht_Mammographie_Final_rev.pdf (accessed 2 August 2015).

5   Moser K, Sellars S, Wheaton M, et al. Extending the age range for breast screening in England: pilot study to assess the feasibility and acceptability of randomisation. *J Med Screen* 2011; 18: 96–102.

6   King's Health Partners (2013). *NHS breast screening. Helping you decide.* Available from: www.cancerscreening.nhs.uk/breastscreen/publications/ia-02.html (accessed 2 August 2015).

7   Forbes LJ, Ramirez AJ; Expert Group on Information about Breast Screening. Offering informed choice about breast screening. *J Med Screen* 2014; 21: 194–200.

8   Wilson JM, Jungner YG. Principles and practice of mass screening for disease [in Spanish]. *Bol Oficina Sanit Panam* 1968; 65: 281–393.

9   Schröder FH, Hugosson J, Roobol MJ, *et al.* Screening and prostate cancer mortality: results of the European Randomised Study of Screening for Prostate Cancer (ERSPC) at 13 years of follow-up. *Lancet* 2014; 384: 2027–35.

10 Schröder FH, Hugosson J, Carlsson S, *et al.* Screening for prostate cancer decreases the risk of developing metastatic disease: findings from the European Randomized Study of Screening for Prostate Cancer (ERSPC). *Eur Urol* 2012; 62: 745–52.

11 Van der Kwast TH, Roobol MJ. Defining the threshold for significant versus insignificant prostate cancer. *Nat Rev Urol* 2013; 10: 473–82.

12 Cooper CS, Eeles R, Wedge DC, *et al.* Analysis of the genetic phylogeny of multifocal prostate cancer identifies multiple independent clonal expansions in neoplastic and morphologically normal prostate tissue. *Nat Genet* 2015; 47: 367–72.

13 Gundem G, Van Loo P, Kremeyer B, *et al.* The evolutionary history of lethal metastatic prostate cancer. *Nature* 2015; 520: 353–7.

14 Lane JA, Donovan JL, Davis M, *et al.* Active monitoring, radical prostatectomy, or radiotherapy for localised prostate cancer: study design and diagnostic and baseline results of the ProtecT randomised phase 3 trial. *Lancet Oncol* 2014; 15: 1109–18.

15 Turner EL, Metcalfe C, Donovan JL, *et al.* Design and preliminary recruitment results of the Cluster Randomised Trial of PSA Testing for Prostate Cancer (CAP). *Br J Cancer* 2014; 110: 2829–36.

16 Eeles R, Goh C, Castro E, *et al.* The genetic epidemiology of prostate cancer and its clinical implications. *Nat Rev Urol* 2014; 11: 18–31.

17 Rosario DJ, Lane JA, Metcalfe C, *et al.* Short term outcomes of prostate biopsy in men tested for cancer by prostate specific antigen: prospective evaluation within ProtecT study. *BMJ* 2012; 344: d7894.

18 Murphy G, Haider M, Ghai S, Sreeharsha B. The expanding role of MRI in prostate cancer. *Am J Roentgenol* 2013; 201: 1229–38.

19 Moore CM, Robertson NL, Arsanious N, *et al.* Image-guided prostate biopsy using magnetic resonance imaging-derived targets: a systematic review. *Eur Urol* 2013; 63: 125–40.

20 Roobol MJ, Steyerberg EW, Kranse R, *et al.* A risk-based strategy improves prostate-specific antigen-driven detection of prostate cancer. *Eur Urol* 2010; 57: 79–85

21 Vertosick EA, Poon BY, Vickers AJ. Relative value of race, family history and prostate specific antigen as indications for early initiation of prostate cancer screening. *J Urol* 2014; 192: 724–8.

22 Vickers A, Carlsson S, Laudone V, Lilja H. It ain't what you do, it's the way you do it: five golden rules for transforming prostate-specific antigen screening. *Eur Urol* 2014; 66: 188–90.

23 Carlsson S, Assel M, Sjoberg D, *et al.* Influence of blood prostate specific antigen levels at age 60 on benefits and harms of prostate cancer screening: population based cohort study. *BMJ* 2014; 348: g2296.

24 Bryant RJ, Sjoberg DD, Vickers AJ, *et al.* Predicting high-grade cancer at ten-core prostate biopsy using four kallikrein markers measured in blood in the ProtecT study. *J Natl Cancer Inst* 2015; 107: pii: djv095.

25 Espaldon R, Kirby KA, Fung KZ, *et al.* Probability of an abnormal screening prostate-specific antigen result based on age, race, and prostate-specific antigen threshold. *Urology* 2014; 83: 599–605.

26 International Consultation on Urological Diseases (2013). *Incontinence.* 5th ed. Available from: www.icud.info/incontinence.html (accessed 2 August 2015).

27 Teoh JY, Yuen SK, Tsu JH, *et al.* Prostate cancer detection upon transrectal ultrasound-guided biopsy in relation to digital rectal examination and prostate-specific antigen level: what to expect in the Chinese population? *Asian J Androl* doi: 10.4103/1008-682X.144945.

28 Oh JJ, Jeong SJ, Jeong CW, *et al.* Is there any association between the severity of lower urinary tract symptoms and the risk of biopsy-detectable prostate cancer in patients with PSA level below 20 ng/ml in multi-core prostate biopsy? *Prostate* 2013; 73: 42–7.

29 Shapiro S, Venet W, Strax P, *et al.* Ten- to fourteen-year effect of screening on breast cancer mortality. *J Natl Cancer Inst* 1982; 69: 349–55.

30 Zackrisson S, Andersson I, Janzon L, *et al.* Rate of overdiagnosis of breast cancer 15 years after end of Malmo mammographic screening trial: follow-up study. *BMJ* 2006; 332: 689–92.

31 Tabar L, Gad A. Screening for breast cancer: the Swedish trial. *Radiology* 1981; 138: 219–22.

32 Arnesson LG, Vitak B, Manson JC, *et al.* Diagnostic outcome of repeated mammography screening. *World J Surg* 1995; 19: 372–7.

33 Miller AB, To T, Baines CJ, Wall C. The Canadian National Breast Screening Study-1: breast cancer mortality after 11 to 16 years of follow-up. A randomized screening trial of mammography in women age 40 to 49 years. *Ann Intern Med* 2002; 137 (5 part 1): 305–12.

34 Miller AB, To T, Baines CJ, Wall C. Canadian National Breast Screening Study-2: 13-year results of a randomized trial in women aged 50–59 years. *J Natl Cancer Inst* 2000; 92: 1490–9.

35 Frisell J, Eklund G, Hellstrom L, *et al.* Randomized study of mammography screening – preliminary report on mortality in the Stockholm trial. *Breast Cancer Res Treat* 1991; 18: 49–56.

36 Bjurstam N, Bjorneld L, Duffy SW, *et al.* The Gothenburg breast screening trial: first results on mortality, incidence, and mode of detection for women ages 39-49 years at randomization. *Cancer* 1997; 80: 2091–9.

37 Moss SM, Cuckle H, Evans A, *et al.*; Trial Management Group. Effect of mammographic screening from age 40 years on breast cancer mortality at 10 years' follow-up: a randomised controlled trial. *Lancet* 2006; 368: 2053–60.

13 The Nursing Perspective

Natalie Doyle, Richard Henry

Background

Cancer is predominantly a disease of the older person: there are currently 1.3 million older people living with cancer in the UK.[1] Overall, they report a positive experience of their cancer treatment and care.[2]

Nursing needs

There is compelling evidence that older people with cancer have specific nursing needs[3] that may not all be addressed by the generalist or specialist workforce. This remains a central problem for the design and delivery of cancer services; however, increasing emphasis upon person-centred approaches to care would seem to offer a means of addressing this problem.

Nursing care in the general setting

The majority of older people with cancer in the UK are cared for by nurses in general settings such as acute hospital wards, care homes and the community who do not necessarily have any specialist knowledge or training.[4,5] The complexity of care in the general settings can be marked:[6] Corner[7] identified the need for advanced communication skills together with specific theoretical and practical knowledge of cancer. Yet there is evidence that these needs are often inadequately met,[8–10] and nurses themselves concede that there is a requirement for ongoing professional development in treating and caring for older people with cancer.[11] Meeting the educational and developmental needs of these nurses arguably represents the greatest contemporary challenge to the oncology nursing community.

Nurses working in specialist oncology settings

Specialist cancer care in the UK is provided by multiple professional teams in cancer units and cancer centres, or by specialist cancer services in the community. Nurses are required, as a minimum, to have an understanding of cancer and its treatment as well as skills in assessment, communication and care delivery. Whilst evidence suggests that the experience of older people is largely positive and they report confidence in their ward nurses,[2] there are circumstances where nurses appear poorly equipped to respond to the wider health needs of older people.[12]

Person–centred practice

Person-centred approaches reflect changes in nursing practice and are consistent with the observation by Macmillan Cancer Support that older people are not a homogenous group,[1] which was in response to the demonstration by Esbensen *et al.*[13] of a wide variation in patterns of change in the functional ability of older people throughout their cancer experience.

Nursing the person with cancer

The nursing care of people with cancer can be stressful, challenging and emotionally demanding.[7] The Nursing and Midwifery Council acknowledges that the same is true of the care of older people and emphasizes the importance of:

- People (focusing on nursing competence, motivation and values).
- Process (highlighting respect, teamwork, communication and assessment).
- Place (appropriateness of place of care and resources, underlining a commitment to equality and diversity).[14]

This is consistent with the publication of the 'six C's' by NHS England[15] (Table 13.1), which focus on helping people to stay independent whilst maximizing well-being and improving health outcomes. This document stresses the importance of building and strengthening leadership, and additionally highlights the need for quality of care, positive experience of care and measurement of its impact.

Table 13.1 The six C's of NHS England.[15]

- Care
- Compassion
- Competence
- Communication
- Courage
- Commitment

Similarly, guidance by the Royal College of Nursing[16] offers a number of key concepts (Table 13.2) to assist nurses in their practice.

Table 13.2 Royal College of Nursing guidance.[16]

- Respect and holism
- Power and empowerment
- Choice and autonomy
- Empathy and compassion

Holistic nursing

Effective nursing of older people with cancer should recognize the difference between chronological, biological and functional ageing and be underpinned by a holistic approach to care. This can be facilitated by a thorough assessment which necessarily takes account of the person's unique situation and experience. The National Cancer Action Team defines Holistic Needs Assessment (HNA) as 'a process of gathering information from the patient and/or carer in order to inform discussion and develop a deeper understanding of what the person understands and needs'.[17] It is concerned with the whole person and incorporates their physical, psychosocial, spiritual and emotional well-being into the assessment process. The National Cancer Action Team suggests a number of key time points (Table 13.3) when an HNA should be conducted.[17] These can be used to generate a plan of care that can be used across the boundaries of general and specialist care.

The HNA and care plan are integral parts of the recovery package outlined by the National Cancer Survivorship Initiative[18] (Table 13.4). The recovery package is a series of interventions that, when delivered together, can improve care and support for people living with and beyond cancer. Such care plans and interventions are particularly pertinent to the care of older people, whose needs may be more complex.

Table 13.3	Key time points for undertaking an HNA.[17]

- Around the time of diagnosis
- Commencement of treatment
- Completion of the primary treatment plan
- Each new episode of disease recurrence
- The point of recognition of incurability
- The beginning of end of life
- The point at which dying is diagnosed
- At any other time that the patient may request
- At any other time that a professional carer may judge necessary

Table 13.4	The National Cancer Survivorship Initiative recovery package.[18]

- HNA and care plan (at key points of care pathway)
- Treatment summary (completed at end of each acute phase and sent to GP)
- Cancer care review (completed by GP or practice nurse)
- Attendance at a patient education and support event

Developing the nursing role

Arguably the success of cancer nursing practice depends on the continued introduction of person-centred nursing.[19] The central tenet behind person-centred nursing is the need to develop greater insights into the person behind the patient. In this way, the person's needs and goals become central to the nursing process. The importance of strong leadership, the development of the requisite skills and knowledge, as well as organizational and environmental support to work in this manner, are paramount.[19] The practice of person-centred nursing is predicated on supporting people to participate in decision making and to self-manage their condition wherever possible. It has been suggested that older people are less likely to be given information on the side effects of their treatment.[2] The use of HNA and a treatment summary, which are component parts of the recovery package,[18] offers a means of sharing information whilst facilitating a more person-centred approach to care.

Although the HNA addresses a number of needs for older people with cancer, it may be augmented by the addition of evidence-based Comprehensive Geriatric Assessment (CGA). Certain elements of the HNA and CGA overlap, but there are a number of important differences. HNA is an assessment process which focuses on assessing physical, psychosocial, spiritual and emotional well-being, usually in the context of the patient's cancer or cancer treatment. Appropriate referrals would be made as a consequence of difficulties identified by the HNA. By contrast, CGA is not an assessment (although its name would imply this): it is in fact a complex intervention that includes screening, assessment, intervention and follow-through. Validated tools may be used to assist screening or to supplement clinical assessment but are not crucial to performing CGA. CGA includes assessing and intervening in domains included in the HNA but also additional aspects identified through clinical history taking and physical examination (e.g. clinical review of comorbidities and geriatric syndromes, identifying previously undiagnosed medical problems, reviewing/adjusting polypharmacy, mental health review, function and social support assessment). Critically, CGA is an iterative process whereby interventions are put in place and re-reviewed and further adjustments made as required.

In the care of older people, nurses undertake a number of roles in performing CGA. These may include completing validated tools to facilitate the screening part of CGA, which are subsequently used to support geriatrician-led assessment and intervention. In some CGA services, nurses complete the whole complex intervention after specialist training in its use and are usually supported in this by a geriatrician.

In the oncology setting, nurse-led CGA results in improved survival following cancer surgery.[20] CGA is not currently widely used in cancer medical or nursing practice in the UK[21] but is recommended in this setting by the Department of Health and Macmillan Cancer Support.[22] Ensuring that cancer nurses have the necessary skills and knowledge to incorporate at least CGA screening to identify those needing in-depth review could be regarded as a priority in the care of older people with cancer.

The clinical nurse specialist

It is perhaps the clinical nurse specialist who seems closest to realizing the full potential of person-centred approaches to care. This role acknowledges that, for many older people, the cancer pathway can be lengthy, complex and often disjointed, with patients' needs varying from the point of diagnosis to the post-treatment phases.[23] The fact that this complexity is often compounded by a range of comorbidities and/or geriatric syndromes[24] underlines the importance of the key worker role (typically undertaken by a clinical nurse specialist) with specific skills and specialist knowledge in cancer.[25] There may be a role for extending the skill-set to include specialist knowledge in assessing and managing the wider needs of older people by using CGA in the oncology setting.

The cancer reform strategy describes the main function of the clinical nurse specialist as technical, providing information, emotional support and coordination, whereas the National Cancer Action Team extends the role to proactive management, care coordination and ensuring the responsiveness and appropriateness of services.[26] Willard and Luker[27] stress the importance of information giving, symptom control, psychological care and social support, as well as being a patient advocate and expert caregiver. Evaluations of this role are consistently positive:[28] the value and contribution of the clinical nurse specialist are widely acknowledged.[29] For older people, the benefits of this role can be significant.[30] The role is usually treatment- or disease-specific.[31] Management of side effects by a treatment-specific chemotherapy nurse specialist may help to avoid dose reductions, delays and omissions and consequently improve the likely efficiency and efficacy of treatment.[32] Those receiving disease-specific specialist nurse-led follow-up have fewer medical consultations following cancer treatment compared with conventional medical follow-up.[33]

Access to a clinical nurse specialist, however, varies across the UK and according to tumour site, resulting in inconsistent provision of this service.[34] As a result, older people are less likely to have access to a clinical nurse specialist,[35] which could lead to unmet needs and an increase in the risk of emergency admissions.[34]

Conclusion

The nursing contribution to older people affected by cancer is widely recognized and valued. Evidence suggests that its overall quality can be enhanced by the adoption of a person-centred approach to care delivery. A person-centred approach should be underpinned by effective assessment and knowledgeable practice. For nurses, this means marrying an understanding of cancer and its management with an appreciation of the specific needs of older people.

References

1   Macmillan Cancer Support. *The rich picture of older people with cancer.* Available from: www.macmillan.org.uk/Documents/AboutUs/Research/Richpictures/Richpicture-olderpeoplewithcancer.pdf (accessed 10 February 2015).

2   National Cancer Intelligence Network, Public Health England (2015). *Older people and cancer.* Available from: www.ncin.org.uk/publications/older_people_and_cancer (accessed 10 February 2015).

3   Bellury LM, Ellington E, Beck SL, *et al.* Elderly cancer survivorship: an integrative review and conceptual framework *Eur J Oncol Nurs* 2011; 15: 233–42.

4   Bourbonniere M, Van Cleave J. Cancer care in nursing homes *Semin Oncol Nurs* 2006; 22: 51–7.

5   Wood C, Ward J. A general overview of the cancer education needs of non-specialist staff. *Eur J Cancer Care* 2000; 9: 191–6.

6   Henke-Yarbro C. The history of cancer nursing. In: McCorkle R, Grant M, Frank-Stromberg M, Baird S, eds. *Cancer nursing: a comprehensive textbook.* 2nd ed. Philadelphia, PA: Saunders, 1994; 12–24.

7   Corner J. Nurses' experiences of cancer. *Eur J Cancer Care* 2002; 11: 193–9.

8   Gill F, Duffy A. Caring for cancer patients in non specialist wards. *Br J Nurs* 2010; 19: 760–7.

9   Hicks C, Fide J. The educational needs of non specialist breast care nurses *Nurse Educ Today* 2003; 23: 509–21.

10 McCaughan E, Parahoo K. Medical and surgical nurses' perceptions of their level of competence and educational needs in caring for patients with cancer. *J Clin Nurs* 2000; 9: 420–8.

11 Mohan S, Wilkes LM, Ogunsiji O, Walker A. Caring for patients with cancer in non-specialist wards: the nurse experience. *Eur J Cancer Care* 2005; 14: 256–63.

12 Wedding U, Rohrig B, Klippstein A, *et al.* Co-morbidity and functional deficits independently contribute to quality of life before chemotherapy in elderly cancer patients. *Support Care Cancer* 2007; 15: 1097–104.

13 Esbensen B, Thome B, Thomsen T. Dependency in elderly people newly diagnosed with cancer – a mixed method study. *Eur J Oncol Nurs* 2012; 16: 137–44.

14 Nursing and Midwifery Council (2009). *Guidance for the care of older people.* Available from: www.erskine.org.uk/sites/default/files/Guidance_for_the_care_of_older_people_date%5B1%5D.pdf (accessed 10 July 2015).

15 Commissioning Board Chief Nursing Officer, DH Chief Nursing Adviser (2012). *Compassion in practice. Nursing, midwifery and care staff. Our vision and strategy.* Available from: www.england.nhs.uk/wp-content/uploads/2012/12/compassion-in-practice.pdf (accessed 10 July 2015).

16 Royal College of Nursing. *Person-centred care.* Available from: www.rcn.org.uk/development/practice/cpd_online_learning/dignity_in_health_care/person-centred_care (accessed 10 February 2015).

17 National Cancer Action Team. *Holistic common assessment of supportive and palliative care needs for adults with cancer.* London: National Cancer Action Team, 2007.

18 National Cancer Survivorship Initiative (2012). *The recovery package.* Available from: www.ncsi.org.uk/what-we-are-doing/the-recovery-package (accessed 10 February 2015).

19 Draper J, Tetley J (2013). *The importance of person-centred approaches to nursing care.* Available from: www.open.edu/openlearn/body-mind/health/nursing/the-importance-person-centred-approaches-nursing-care (accessed 10 February 2015).

20 McCorkle R, Strumpf NE, Nuamah IF. A specialised home care intervention improves survival among older post-surgical cancer patients. *J Am Geriatr Soc* 2000; 48: 1707–13.

21 Duffin C. Tackling ageism in cancer treatment. *Nurs Older People* 2013; 25: 14–17.

22 Macmillan Cancer Support, Department of Health, Age UK (2012). *Cancer services coming of age: learning from the Improving Cancer Treatment Assessment and Support for Older People Project.* Available from: www.macmillan.org.uk/Documents/AboutUs/Health_professionals/OlderPeoplesProject/CancerServicesComingofAge.pdf (accessed 13 June 2015).

23 de Vries M, van Weert J, Jansen J, *et al.* Step by step development of clinical care pathways for older cancer patients: necessary or desirable? *Eur J Cancer* 2007; 43: 2170–8.

24 Hurria A. Assessment of the older adult with cancer. *J Support Oncol* 2008; 6: 80–1.

25 Jennings Sanders A, Anderson E. Older women with breast cancer: perceptions of the effectiveness of nurse case managers. *Nurs Outlook* 2007; 51: 108–14.

26 Department of Health (2007). *Cancer reform strategy.* Available from: www.nhs.uk/NHSEngland/NSF/Documents/Cancer%20Reform%20Strategy.pdf (accessed 10 February 2015).

27 Willard C, Luker K. Working with the team strategies employed by hospital cancer nurse specialists to implement their role. *J Clin Nurs* 2007; 16: 716–24.

28 Quality Health (2014). *2014 National cancer patient experience survey.* Available from: www.quality-health.co.uk/resources/surveys/national-cancer-experience-survey/2014-national-cancer-patient-experience-survey (accessed 10 July 2015).

29 Department of Health (2011). *Improving outcomes: a strategy for cancer.* Available from: www.gov.uk/government/uploads/system/uploads/attachment_data/file/213785/dh_123394.pdf (accessed 10 February 2015).

30 Farrell C, Molassiotis A, Beaver K, Heaven C. Exploring the scope of oncology specialist nurses' practice in the UK. *Eur J Oncol Nurs* 2011; 15: 160–6.

31 Amir Z, Scully J, Borrill C. The professional role of breast cancer nurses in multi-disciplinary breast cancer care teams *Eur J Oncol Nurs* 2004; 8: 306–14.

32 National Cancer Action Team (2010). *Excellence in cancer care: the contribution of the clinical nurse specialist.* Available from: www.macmillan.org.uk/Documents/AboutUs/Commissioners/ExcellenceinCancerCaretheContributionoftheClinicalNurseSpecialist.pdf (accessed 10 February 2015).

33 Cox K, Wilson E. Follow up for people with cancer: nurse led services and telephone interventions *J Adv Nurs* 2003; 43: 51–61.

34 Macmillan Cancer Support. *Cancer clinical nurse specialists.* Available from: www.macmillan.org.uk/Documents/AboutUs/Commissioners/ClinicalNurseSpecialistsAnEvidenceReview2012.pdf (accessed 10 February 2015).

35 Royal College of Nursing (2010). *Guidance on safe nurse staffing levels in the UK.* Available from: www.rcn.org.uk/__data/assets/pdf_file/0005/353237/003860.pdf (accessed 10 February 2015).

14 Allied Health Professional Perspective

Karen Hargreaves, Thangaraj Senniappan, Margot Gosney

Introduction

This chapter gives an overview of the range of roles of allied health professionals (AHPs) and how they can support older people, their relatives and carers at different stages of their cancer journey. AHPs include: dietitians, lymphoedema therapists, occupational therapists, orthotists, physiotherapists, podiatrists, radiographers, and speech and language therapists.

AHPs working with cancer patients may specialize in the field of cancer care or remain generalists throughout their career, with intermittent contact with cancer patients. The aim of the specialist AHP role is to undertake holistic assessments, and from these assessments provide tailored advice and support to individuals affected by cancer and those closest to them. AHPs act as a referral point for others working in a variety of settings: from hospitals to the voluntary sector. They support people to adapt their lives to meet the challenges they face. Rehabilitation, to a greater or lesser extent, is a common theme. Effective rehabilitation requires different professionals to work as part of well-integrated teams to achieve the best outcomes. Good communication between these teams is essential.[1] The support should always be person-centred and take account of the potential for additional sensory deficits that can impede communication: hearing loss, for example, can be improved by simple interventions such as ensuring that the AHP gains the patient's attention and faces the patient when speaking, and remains mindful of providing information in an accessible way.[2] People may benefit from rehabilitation at diagnosis prior to any treatment, to optimize their condition, and throughout their treatment, to minimize symptom effects. Several studies have identified unmet needs of cancer patients in psychosocial, physical, sexual and occupational domains.[3] AHPs are well placed to identify and support patients with their needs. Older patients may already be challenged by daily activities before a cancer diagnosis, and need additional support to make adjustments to regain or maintain a quality of life that is acceptable to them. AHPs contribute to a person's quality of life and work to improve outcomes, e.g. by improving nutritional support to preserve strength and reduce the hospital stay.[4] It is not the responsibility of any one group of professionals to enable people to reach their potential despite having had a diagnosis of cancer, but rather a combination of the varied skills provided by AHPs at the right time.

What do the different AHP services offer?

The blurring of boundaries between professionals can cause confusion for the referrer. Different geographical areas will have different systems in place and it is important that referrers take time to familiarize themselves with the services in their location and be clear about what they wish to achieve from any referral. The National Cancer Action Team published care pathways for several cancer sites.[5] Local cancer networks were then tasked with defining interventions for the AHP (Table 14.1). Reference to these pathways may aid a clinician to make appropriate referrals. Rehabilitation and care needs should be checked at key points along the patient pathway to ensure the correct AHP is involved in a timely fashion.

As the number of older people living with cancer rises,[6] so does the complexity of their needs.

Table 14.1 The role of AHPs in the cancer pathway.[9]

AHP	Summary of role	Involvement in cancer pathway
Art, music and drama therapists	Work with cancer patients and use the psychological and social potentials of the arts to support patients with a wide range of physical, communication and mental health issues	A, T, S
Diagnostic radiographers	Employ a range of techniques to produce high-quality images to diagnose an injury or disease including cancer	P, A, T, S
	Responsible for providing safe and accurate high-quality imaging examinations and are increasingly involved in providing first-line reporting results	
	Diagnostic radiographers are also key members of the breast screening programme	
Dietitians	Specialize in the nutritional assessment of cancer patients, which together with other clinical information is used to provide dietary treatment	P, A, T, S
	Malnutrition is the single most common secondary diagnosis in patients with cancer: dietitians advise on achieving optimal nutritional status, improve nutrition throughout the cancer journey and minimize discomfort through appropriate nutritional support	
Lymphoedema practitioners	Health professionals (predominantly nurses, physiotherapists and occupational therapists, and may also include manual lymph drainage therapists) who have specialist postgraduate training in the prevention and management of lymphoedema	A, T, S
	Lymphoedema practitioners provide support and give advice to patients and professionals, obtain and disseminate lymphoedema information and provide lymphoedema patients with a standard of care recognized by the British Lymphology Society, working alongside the recommendations of the International Lymphoedema Framework Project	
Occupational therapists	Assist the patient and carers to maintain the patient's maximum level of function and independence	A, T, S
	They are involved in the care of patients who have problems with functional ability, stress or physical discomfort as a result of cancer and symptom management, and play a pivotal role in vocational rehabilitation	
Orthoptist	Assess, diagnose and treat eye movement defects due to cancer and other clinical conditions	P, A, T, S
Physiotherapists	Help maximize the patient's potential in terms of functional ability and independence, as well as help the patient gain relief from distressing symptoms	A, T, S
	Physiotherapists provide a range of therapies for physical disability and pain	
Podiatrists	Provide assessment, evaluation and foot care for a wide range of patients with a variety of long-term and acute conditions	P, A, T, S
Prosthetists and orthotists	Prosthetists are able to design and fit the most appropriate prosthesis for each patient on an individual basis	T, S
	Orthotists assess, fit and provide education for patients requiring orthotic support	
Speech and language therapists	Specialize in the diagnosis and treatment of patients who have speech and language and/or swallowing problems as a result of cancer	P, A, T, S
	They are also involved in the teaching of alternative methods of communication and symptom management	
Therapeutic radiographers	Play a vital role in cancer radiation therapy	T, S
	Together with medical physicists, they help plan and deliver radiotherapy	
	Therapy radiographers manage the patient pathway through the many radiotherapy processes, providing care and support for patients throughout radiotherapy treatment	
	It is now more common for therapy radiographers to use specialist skills to assess patients on treatment within their own clinics	

A, assessment and diagnosis; P, prediagnosis; S, survivorship; T, treatment.

This group often experiences additional health challenges, so the need for effective, tailored cancer rehabilitation services will increase. Common issues for older people include nutrition, continence, cognition and falls. AHPs are trained to provide interventions in these areas. For example: in patients who are underweight there are implications for treatment, as chemotherapy doses are based on body weight, so optimum doses may not be given; and dietitians are key to the prevention and correction of nutritional depletion and the maintenance of physical strength, which are important in decreasing falls and increasing mobility.[7]

Mobility can be a factor when devising treatment options. Both the person's ability to travel to a treatment centre and his or her functional level should be taken into account: parking, walking long distances in hospitals, and leaving dependents can all have an impact on agreement to proceed or continue with treatment. Access to treatment can be facilitated by provision of equipment, gait and balance training, strength and resistance training,[8] or provision of suitable orthotics. People who are functionally less able may be less likely to be recommended for treatment.

Case study to highlight AHP intervention in fall prevention and mobility

A 79-year-old man, living with his wife who had a diagnosis of dementia, was referred to the emergency department with a fall. He had no children, but a niece lived locally and helped with shopping. He was diagnosed with lung cancer and had falls due to postural hypotension. He was reluctant to attend for treatment because of concerns about how he and his wife would cope if he became less well during treatment.

Actions taken

The patient was reviewed by a physiotherapist and an occupational therapist whilst in the emergency department, and provided with a walking stick. A referral was made to community rehabilitation service for follow-up assessments. An occupational therapy home visit was made and during the visit the patient expressed fears about not being able to cope in the future. The range of services available were explained to him and written information was given to him to review and consider – including a frozen meal delivery system to improve his and his wife's nutrition. A review by social services was requested to assess his wife's needs and a referral made to a voluntary agency for a befriending service to reduce social isolation. Rails were provided to reduce the risk of falls.

Outcome

The patient agreed to a social services review of his wife's needs and accepted a befriender, equipment and a frozen meal delivery service. With these services in place he agreed to have treatment, as he felt better supported.

Why is rehabilitation important?

Rehabilitation is a collaborative process between the person affected by cancer, those close to them and the therapist planning/advising on the treatment option. People's needs should be assessed at various stages during the cancer pathway and provided for as circumstances change.[9] Cancer rehabilitation aims to maximize physical and psychological function, promote independence and help people adapt to their condition. Rehabilitation does not set out to cure people or always return people to full function in all domains. Bray and Cooper[10] identified four types of rehabilitation: preventative, restorative, supportive and palliative. Preventative rehabilitation, such as physiotherapy for breast cancer after surgery, reduces the risk of secondary lymphoedema,[11] and intervention with diet leads to improvement in energy levels, exercise capacity and weight gain.[12]

Case study to highlight a supportive and palliative approach

A 71-year-old woman lived with her husband and had two children who lived locally. She was independent and a very active member of her family, known as the decision-maker by her children. She had previously done all the cooking and taken care of the family. The couple had their own business. She was diagnosed with a brain tumour and had a short life expectancy. Although she was living at home, her family reported that she was 'muddled' and 'unsteady on her feet'.

Actions taken

An occupational therapy and physiotherapy home visit was arranged, during which a cognitive assessment and screen for anxiety and depression were completed. The patient had limited capacity and little insight into her condition but was clear that she wished to remain at home. The therapists established with the family her preferred place of care and likely preferred place of death. This information was shared with the local health team. Mobility was assessed: her balance was impaired, but memory issues would not support the consistent use of walking aids. The therapists jointly assessed with the family where and how she moved within her home: furniture was moved to facilitate safer mobility and reduce the risk of falls whilst facilitating her ability to remain active. The occupational therapist assessed the patient's kitchen skills, which were variable, and advice was given to her family about how to support her with tasks, e.g. she should be involved but not left unsupervised. The home was assessed with regard to future equipment needs, e.g. a hospital bed, and how best to introduce this to her to reduce the stress and trauma of having changes made to her home. A care package was recommended to give the family some time away from their caring responsibilities (a sitting service once a week and night support once a week). Further support for bereavement was identified and a referral made to the community palliative services for psychological support for her husband.

Outcome

The patient died at home among her family, supported by the district nurses and community palliative care. The husband saw a community psychologist for follow-up.

Case study to demonstrate how a supportive and restorative approach can have an impact

A 74-year-old woman had a recent diagnosis of breast cancer. She lived alone and was known to have a history of depressive illness. She underwent a radical mastectomy and chemotherapy with referral to outpatient physiotherapy for treatment to maintain her range of movement and promote mobility, as she had a fear of falling. On outpatient visits she expressed feelings of isolation and depression. She used her computer to keep in touch with her children, who lived abroad. It was noted that she was dehydrated and she admitted she was not drinking much due to her fear of having 'accidents' with her bladder control.

Actions taken

Referral was made to the local continence clinic for a review of the patient's bladder symptoms, and arrangements were made for her to attend a local voluntary day care centre which had access to lymphoedema, art and alternative therapists. In addition, a request was made to a local charity to have a weekly voluntary visitor to reduce her feelings of isolation. She was given written information about online support, as she was confident in using her computer. Her GP was advised of her current emotional state.

Outcome

The patient was seen at the continence clinic and continued to attend her outpatient visits to a physiotherapist and a lymphoedema therapist. She was discharged from the day centre, as she had regained her confidence in going out. She reported that she enjoyed being part of an online support group and was now active in fundraising for a breast cancer charity.

Conclusion

To achieve the best quality of life for a person it is necessary to clarify and understand what is important to that person, assess the normal level of function and ensure that access to specialist services, such as memory clinics or practical help, is available. These resources enable patients to manage their treatment and maintain a quality of life that is acceptable to them.

The National Cancer Action Team[5] recognized that addressing the provision of cancer rehabilitation is cost-effective. People who can return to work or, in the case of the older person, be enabled to live independently by provision of equipment or with a smaller package of care[13] will cost the community less. Well-resourced rehabilitation teams can reduce hospital bed days and even reduce readmission rates by a variety of simple interventions. These might include managing lymphoedema to reduce swelling and prevent damage and infection,[6,9] and teaching patients breathing techniques and pacing to reduce shortness of breath.[14] Patients who have coping strategies to manage their symptoms are likely to spend less time in hospital.[15]

After treatment is completed, many people can have ongoing issues with fatigue, or may express negative feelings or find coping challenging. AHPs work in assorted locations to offer support after cancer.[9] This ongoing support can have a positive effect on quality of life.[16,17] Effective rehabilitation and treatment by AHPs meets government standards of care as aspired to in the NHS Outcomes Framework:[18] 'AHPs are not optional but integral to the necessary treatment of patients. There are clinical and financial risks in patients not receiving AHP input.'[9]

References

1 Compton S. *Fulfilling lives: rehabilitation in palliative care.* London: National Council for Hospice and Specialist Palliative Care, 2000.

2 NHS England, Department of Health (2015). *Action plan on hearing loss.* (Publications gateway reference 03073.) Available from: www.england.nhs.uk/wp-content/uploads/2015/03/act-plan-hearing-loss-upd.pdf (accessed 1 May 2015).

3 Armes J, Crowe M, Colbourne L, *et al.* Patients' supportive care needs beyond the end of cancer treatment: a prospective longitudinal survey. *J Clin Oncol* 2009; 27: 6172–9.

4 Kreuzenga HM, Van Tulder MW, Siedell JC, *et al.* Effectiveness and cost effectiveness of early screening and treatment of malnourished patients. *Am J Nutr* 2005; 82: 1082–9.

5 Macmillan Cancer Support (2013). *Evidence for rehabilitation.* Available from: www.macmillan.org.uk/Aboutus/Healthandsocialcareprofessionals/Newsandupdates/MacVoice/Summer2013/Evidenceforrehabilitation.aspx (accessed 1 May 2015).

6 Macmillan Cancer Support (2010). *Allied health professionals in cancer care. An evidence review.* Available from: www.macmillan.org.uk/Documents/AboutUs/Commissioners/AlliedHealthProfessionalsAnEvidenceReviewOctober2012.pdf (accessed 1 May 2015).

7 Ravesco P, Monteiro-Grillo I, Vidal PM, Camilo ME. Nutritional deterioration in cancer: the role of disease and diet. *Clin Oncol* 2003; 15: 443–50.

8 Strong A, Karavatas SG, Reicherter EA. Recommended exercise protocol to decrease cancer-related fatigue and muscle wasting in patients with multiple myeloma: an evidence-based systematic review. *Top Geriatr Rehabil* 2006; 22: 172–86.

9 NHS London. *Allied Health Professions cancer care toolkit. How AHPs improve patient care and save the NHS money.* (Department of Health gateway reference 17269.) Available from: www.networks.nhs.uk/nhs-networks/ahp-networks/ahp-qipp-toolkits/AHP_ONS_Pathway_final.pdf/view?searchterm=ons%20toolkit (accessed 1 May 2015).

10 Bray J, Cooper J. The contribution to palliative medicine of allied health professionals – the contribution of occupational therapy. In: Doyle D, Banks G, Cherry N, Calman K, eds. *Oxford textbook of palliative medicine.* 3rd ed. Oxford: Oxford University Press, 2000.

11 Lacomba M. Effectiveness of early physiotherapy to prevent lymphoedema after surgery for breast cancer: randomised, single blinded, clinical trial. *BMJ* 2010; 340: 5396.

12 Rueda JR, Sola J, Pascual A, Subirana Casacuberta, M. Non-invasive interventions for improving well-being and quality of life in patients with lung cancer. *Cochrane Database Syst Rev* 2011; 9: CD004282.

13 Hill N. Therapy in an acute front line service. *Occup Ther News* 2010; 18: 25.

14 Bausewein C, Booth S, Gysels M, Higginson IJ. Non-pharmacological interventions for breathlessness in advanced stages of malignant and non-malignant diseases. *Cochrane Database Syst Rev* 2008; 2: CD005623.

15 Wilcock A (2010). *Annual report of Nottingham Macmillan Lung Cancer CARE Service.* Available from: www.macmillan.org.uk/Documents/AboutUs/ Health_professionals/Awards/2012/NottinghamMacmillanLungCancerCAREService.pdf (accessed 1 May 2015).

16 Morey MC, Snyder DC, Sloane R, *et al.* Effects of home-based diet and exercise on functional outcomes among older, overweight long-term cancer survivors. REnEW: a randomized controlled trial. *JAMA* 2009; 301: 1883–91.

17 Reynolds MW, Lim KH. Contribution of visual art-making to the subjective well-being of women living with cancer: a qualitative study. *Arts Psychother* 2007; 34: 1–10.

18 Department of Health (2013). *The NHS outcomes framework 2014/15.* Available from: www.gov.uk/government/uploads/system/uploads/attachment_data/file/256456/NHS_outcomes.pdf (accessed 1 April 2015).

15 Perspectives from a GP on Care of Older People with Cancer

Winnie Kwan

Background

In 2011, patients aged 65 and over accounted for 17% of the population, and those aged 85 and over accounted for 2% of the population.[1] Nearly two-thirds of cancer diagnoses occur in the over-65s and one-third in people aged 75 and over. By 2020, there will be nearly 2 million people aged 65 and over who have survived a diagnosis of cancer.[2]

Consultation rates in primary care are increasing, and the highest rates are among older people. In 2008, estimated rates of GP consultations were reported to be 13.9 per person-year for men and 13.3 per person-year for women in the 85–89 years age group.[3]

Primary care and cancer in older people

The role of the primary care team at a practice level is 'a central and continuing element in cancer care for both the patient and his/her family from primary prevention, pre-symptomatic screening, initial diagnosis through to care and follow up or, in some cases, death and bereavement'.[4] The role has since expanded to include commissioning input and survivorship issues.

The Health and Social Care Act 2012[5] created two new organizations, the NHS Commissioning Board (NHSCB) and Public Health England, and replaced former primary care trusts with clinical commissioning groups (CCGs). CCGs are clinically led groups formed by member general practices in a geographic area to commission services for the population. The commissioning of cancer services is split among these three bodies:

1. The NHSCB commissions specialized services.[6]

2. Public Health England commissions cancer screening services.

3. CCGs commission services for patients with the common cancers, with the exception of radiotherapy, chemotherapy and specialist interventions.

CCGs work with their local authority's health and well-being board to improve cancer outcomes. The local authority, with its responsibility for public health resources, analyses the prevalence and expected rise in cancer incidence (among other health priorities) to produce the Joint Strategic Needs Assessment, which informs the CCG and NHSCB of its commissioning strategy. The CCG has to take into account historic and forecast needs, plus any case for change or opportunities from research evidence/best practice in the commissioning of cancer services. The process is complex, from setting commissioning intentions to contracting and delivery of services, especially in London, where there are wide variations in cancer outcomes and a large heterogeneous population. The London CCGs have to work in partnership with the London-wide Transforming Cancer Services Team, the local integrated cancer system (London Cancer Alliance or London Cancer) and local clinical groups. The focus is on early detection, reducing pathway variations, improving patient experience, and developing strategies for chemotherapy, radiotherapy and end-of-life care.[7]

A major challenge in health services worldwide is the development of an integrated service for the older population with long-term conditions (cardiovascular, respiratory, neurological, musculoskeletal, dementia, etc.), as well as the burden of frailty.[8] The Comprehensive Geriatric Assessment (CGA) approach is the gold standard assessment for older patients with complex needs, whether it is to meet frailty needs or to assess preparation for surgery or chemo- or radiotherapy. Bexley CCG, as an example, is supportive of CGA and is working on how to incorporate the CGA process into the whole range of service provision, from acute to community services.

Prevention is one of the top priorities in the NHS Five Year Forward View addressing the health and well-being gap to tackle avoidable illness.[9] At least one-third of all cancer cases are preventable. Prevention offers the most cost-effective, long-term strategy for the control of cancer.[10] Primary cancer prevention for older people needs to start at a much earlier stage through support for smoking cessation and obesity prevention. In 2012, the percentage of the population in England in the overweight and obese categories of BMI was over 70% from age 45 upwards.[1] Raising awareness of cancer prevention in terms of lifestyle changes through smoking cessation, healthier eating through consumption of more fruit and vegetables, exercise and avoidance of obesity is crucial. Primary care is in an ideal position to promote cancer prevention, but research has identified barriers including time constraint, lack of training and lack of updates (among other factors) to achieving the potential intervention which GPs feel they have the opportunity and the responsibility to deliver.[11] Action is required at the practice and CCG level with strategic direction to address the barriers identified. Practice nursing staff can be effectively deployed in preventive health measures. Commitment, planning and training are essential for success. Screening and early diagnosis are discussed elsewhere in this publication.

The Cancer Patient Experience Survey 2014 highlights the areas for improvement in the hospital as provision of information on financial help, provision of care plans and participation in research. Patients with rarer cancers and those diagnosed via the emergency route tend to have a more negative experience. There is no specific question in the survey on patients' experience of whether care is well coordinated, such as whether they had problems with appointments, travelling, transport, or a long wait for investigation/treatment/results. There is no specific question on patients' out-of–hours experience, as generally neither the clinical nurse specialists nor the GP is available out of hours. Staff in primary care must increase their awareness of the need to support patients with cancer during treatment. The social, emotional and spiritual needs of the patient have to be addressed; hence, a community/hospital cross-boundary multi-professional approach is required.

The score on different professionals working well together to give the patient the best possible care is low at 66%.[12] Improvement in this respect can be achieved by effective, comprehensive and timely inter-professional communication, especially with respect to referrals, outpatient correspondence and hospital discharges. It is important for the GP to include in the 2 week wait referral not only the history of current disease but also a holistic history with all relevant medical and psychosocial background information, including medication, allergies and the patient's premorbid levels of physical, social and cognitive functioning. Electronic or e-referral is now the preferred delivery mode using standardized templates.

Information from the cancer specialist back to primary care is often delivered electronically and either addressed to the patient and copied to the GP or vice versa. The following lists what is essential for the GP to know:

- Cancer diagnosis.
- Investigations results.
- Disease staging.
- Proposed treatment.
- Follow-up arrangements.
- What the patient/family has been told.
- Goal of treatment: curative or palliative.
- Likely adverse effects and their management.
- Any consideration of ceiling of treatment.
- Whether any advance care planning has been initiated.

For patients with advanced disease, it is crucial to inform the GP whether an end-of-life discussion has taken place, whether a 'Do Not Attempt Cardiopulmonary Resuscitation' has been signed, and whether the patient and family are aware of imminent death.

Whilst palliative care is discussed in a separate chapter, meaningful communication with the patient is the foundation of care with compassion. A therapeutic relationship involves understanding the patient's perspective; hence, it is necessary to elicit the older cancer patient's understanding of his/her condition, worst fears, goals if the condition deteriorates and what trade-offs he/she is or is not willing to make. These fit-for-purpose questions are what Dr Atul Gawande has learnt to ask his patients in the shared decision process when they are faced with a poor prognosis. These were good enough questions for him to ask his father in his personal experience. The limits of medicine and the inadequacy of the doctor's paternalistic or informative approach to patients with advanced cancer are exposed in Dr Gawande's book.[13]

Helping patients to face mortality and giving them the insight and opportunity to make the best of their remaining life is a challenge to the medical profession. The converse is iatrogenic harm with futile treatment, depriving the patient of the precious remaining time to fulfil outstanding ambitions, however great or small. The skill of the doctor is to balance this risk against the potential benefit of treatment.

Conclusion and learning points

- The NHS is facing the huge challenge of an increasingly older population. CGA needs to be more widely available to address complex needs.
- Prevention needs to start early: in particular, smoking cessation and obesity avoidance.
- Supporting patients/carers through the cancer journey until the end of life demands an integrated approach.
- Local cancer stakeholders should seize initiatives to foster effective and mutually supportive working relationships to aim for seamless patient care.
- Patients' feedback about understanding, fears, goals and priorities needs to be elicited and addressed.

References

1 Health and Social Care Information Centre (2014). *Focus on the health and care of older people.* Available from: www.hscic.gov.uk/catalogue/PUB14369/focu-on-hac-op-main-pub-doc%201.1.pdf (accessed 30 June 2015).

2 National Cancer Intelligence Network. *Older people and cancer.* Available from: www.ncin.org.uk/publications/older_people_and_cancer (accessed 30 June 2015).

3 Hippisley-Cox J, Vinogradova Y (2009). *Trends in consultation rates in general practice 1995/1996 to 2008/2009: analysis of the QResearch database.* Available from: www.hscic.gov.uk/catalogue/PUB01077/tren-cons-rate-gene-prac-95-09-95-09-rep.pdf (accessed 30 June 2015).

4 Calman K, Hine D; Expert Advisory Group on Cancer to the Chief Medical Officers of England and Wales (1995). *A policy framework for commissioning cancer services.* Available from: http://webarchive.nationalarchives.gov.uk/20080814090336/dh.gov.uk/en/Publicationsandstatistics/Publications/PublicationsPolicyAndGuidance/DH_4071083 (accessed 30 June 2015).

5 Department of Health (2012). *Health and Social Care Act 2012: fact sheets.* Available from: www.gov.uk/government/publications/health-and-social-care-act-2012-fact-sheets (accessed 30 June 2015).

6 Specialised Services Commissioning Transition Team (2012). *Manual for prescribed specialised services.* Available from: www.england.nhs.uk/wp-content/uploads/2012/12/pss-manual.pdf (accessed 30 June 2015).

7 NHS England. *Transforming cancer services for London. Commissioning cancer survivorship: an overview.* Available from: www.ncsi.org.uk/wp-content/uploads/Transforming-Londons-Cancer-services-v0-6-181013PDF.pdf (accessed 30 June 2015).

8 Goodwin N, Dixon A, Anderson G, Wodchis W (2014). *Providing integrated care for older people with complex needs. Lessons from seven international case studies.* Available from: www.kingsfund.org.uk/sites/files/kf/field/field_publication_file/providing-integrated-care-for-older-people-with-complex-needs-kingsfund-jan14.pdf (accessed 30 June 2015).

9 NHS (2014). *Five Year Forward View.* Available from: www.england.nhs.uk/wp-content/uploads/2014/10/5yfv-web.pdf (accessed 30 June 2015).

10 World Health Organization. *Cancer prevention.* Available from: www.who.int/cancer/prevention/en/ (accessed 30 June 2015).

11 Cancer Focus Northern Ireland. *Investigating the actual and potential role of the general practitioner, practice nurse and nurse practitioner in the prevention of cancer.* Available from: www.cancerfocusni.org/wp-content/uploads/Cancer-Focus-Research-Report-Actual-Potential-Roles-of-the-GP-PCN-in-the-prevention-of-cancer.pdf (accessed 30 June 2015).

12 Quality Health (2014). *2014 National cancer patient experience survey.* Available from: www.quality-health.co.uk/resources/surveys/national-cancer-experience-survey/2014-national-cancer-patient-experience-survey (accessed 30 June 2015).

13 Gawande A. *Being mortal. Illness, medicine, and what matters in the end.* London: Profile Books/Wellcome Collection, 2014.

16 Anaesthetic Perspective

Stephen Alcorn, Irwin Foo

Introduction

The older cancer patient who requires operative intervention poses several specific problems to the anaesthetist. While age in and of itself is not a predictor of long-term survival in the critically unwell older person,[1] the higher incidence of comorbidities coupled with the pathophysiological effects of the malignant process and its treatment often render older people at higher risk of morbidity and mortality in the perioperative period. A careful assessment of functional reserve should be undertaken by the anaesthetist to ascertain whether the patient is able to cope with the stress of radical surgery, to plan postoperative care and to allow for informed discussion preoperatively.

Assessment and anaesthetic approach to the older cancer patient

Assessment of cardiorespiratory functional reserve

One of the cornerstones of predicting perioperative risk is the assessment of cardiorespiratory functional reserve. Cardiovascular comorbidities and obesity may cause further respiratory compromise as well as physical deconditioning.

A simple and practical tool to assess a patient's ability to meet the cardiorespiratory demands of the stress of surgery is the concept of metabolic equivalents of task (METs). One MET equates to the oxygen consumption of a 70 kg 40-year-old male in the resting state, and activities which require higher oxygen consumption are described as multiples of this baseline[2] (Table 16.1). Studies have suggested that if patients are unable to participate in activities requiring approximately 4 METs they are more likely to experience perioperative cardiovascular complications,[3] an increased length of hospital stay, and mortality.[4] Such patients should undergo more formal cardiovascular assessment, e.g. cardiopulmonary exercise testing. This is particularly important for high-risk invasive surgery, e.g. intrathoracic and intraperitoneal procedures or operations where anticipated blood loss may exceed 1500 ml. Cardiopulmonary exercise testing calculates several variables including the level of exertion beyond which oxygen supply is limited and therefore anaerobic metabolism becomes significant. This is termed the anaerobic threshold. An anaerobic threshold below 11 ml/min/kg has been shown to be

Table 16.1 METs (adapted from Jetté *et al.*[2]).

MET score	Example activities
1	Eat and dress, walk indoors around the house
2	Walk a block on the level, do light work around the house
4	Climb a flight of stairs or walk uphill, heavy domestic work, run a short distance
6	Moderate recreational activities, e.g. dancing, golf, doubles tennis
10	Strenuous sports, e.g. swimming at 3 km/h

Table 16.2 Chemotherapeutic agents and organ toxicity (modified from Allan *et al.*[6]).

Organ toxicity	Examples of chemotherapeutic drugs responsible
Pulmonary	Cytotoxic antibiotics (e.g. bleomycin, mitomycin C, doxorubicin), nitrosureas (e.g. lomustine), alkylating agents (e.g. cyclophosphamide, chlorambucil), antimetabolites (e.g. methotrexate), plant alkaloids (e.g. vincristine, etoposide)
Cardiac	Cytotoxic antibiotics, alkylating agents, plant alkaloids, others (e.g. fluorouracil, cisplatin)
Hepatic	Nitrosureas, antimetabolites, cytotoxic antibiotics, others (e.g. fluorouracil, vincristine)
Renal	Nitrosureas, others (e.g. bleomycin, cisplatin, cyclophosphamide, vincristine)

predictive of cardiac morbidity and mortality[5] and to correlate well with a MET level <4. It should prompt more intense perioperative monitoring and support, e.g. intraoperative inotropes, postoperative HDU or ITU care and 24–48 h postoperative ventilation to reduce the work of breathing and the burden on the myocardium. Older patients unable to be tested on a bicycle ergometer or a treadmill because of lower limb arthritis or peripheral vascular disease may require other specialist dynamic testing, e.g. dobutamine stress echocardiography.

Influence of chemotherapeutic agents

The management of some cancers involves neoadjuvant chemotherapy and radiation therapy before definitive surgery. Prior treatment with these modalities may have cardiorespiratory toxicity, compounding background heart and lung disease. Of particular importance for the anaesthetist are the anthracyclines, which cause cardiotoxicity and QT prolongation, and bleomycin, which may cause pulmonary toxicity especially in combination with high inspired concentrations of oxygen (Table 16.2).[6] Any unexplained symptoms such as increasing breathlessness or new-onset chest pain should be investigated further. Indications for preoperative echocardiography[7] are listed in Table 16.3, while pulmonary function tests should be carried out in patients who are given chemotherapeutic agents known to cause pulmonary toxicity.

Assessment of frailty

It is becoming evident that frailty in this age group determines outcome after surgery. The *Age old problem* report[8] showed that 66% of older patients who died postoperatively were identified as frail. An assessment of frailty performed preoperatively is helpful for the anaesthetist to quantify perioperative risk and to make a more informed assessment of the patient. A recent study[9] confirmed that frailty was not only an independent risk predictor for postoperative

Table 16.3 Indications for preoperative echocardiogram (adapted from British Society of Echocardiography guidelines[7]).

Indication
Documented ischaemic heart disease with reduced functional capacity (<4 METs)
Unexplained shortness of breath (in absence of clinical heart failure and normal ECG/chest x-ray)
Murmur in presence of cardiac or respiratory symptoms
Murmur in asymptomatic individual with suspected severe structural heart disease

complications, increasing length of hospital stay and discharge to a skilled nursing facility, but it also enhanced the predictive ability of commonly used operative risk models, e.g. the American Society of Anesthesiologists (ASA) grading (used universally in the UK as a measure of perioperative risk) (Figure 16.1). It is likely that frailty assessment will become part of the preoperative routine in the future.

Prehabilitation

Prehabilitation is a growing field in both cancer therapy and management of the older surgical patient. The aims include improving patients' physical and psychological health and optimizing their cardiovascular fitness: therefore, diminishing their perioperative risk while potentially opening a wider range of treatment options. Strategies may involve aerobic fitness training, weight reduction, dietary interventions and psychological therapies. A recent pilot study in rectal cancer patients demonstrated that neoadjuvant chemoradiotherapy prior to definitive surgery reduced physical fitness, but, with a structured exercise training programme before surgery, physical fitness was restored to baseline level.[10]

Preoperative medications and interaction with anaesthesia

In addition to treatment for their cancer, older patients are frequently taking a plethora of prescribed and non-prescribed medications. In the context of anaesthesia, potential drug interactions are common. This patient, for example, is likely to be taking at least one antihypertensive agent, which has the potential to cause life-threatening hypotension or organ ischaemia when combined with general anaesthesia. It is essential to discuss with the anaesthetist which of these medicines should be continued in the perioperative period. However, as a general rule of thumb, ACE inhibitors and angiotensin II receptor antagonists should be withheld on the

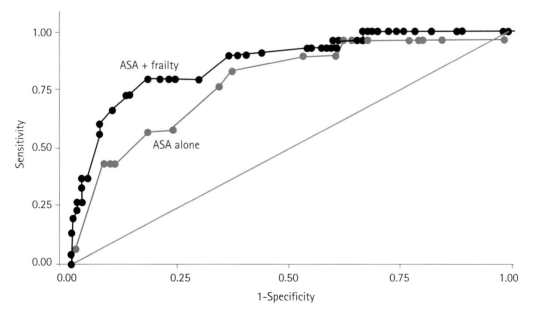

Figure 16.1 Receiver operating characteristics (ROC) curve showing the ability of the ASA risk index to predict surgical complications and discharge to an assisted or skilled nursing facility. Frailty was added to the ASA risk index to demonstrate the combined ability of these indices to predict discharge disposition. The area under the ROC curve is 0.8694. Redrawn from Makary et al.[9]

day of surgery unless prescribed for congestive cardiac failure, while beta-blockers should generally be continued throughout. Furthermore, antiplatelet and anticoagulant therapies should be discussed with the anaesthetist, especially if a regional anaesthetic technique is planned. Renal and/or hepatic impairment may also influence anaesthetic and analgesic drug choice, as impaired metabolism and excretion can significantly prolong drug action and enhance drug interactions.

It is also important to establish whether patients are taking any herbal medications, as these may contain a variety of chemicals which may potentially interact with other drugs or have their own potentially noxious side effects in the perioperative period. For example, St John's Wort may precipitate serotoninergic crisis, while garlic supplements may have antiplatelet effects and increase perioperative bleeding. The ASA recommends that all herbal remedies be stopped 2–3 weeks prior to elective surgery.

Nutritional status

Older cancer patients may present in various nutritional states. The obese patient has a higher risk of difficult venous access, difficult intubation and ventilation, perioperative pressure sores, difficult surgical access prolonging surgical time and potentially increasing blood loss, prolonged duration of fat-soluble drugs such as volatile anaesthetic agents, and poor wound healing. Conversely, the malnourished patient has a higher risk of electrolyte imbalance and vitamin deficiency, perioperative nerve injury, hypothermia and impaired recovery and rehabilitation. Enhanced recovery programmes, which are multimodal, evidence-based pathways aimed at involving patients in their own care and minimizing the physiological stress response to surgery (Figure 16.2), have led to a reduction in postoperative complications and length of hospital stay.[11] The important components of enhanced recovery programmes, which include optimization of preoperative comorbidities, patient education, preoperative carbohydrate loading, minimally invasive surgery, avoidance of systemic-based opioid techniques where possible, individualised goal-directed fluid therapy and planned early mobilization, are now recommended in all surgical specialities. The use of carbohydrate loading prior to surgery in order to attenuate insulin resistance and negative nitrogen balance has resulted in improved patient comfort and a reduction in hospital stay.[12]

Temperature regulation

Older patients in general are at greater risk of perioperative hypothermia, with potential negative implications such as increased oxygen requirements due to shivering, impaired coagulation and reduced peripheral perfusion resulting in poor wound healing. It is essential, therefore, to monitor patient temperature closely during the perioperative period. Steps should be taken to decrease this risk by simple measures, e.g. provision of additional blankets as well as consideration of pre-warming the patient on the ward using a forced air warming system for at least 30–60 min prior to surgery.

Fluid management

Fluid management is another area that can present multiple challenges in the perioperative period, particularly in older patients undergoing major procedures. During major surgery, where large fluid shifts are likely to occur, additional monitoring may be required. Intra-arterial BP monitoring, central venous pressure monitoring and the use of cardiac output monitoring devices such as the oesophageal Doppler,[13] which allows real-time stroke volume estimations, will help guide fluid management. A urinary catheter allowing hourly urine measurements postoperatively may aid management, with a reduction in urine output triggering a fluid challenge and reassessment.

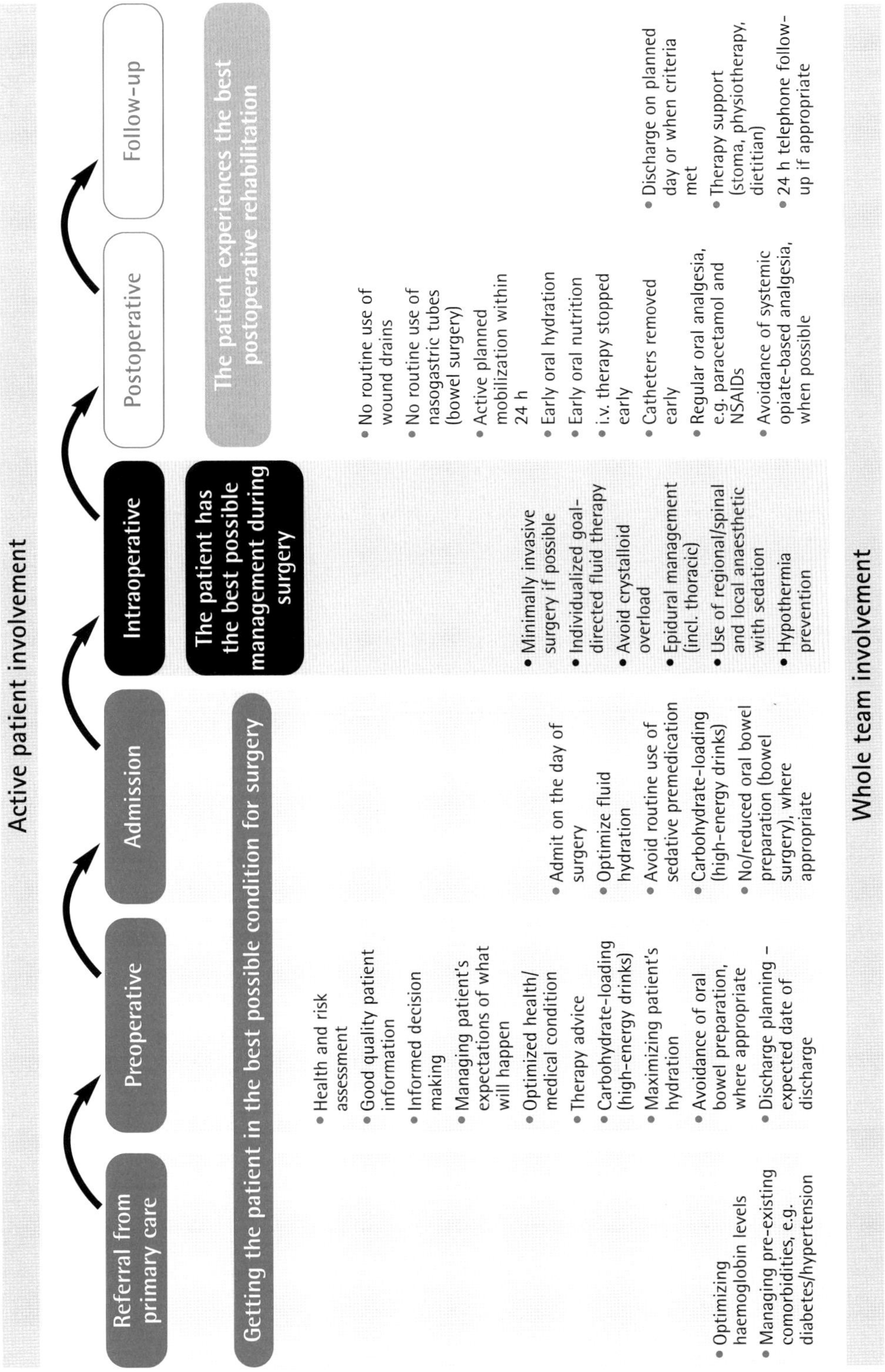

Active patient involvement

| Referral from primary care | Preoperative | Admission | Intraoperative | Postoperative | Follow-up |

Getting the patient in the best possible condition for surgery

The patient has the best possible management during surgery

The patient experiences the best postoperative rehabilitation

- Optimizing haemoglobin levels
- Managing pre-existing comorbidities, e.g. diabetes/hypertension

- Health and risk assessment
- Good quality patient information
- Informed decision making
- Managing patient's expectations of what will happen
- Optimized health/medical condition
- Therapy advice
- Carbohydrate-loading (high-energy drinks)
- Maximizing patient's hydration
- Avoidance of oral bowel preparation, where appropriate
- Discharge planning – expected date of discharge

- Admit on the day of surgery
- Optimize fluid hydration
- Avoid routine use of sedative premedication
- Carbohydrate-loading (high-energy drinks)
- No/reduced oral bowel preparation (bowel surgery), where appropriate

- Minimally invasive surgery if possible
- Individualized goal-directed fluid therapy
- Avoid crystalloid overload
- Epidural management (incl. thoracic)
- Use of regional/spinal and local anaesthetic with sedation
- Hypothermia prevention

- No routine use of wound drains
- No routine use of nasogastric tubes (bowel surgery)
- Active planned mobilization within 24 h
- Early oral hydration
- Early oral nutrition
- i.v. therapy stopped early
- Catheters removed early
- Regular oral analgesia, e.g. paracetamol and NSAIDs
- Avoidance of systemic opiate-based analgesia, when possible

- Discharge on planned day or when criteria met
- Therapy support (stoma, physiotherapy, dietitian)
- 24 h telephone follow-up if appropriate

Whole team involvement

Figure 16.2 The enhanced recovery pathway.[11]

Pain management

Older patients may also be at increased risk of poor pain management due to impaired communication or cognition, stoic attitudes, and the potential for drug interactions and toxicity. As in any postoperative patient, an integrated polymodal approach involving simple analgesia (paracetamol), with enteral or parenteral opioids, and/or opioid-sparing techniques such as regional anaesthesia, wound catheters or antineuropathic agents (e.g. gabapentin, pregabalin) will be of maximum benefit. In some older patients, opioid side effects are almost as distressing as the pain itself, and close attention should be paid to early treatment of constipation, nausea or delirium.

Perioperative cognitive disorders

There is increasing awareness of the potential for postoperative delirium or even cognitive impairment amongst older people undergoing surgery and anaesthesia. As postoperative delirium is associated with increased complications (falls, pneumonia), a prolonged hospital stay and increased mortality, early recognition and management are important. A recent development in this area is the more frequent screening of patients for delirium in the recovery room. Recovery room delirium is a strong predictor of postoperative delirium,[14] and patients screened positive should be targeted for early intervention, e.g. the use of prophylactic low-dose intravenous haloperidol[15] and proactive geriatrics consultation.[16]

Conclusion

Older cancer patients undergoing a surgical procedure present multiple challenges for the anaesthetist. The combination of multiple comorbidities, frailty, polypharmacy, malignancy and surgery necessitates careful preoperative assessment to plan the optimal pre-, peri- and postoperative investigations and interventions to ensure a successful outcome.

References

1 Chelluri L, Pinsky MR, Donahoe MP, Grenvik A. Long-term outcome of critically ill elderly patients requiring intensive care. *JAMA* 1993; 269: 3119–23.

2 Jetté M, Sidney K, Blümchen G. Metabolic equivalents (METs) in exercise testing, exercise prescription, and evaluation of functional capacity. *Clin Cardiol* 1990; 13: 555–65.

3 Reilly DF, McNeely MJ, Doerner D, *et al.* Self-reported exercise tolerance and the risk of serious perioperative complications. *Arch Intern Med* 1999; 159: 2185–92.

4 Snowden CP, Prentis J, Jacques B, *et al.* Cardiorespiratory fitness predicts mortality and hospital length of stay after major elective surgery in older people. *Ann Surg* 2013; 257: 1097–104.

5 Older P, Hall A, Hader R. Cardiopulmonary exercise testing as a screening test for perioperative management of major surgery in the elderly. *Chest* 1999; 116: 355–62.

6 Allan N, Siller C, Breen A. Anaesthetic implications of chemotherapy. *Contin Educ Anaesth Crit Care Pain* 2012; 12: 52–6.

7 British Society of Echocardiography. *Indications for echocardiography.* Available from: www.bsecho.org/indications-for-echocardiography (accessed 1 April 2015).

8 Wilkinson K, Martin IC, Gough MJ, *et al. An age old problem. A review of the care received by elderly patients undergoing surgery.* London: National Confidential Enquiry into Patient Outcomes and Death, 2010.

9 Makary MA, Segev DL, Pronovost PJ, *et al.* Frailty as a predictor of surgical outcomes in older patients. *J Am Coll Surg* 2010; 210: 901–8.

10 West MA, Loughney L, Lythgoe D, *et al.* Effect of prehabilitation on objectively measured physical fitness after neoadjuvant treatment in preoperative rectal cancer patients: a blinded interventional pilot study. *Br J Anaesth* 2015; 114: 244–51.

11 NHS Enhanced Recovery Partnership Programme (2010). *Delivering enhanced recovery. Helping patients to get better sooner after surgery.* Available from: www.nesra.co.uk/files/training/education/Delivering%20enhanced%20recovery.pdf (accessed 5 May 2015).

12 Kratzing C. Pre-operative nutrition and carbohydrate loading. *Proc Nutr Soc* 2011; 70: 311–15.

13 National Institute for Health and Care Excellence. *CardioQ-ODM oesophageal Doppler monitor. NICE medical technologies guidance 3.* London: NICE, 2011.

14 Radtke FM, Franck M, MacGuill M, *et al.* Duration of fluid fasting and choice of analgesic are modifiable factors for early postoperative delirium. *Eur J Anaesthesiol* 2010; 27: 403–5.

15 Wang W, Li HL, Zhu X, *et al.* Haloperidol prophylaxis decreases delirium incidence in elderly patients after noncardiac surgery: a randomized controlled trial. *Crit Care Med* 2012; 40: 731–9.

16 Marcantonio ER, Flacker JM, Wright RJ, Resnick NM. Reducing delirium after hip fracture: a randomized trial. *J Am Geriatr Soc* 2001; 49: 516–22.

Further reading

- White SM, Dhesi JK, Foo ITH, eds. Anaesthesia for the elderly. *Anaesthesia* 2014; 69 (suppl 1): 1–98.

17 Ethics, Consent and Capacity in the Older Cancer Patient

Matthew Appleby, Margot Gosney

Introduction

As advances in the investigation and treatment of cancer progress, there is good evidence indicating a significant disparity in the treatment of older cancer patients.[1,2] National Cancer Intelligence Network data indicate that rates of certain definitive treatments, such as surgery and radiotherapy, are less likely to occur in older patients.[3,4] This chapter aims to outline the ethical dilemmas of 'suitability' and 'appropriateness' in the treatment of older cancer patients. The process of consent, in accordance with the Mental Capacity Act (MCA) 2005,[5] is defined, with clear explanations given of capacity assessment to help guide the treating team when attempting best interest decisions.

Ethics in the older patient

There are four overarching principles in medical ethics: (1) non-maleficence, (2) beneficence, (3) respect for autonomy and (4) justice, but these can often appear to conflict in approaches to older cancer patients.

Non–maleficence

Ageing undeniably affects patient fitness but not necessarily the appropriateness of treatment, and these are too often conflated: 'suitability' and age are not equivalent. All medical treatments may do harm, and some may kill. This is no more evident than in chemoradiation, where the burden of treatment may be too toxic for the ageing physiology. Efforts have been made to support oncological decision making with measures such as the Karnofsky and Eastern Cooperative Oncology Group performance status; however, evidence indicates significant interobserver variability. Therefore, many elderly care physicians have championed the development of Comprehensive Geriatric Assessment (CGA), which encompasses a wider range of domains to assess appropriateness and suitability for treatment:

- Functional status.
- Falls.
- Cognitive status.
- Depression.
- Nutrition.
- Comorbidity.

For full information on the use of CGA in cancer care please see the International Society of Geriatric Oncology practice guideline.[6]

Beneficence

In the current paradigm of NHS cancer services, weighing the possible benefits against the known risks of treatment rests with the multidisciplinary team (MDT). When the risks are almost certain, and the benefits are unlikely, the balance is easily weighed against treatment. But too often in the older cancer patient beneficence may be considered simply as removing the 'risk of harm' caused by actual treatment. The morality of palliating pain and suffering is undermined if appropriate investigations and treatment are withheld by virtue of age. Prolonging a poor quality of life is unlikely to benefit the patient, but rarely is this distinction made in younger patients, where radical treatments are frequently justified. By providing informed consent, and respecting autonomy, it is the older cancer patient who can ultimately assign his or her own weight to the risks and benefits of treatment.

Respect for autonomy

In the UK, a capacitous patient always has the right to refuse treatment, but there is no such right to demand it. Therefore, autonomy is constrained by the choices and recommendations offered by the oncology MDT. Quality of life from the perspective of the MDT may presuppose the patient's best interests despite full capacity. To not offer a patient surgery for breast cancer with bone metastases would seem appropriate *prima facie*, but not even to offer the patient the option of chemotherapy requires clear evidence of futility, absent benefit or clear harm. The value of patient autonomy has been indicated by Appleby and Gosney,[7] who, by comparing the same oncology MDT decisions, showed that 26% of cognitively impaired patients did not have their malignancy confirmed by histopathology, as opposed to only 5% in the unimpaired group. Basic palliation was given to 64% of the cognitively impaired patients as opposed to only 23% of the unimpaired group.

Justice

Treating patients with equity, irrespective of age, is contingent on societal values. The 'fair innings' argument is repeatedly put forward as a justification for denying treatment to older people that would be deemed appropriate for younger patients. The NHS constitution pledges a 'comprehensive service to all, irrespective of age', and, in the UK, the statutory right to receive equal medical treatment is established in the Equality Act 2010.[8] For the ageing process to be embraced rather than feared, the law has made provision for concern about discriminatory behaviour towards older patients to be redressed.

Consent

Integral to the notions of ethical treatment are the fundamentals of capacity and consent. In the UK, the General Medical Council[9] gives clear guidance on consent and the importance of person-centred treatments made *with* the patient, rather than *for* the patient. There are many different types of consent depending on the procedure being performed, but what follows is the framework within which all consent is based.

For consent to be valid, three core requirements must be satisfied (Figure 17.1).

Non-coercion

Consent must be given voluntarily and without fear or pressure. Older cancer patients may feel intimidated by the clinical environment and with decisions being made at the clinician's pace, rather than their own. For consent to be valid, medical decisions must be made with a patient who feels he or she has the right to agree or decline treatment without suffering displeasure not limited just to the clinician but also to the family, friends and carers. Older patients may be vulnerable to the expectations of those assumed to be in supporting roles, and the clinician has a duty to ensure decisions are the patient's own. The doctor may recommend a particular treatment but should not put pressure on the patient to accept that advice.

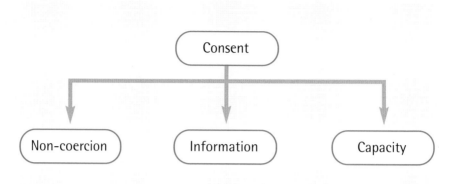

Figure 17.1 The three core requirements of consent.

Information

Although physicians have specialist knowledge, they are expected to be able to explain the consequences of agreeing to or refusing treatment in terminology that allows the patient to make an informed decision. This does not necessitate describing every possible risk and variable, but the expectation is that an appropriate scope of outcomes is concisely explained in simple terminology. Cancer therapies are daunting and often have a great array of side effects that need to be explored. This is best done with the support of cancer nurse specialists who can revisit information after initial consultations. Appropriate adjustments should be made, including catering for the visually impaired and hard of hearing at consultations, without requiring consultants to shout details or asking next of kin to 'explain it later'.

Capacity

Mental capacity is the ability individuals have to make decisions for themselves. In the UK, assessment of mental capacity is outlined in the MCA,[5] which is underpinned by five key principles:

Presume capacity

Every adult has the right to make his or her own decisions. Unlike consent, a capacity assessment does not need to be sought at each interaction: capacity should be assumed unless there is good reason to believe it is impaired. No one else can make a decision on behalf of an adult who has capacity.

Supported decision making

Patients should be given all appropriate help before it is concluded that they lack capacity. As with giving information for consent, treatments can be explained in a number of ways to assist those with hearing or visual impairment. It is easy to suppose that a patient lacks capacity just because they cannot hear questions during busy ward rounds: attempts should always be made to present decisions and information in an environment that supports the patient.

Unwise decisions

Individuals have the right to make what appear to be strange or unwise decisions. Values and beliefs differ and may stray far from what the medical team think is appropriate. However, patients have the right to make treatment decisions based on their own perspectives and do not need to justify them, but they may be asked to explain their reasoning.

Best interests

A patient who lacks capacity should be treated in his or her best interests. To work out what is in the person's best interests, the decision maker must:

- Not assume best interests based on merely the person's age, appearance or condition.
- Consider whether the decision can be postponed until a time when the patient might have regained capacity.
- Involve the person who lacks mental capacity in the decision as much as possible.
- Decisions should be based on the patient's past and present beliefs and values and on any previous expression of his or her views, verbal or written, when capacity was present. The MCA[5] has recommended the use of the 'advanced statement' and 'advanced decision to refuse treatment', to help doctors with decision making in the event of a person becoming incapacitated.
- Consider the views of others, such as family, friends and carers who knew the patient best and can help when outlining the patient's wishes when capacity was present.
- Not be motivated by a wish to bring about the person's death.

Confidentiality should not be breached simply because a patient lacks capacity. A patient lacking capacity has equal right to confidentiality: breaching confidentiality, with, say, next of kin, should only be done if the clinician believes it is in an attempt to ascertain the patient's best interests.

Least restrictive intervention

Anything done for or on behalf of a person without capacity should be the least restrictive of that person's rights and freedoms. Distressed or delirious patients may be unable to understand treatment that has been initiated in their best interests, such as blood tests or medications. However, every attempt should be made to use interventions that use minimal force, and these should always be for the benefit of the patient rather than for that of the treating staff. Restraint and the use of force are only permitted if the person using them reasonably believes it is necessary to prevent further harm to the incapacitated patient. If restraint is used it must be proportionate to the likelihood and seriousness of the harm posed. All practitioners should be able to defend any decision to use restraint or treat a patient against his or her will. Best practice is for best interest decisions to be made collectively as part of a treating team.

Capacity assessment

The MCA[5] establishes the legal basis for assessing whether a person lacks the capacity to make a particular decision at a particular time: this is known as 'decision-specific' capacity. No person may be labelled unable or incapable of making decisions as a result of a medical condition, as decisions range vastly in their complexity and the capacity required to make them.

To test whether the person has capacity, first ask whether he or she has an impairment of the mind or brain, or a disturbance of mental function. If this is the case, ask whether that impairment or disturbance means that the person is unable to make the decision in question at the time it needs to be made. If these two conditions are satisfied then a capacity assessment should be performed (Figure 17.2). For a patient to have capacity he or she must be able to complete all of the following requirements:

- Understand the information relevant to the decision being presented.
- Retain the information.

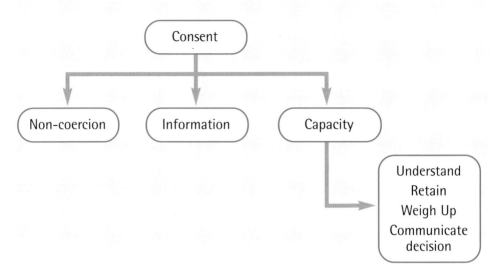

Figure 17.2 Capacity as part of the consent process.

• Weigh up that information as part of the process of making the decision.

• Reach a decision and communicate it by any means.

If it is believed that a patient is incapacitated by virtue of being unable to perform one or more of these requirements, then this must be documented and explained clearly. For example, if the clinician believes the person is refusing treatment due to lack of understanding of the risks, the clinician should ask him or her to explain the risks back. If the patient is too distressed to react to questions being asked, attempts should be made to alleviate pain or agitation so that the decision may be considered when the patient is better able to process the information.

Conclusion

 The literature has indicated a significant difference in the investigation and treatment of older cancer patients. Too often older patients may be presumed incapacitous, or treated in their best interests, without any documented assessment of their physical or mental health. Consequently, suitability and appropriateness may be based on a brief clinical history in the MDT, which may be overly influenced by the mention of age or dementia, or a suspicion thereof. Such decisions challenge notions of equality, autonomy and justice as outlined in this chapter.

Cancer specialists are justifiably cautious not to cause further distress and suffering as a consequence of their treatments, and this should not be underestimated in patients lacking capacity. Best interest decisions may often favour procedures that are not curative, but are very likely less painful and distressing. However, the assumption that older cancer patients would be unable to participate in decisions about their treatment is unacceptable, as is the suggestion that these patients are *prima facie* inappropriate for intensive treatment of malignancy. Therefore, it is argued that a more comprehensive assessment of physical and mental health be performed by the MDT before discussion of appropriateness, to present a more justifiable and clearly documented treatment decision.

References

1 Moller H, Flatt G, Moran A. High cancer death rates in the elderly in the UK. *Cancer Epidemiol* 2011; 35: 407–12.

2 Turner N, Haward R, Mulley G, Selby P. Cancer in old age – is it inadequately investigated and treated? *BMJ* 1999; 319: 309–12.

3 National Cancer Intelligence Network (2010). *Breast cancer in the elderly – NCIN data briefing.* Available from: www.ncin.org.uk/publications/data_briefings/breast_cancer_elderly (accessed 21 February 2015).

4 Department of Health. *Reducing cancer inequality: evidence, progress and making it happen: a report by the National Cancer Equality Initiative.* London: HMSO, 2010.

5 Department of Health. *Mental Capacity Act 2005.* London: HMSO, 2005. Available from: www.legislation.gov.uk/ukpga/2005/9/pdfs/ukpga_20050009_en.pdf (accessed 26 February 2015).

6 International Society of Geriatric Oncology (2011). *Practice guideline. Comprehensive Geriatric Assessment (CGA) in oncological patients.* Available from: www.siog.org/images/SIOG_documents/cga_practice_guideline_wildiers_jul2011.pdf (accessed 26 February 2015).

7 Appleby M, Gosney M. Differences in the investigation and treatment of elderly patients with cancer when cognitive impairment is present. *J Geriatr Oncol* 2014; 5 (suppl 2): S39–40.

8 Equality and Human Rights Commission. *Equality Act 2010.* London: HMSO, 2010. Available from: www.gov.uk/government/publications/equality-act-guidance (accessed 27 February 2015).

9 General Medical Council. *Consent: patients and doctors making decisions together.* London: GMC, 2008. Available from: www.gmc-uk.org/guidance/ethical_guidance/consent_guidance_index.asp (accessed 21 February 2015).

18 Palliative Care in Older Cancer Patients

Lucy Adkinson, Michael I. Bennett

Introduction

Palliative care aims to relieve the suffering of patients with life-limiting illnesses, and that of their carers, and is applicable at all stages of disease, not simply limited to end-of-life care. It incorporates thorough symptom assessment and management, as well as psychosocial and spiritual support, and aims to establish the goals of care for patients and plan for their future. The purpose of this chapter is to review the issues specific to the older cancer patient in palliative care. It discusses where special care is needed; it is therefore not a comprehensive overview of general palliative care, symptom control and advance care planning.

In the older population with cancer there are additional challenges to symptom control. As well as their primary cancer diagnosis, patients are more likely to have multiple comorbidities, and these conditions, such as heart failure and chronic obstructive pulmonary disease (COPD), present their own symptom challenges and are life-limiting conditions in their own right. In a study of 226 people aged over 60 with advanced COPD, heart failure or cancer, it was found that symptom prevalence such as pain (27%), fatigue (47%) and depression (11%) was the same across all three conditions.[1] Furthermore, older people are less likely to die in their usual place of care or hospice and more likely to die in hospital,[2] meaning that hospital physicians need to be able to provide palliative care and refer to specialist services when needed. Finally, older patients are more likely to have older spouses as carers who have their own health issues, or have no informal carers because they live alone. These factors all contribute to the complexity of the palliative management of older patients with cancer.

Symptom assessment in the older cancer patient

In the older patient with cancer the spectrum of symptoms is different from that of their younger counterparts. Frailty is much more common, and this can lead to restricted mobility, urinary incontinence, falls and delirium. However, common malignant symptoms such as pain are just as prevalent in this population and will be discussed in more detail.

Additional difficulties in assessing this population arise from the increased likelihood of significant sensory or cognitive impairment, and this must be incorporated into the selection and prescription of any medications. This poses a challenge to assessment and may therefore require more frequent reassessment or use of pain and symptom assessment tools to monitor symptom management, as recall of symptoms and assessment of benefit of interventions may be poor.[3] If the patient has significant cognitive impairment, subjective symptom assessment may be impossible and objective assessment such as observing changes in behaviour and body language will be required.

Pain management

There is discrepancy in the management of symptoms between the older and younger population. Pain is often overlooked and under-assessed in the older population, especially if the patient has cognitive impairment.[3] However, the intensity and frequency of cancer pain is the same for cancer patients of all ages.[4] Thus, concerns exist that older patients experience less effective pain control compared with their younger counterparts.

There are several reasons for this discrepancy, both on the part of the patient and of the health professional. Evidence suggests that older people may report pain less, potentially because they believe the myth that it is a 'natural' part of the ageing or cancer process and that it cannot be alleviated. They may also have concerns about opioid medications and fears of addiction. There may also be an increased stoicism and reluctance to discuss pain. Sensory and cognitive impairment can also lead to difficult communication and assessment.[3,5]

A review of opioid prescription practice for cancer patients in the UK found that as patients got older they were less likely to receive opioids,[6] despite evidence that pain intensity is similar to that in younger patients.[4] If they did receive opioid prescriptions then they were for smaller doses and prescribed when the patient was closer to death. When opioids are titrated carefully there are similar rates of side effects, dose escalation and opioid switching[7,8] between younger and older patients. Not managing pain can have significant consequences for the patient and health service. Poor pain control can lead to low mood, social isolation and increased hospitalization and resource use.[9]

Prescription of medications relevant to palliative care: things to consider

The management of symptoms and provision of palliative care is overall the same for older patients as for younger patients. There are more comprehensive texts available on symptom management; here, however, we detail prescription issues specific to the older cancer patient.

Compliance and concordance

Misunderstanding medicines is common in older patients; therefore, written or verbal information can help concordance. This should be supplemented by addressing any concerns regarding side effects or by seeking a review. If sensory or cognitive impairment is an issue, the use of additional supportive measures is needed, such as providing medication prompts, using dosette medication boxes and involving carers in administering medicines. A thorough medication review and stopping any unnecessary medications are also helpful.

Opioids

Changes in drug metabolism occur with ageing, such as decreased volume of distribution of drugs, because of lower body fat, and increased renal and hepatic impairment, leading to reduced drug excretion and metabolism. These changes impact on older patients' response to common palliative care drugs. Oral morphine is still the first choice of opioid in the older patient, unless there is renal failure. NICE guidance on initiating and titrating strong opioids should be followed.[10]

Opioids in renal failure

Morphine and its active and toxic metabolites are renally excreted and accumulate in renal failure leading to significant toxicity. In moderate renal impairment (glomerular filtration rate 30–59 ml/min/1.73 m^2), oxycodone should be considered. This is a strong opioid with a potency ratio of 1.5:1 compared with oral morphine. Therefore, 10 mg oxycodone is equivalent to 15 mg morphine. It is predominantly metabolized in the liver but still has reduced clearance in renal failure, so caution is needed with reduced doses and longer dosing intervals.

In severe renal failure the 'safe' opioids are alfentanil, fentanyl and buprenorphine. Alfentanil is injectable-only and appropriate in a continuous subcutaneous infusion but not as breakthrough analgesia, as its half-life is brief and it has a short duration of action. It is 20–30 times more potent than oral morphine, and specialist advice on its prescription should be sought.

Transdermal opioid patches

The opioid patches available are fentanyl and buprenorphine. These have the advantage over oral opioids of being safe in renal failure, aiding compliance and concordance, as they are changed every 3 or 7 days, and being helpful in patients with no oral route for medication, for example dysphagia caused by head and neck cancer. However, there are also significant cautions with their use. An appreciation of the strength of opioid patches is required: a 12 µg/h fentanyl patch is roughly equivalent to 30–45 mg oral morphine; it is therefore inappropriate to prescribe it in an opioid-naive older patient. It can take 12–24 h to reach a steady state of drug after first application, meaning that the patient's 'as required' medication will be needed during this time. Dose titration with patches is difficult and potentially unsafe; therefore, the use of patches should be restricted to patients with stable pain on stable opioid doses.

Neuropathic agents

In cancer-related neuropathic pain, adjuncts to opioids, such as amitriptyline, pregabalin or gabapentin, can be effective in older patients. Starting doses should be lower and titration slower: 100 mg for gabapentin (rather than 300 mg) and 25 mg for pregabalin (rather than 75 mg). These also accumulate in renal impairment, causing dizziness and drowsiness, which can be particularly disabling for older patients.

Amitriptyline can be an effective adjuvant analgesic when used in low doses such as 10–20 mg at night. However, antimuscarinic and antihistaminergic side effects mean it should be used with caution in those with urinary hesitancy, narrow-angle glaucoma and cardiac disease. These side effects can also lead to postural hypotension and drowsiness, which leads to an increased risk of falls and hip fractures.[11]

Antiemetics

The common antiemetics used in palliative care all have cautions with use in the older population. Metoclopramide, haloperidol and levomepromazine are all dopamine antagonists. This prohibits their use in those with Parkinson's disease or parkinsonism. The risk of associated extrapyramidal side effects is more pronounced in older people and those with dementia. Therefore, use the smallest possible dose for the shortest duration possible (for example 1.5 mg haloperidol once or twice daily). Domperidone is a dopamine antagonist that does not cross the blood–brain barrier and so is safer in this respect. It is, however, associated with QT prolongation.

If dopamine antagonists are contraindicated or ineffective, cyclizine can be used in a dose of 25 mg three times daily. It shares similar side effects and risks to those of amitriptyline.

Conclusion

Older cancer patients experience a similar range and intensity of symptoms to those of younger cancer patients, but their care is complicated by increased frailty. Despite this, older patients are less likely to be referred to palliative care services. More skilful assessment and prescribing are therefore needed to ensure their needs are met alongside oncological management.

References

1 Walke L, Gallo W, Tinetti M, *et al.* The burden of symptoms among community-dwelling older persons with advanced chronic disease. *Arch Intern Med* 2004; 164: 2321–4.

2 Public Health England (2013). *What we know now 2013. New information collated by the National End of Life Intelligence Network.* Available from: www.endoflifecare-intelligence.org.uk/resources/publications/what_we_know_now_2013 (accessed 9 June 2015).

3 Hadjistavropoulos T, Herr K, Turk D, *et al.* An interdisciplinary expert consensus statement on assessment of pain in older persons. *Clin J Pain* 2007; 23 (1 suppl): S1–43.

4 Bennett MI, Closs SJ, Chatwin J. Cancer pain management at home (I): do older patients experience less effective management than younger patients? *Support Care Cancer* 2009; 17: 787–92.

5 Closs SJ, Chatwin J, Bennett MI. Cancer pain management at home (II): does age influence attitudes towards pain and analgesia? *Support Care Cancer* 2009; 17: 781–6.

6 Higginson IJ, Gao W. Opioid prescribing for cancer pain during the last 3 months of life: associated factors and 9-year trends in a nationwide United Kingdom cohort study. *J Clin Oncol* 2012; 30: 4373–9.

7 Loick G, Radbruch L, Sabatowski R, *et al.* Morphine dose and side effects: a comparison of older and younger patients with tumor pain [article in German]. *Dtsch Med Wochenschr* 2000; 125: 1216–21.

8 Mercadante S, Ferrera P, Villari P, Casuccio A. Opioid escalation in patients with cancer pain: the effect of age. *J Pain Symptom Manage* 2006; 32: 413–19.

9 Mercadante S, Arcuri E. Pharmacological management of cancer pain in the elderly. *Drugs Aging* 2007; 24: 761–76.

10 Bennett MI, Graham J, Schmidt-Hansen M, *et al.* Prescribing strong opioids for pain in adult palliative care: summary of NICE guidance. *BMJ* 2012; 344: e2806.

11 Ruxton K, Woodman R, Mangoni A. Drugs with anticholinergic effects and cognitive impairment, falls and all-cause mortality in older adults: a systematic review and meta-analysis. *Br J Clin Pharmacol* doi: 10.1111/bcp.12617.

01 A Patient with Lung Cancer, Chronic Obstructive Pulmonary Disease, Hypertension and Dizziness

Aspasia Soultati, Sasi Pathmanathan, Matt Sweeting, Ana Montes

Case history

A 71-year-old man presented with increasing shortness of breath, productive cough, lethargy, weight loss and haemoptysis. CT was suggestive of stage IV lung cancer (T4N3M1a), and bronchial biopsies confirmed squamous cell carcinoma. Past medical history included peripheral vascular disease, hypertension and chronic obstructive pulmonary disease (COPD). His medications included: salbutamol inhaler (as required), simvastatin, clopidogrel, bisoprolol, amlodipine and ramipril. He had been a lifelong smoker (60 pack-year history) and drank 24 units alcohol/week. He lived with his son in a first floor flat and mobilized independently with a stick.

A Barthel Index of activities of daily living (ADL) was used to assess his functional ability and revealed he needed assistance with bathing and using stairs. He also reported intermittent dizziness on standing and two falls (one associated with syncope) in the last 6 months. His lying BP was 130/90 mmHg, with a BP of 105/65 mmHg at 1 min, which improved to 120/75 mmHg at 3 min. His ECG showed sinus rhythm with a rate of 70 bpm and no ischaemic change. He was urgently referred to a falls clinic.

In view of metastatic non-small-cell lung carcinoma (NSCLC) he was offered palliative chemotherapy and opted for treatment to preserve his quality of life. Because of his respiratory and vascular comorbidities he received carboplatin AUC 5 and gemcitabine 1000 mg/m² with prophylactic antibiotics. He experienced severe nausea and required a dose reduction. He completed four cycles with no further complications and achieved partial response. Nine months later he progressed locally and proceeded to second-line chemotherapy with docetaxel 60 mg/m², with partial response. He progressed 4 months later with liver metastases and at this point his performance status (PS) had deteriorated significantly and he was offered best supportive care (BSC) by his community palliative team. He died at home approximately 18 months after the initial diagnosis.

What is the goal of cancer treatment for this patient?

What is the evidence base for treatment options in metastatic NSCLC?

What is the evidence base for treatment options in this patient?

How should this patient be optimized prior to starting cancer treatment?

What is the goal of cancer treatment for this patient?

The treatment aim in metastatic NSCLC is to control symptoms, preserve functional status and prolong survival. The patient wanted to stay at home with his son and was willing to accept additional support. With appropriate tailored chemotherapy he achieved 18 months' survival with a good quality of life.

What is the evidence base for treatment options in metastatic NSCLC?

Treatment decisions should be directed by a multidisciplinary cancer team and will depend on histology, molecular pathology, age, PS, comorbidities and patient preference. Four cycles of platinum-based doublet chemotherapy are recommended for patients with PS 0–2. In the presence of *EGFR* mutation, tyrosine kinase inhibitors (TKIs) should be offered as first-line agents in patients with PS 0–3. Second-line agents include taxanes and erlotinib. Enrolment into clinical trials should be considered. Patients with *ALK* rearrangement should be offered crizotinib. In patients unfit for systemic therapy, BSC should be offered.[1]

What is the evidence base for treatment options in this patient?

NSCLC is a disease of older adults (median age at diagnosis 69 years; 47% diagnosed ≥70 years). As the population ages, an increasing number of patients with lung cancer are referred for treatment. Appropriate treatment depends on a comprehensive assessment to determine the patient's likelihood of dying from cancer rather than from other comorbidities, and also potential toxicity based on physiological function. Older patients can be categorized into those who are fit and will benefit from standard regimens, those who are vulnerable and need adjusted regimens, and those who are frail and should be offered BSC. This patient falls into the vulnerable category; therefore, carboplatin was used to avoid fluid overload and protect the kidneys, and doses were reduced and prophylactic antibiotics given in view of his COPD, as there is evidence that this decreases infection and mortality.

Randomized trials assessing first-line chemotherapy for older patients with metastatic NSCLC are limited (Table 1.1).[2–9] The Elderly Lung Cancer Vinorelbine Italian Study (ELVIS)[2] established survival (21 vs 28 weeks; $p=0.03$) and symptomatic benefit with vinorelbine compared with BSC in patients with PS 0–2, but stopped early due to a low enrolment rate. Several trials have compared platinum doublets versus monotherapy. Quoix *et al.*[7] demonstrated that carboplatin combined with paclitaxel was superior to single-agent gemcitabine or vinorelbine (overall survival [OS] 10.3 vs 6.2 months; $p<0.0001$) despite higher toxicity rates. Yet, in a recent trial,[8] docetaxel combined with weekly cisplatin was inferior to docetaxel alone. In a series of age-based analyses of prospective trials, the feasibility and superiority of the doublets was established among the older subpopulation.

A comprehensive meta-analysis comparing doublets with single third-generation agents included 2510 older patients across 10 trials and demonstrated the superiority of platinum-based doublets in terms of 1 year survival ($p=0.009$) and responses ($p=0.000$), with worse haematological and neurotoxicity.[9] To decrease toxicity, several trials have proposed non-platinum doublets versus monotherapy but have shown inconsistent results.

The TKIs gefitinib, erlotinib and afatinib are recommended in older patients either as first line in the presence of *EGFR* mutation or as second line in non-mutated patients (erlotinib), based on subgroup analysis of phase III trials. Older patients experience significantly more grade ≥3 toxicity with TKIs (35% vs 19%; $p<0.001$), including rash, fatigue and dehydration.

For vulnerable patients, either a single third-generation agent (gemcitabine, vinorelbine,

Table 1.1 Randomized trials assessing first-line chemotherapy in older patients with NSCLC.

Trial	N	Age (years)	Chemotherapy	RR	PFS	OS	p-value
Monotherapy							
ELVIS[2]	161	>70	Vinorelbine vs BSC	19.7 vs 0	NR	6.9 vs 4.9	0.03
Kudoh et al.[3]	182	>70	Vinorelbine vs docetaxel	9.9 vs 22.7	3.1 vs 5.5	9.9 vs 14.3	0.138
Non-platinum doublets							
MILES[4]	698	>70	Vinorelbine vs gemcitabine vs vinorelbine + gemcitabine	18 vs 16 vs 21	4.2 vs 4.4 vs 4.4	8.4 vs 6.9 vs 7.0	0.93 0.65
SICOG[5]	120	>70	Vinorelbine vs gemcitabine + vinorelbine	15 vs 22	NR	4.2 vs 6.8	
Comella et al.[6]	264 (220)[a]	>70	Gemcitabine vs paclitaxel vs gemcitabine + vinorelbine vs gemcitabine + paclitaxel	18 vs 13 vs 23 vs 32	3.3 vs 3.7 vs 4.1 vs 4.5	5.1 vs 6.4 vs 9.7 vs 9.2	0.028
Platinum doublets							
Quoix et al.[7]	451	>70	Gemcitabine or vinorelbine vs carboplatin + paclitaxel	10.2 vs 27.1	2.8 vs 6.0	6.2 vs 10.3	<0.0001
Abe et al.[8]	276	>70	Docetaxel vs docetaxel + cisplatin	24.6 vs 34.4	4.4 vs 4.7	14.8 vs 13.3	NR
Meta-analysis							
Qi et al.[9]	2510 (10 trials)	>70	Doublet vs single third-generation agent	1.54 95% CI 1.36–1.73 p=0.000	TTP HR 0.76 95% CI 0.60–0.96 p=0.022	HR 0.84 95% CI 0.71–1.00 p=0.053	0.053

[a]220 patients were >70 years old.
NR, not reported; PFS, progression-free survival; TTP, time to progression.

taxane) or a weekly platinum doublet has been suggested despite the absence of evidence from phase III trials.

As the trials indicate that chemotherapy can improve survival when given to fit, older patients, standard platinum doublet chemotherapy should be discussed in patients with PS 0–1. Single-agent chemotherapy may be offered to vulnerable patients (Figure 1.1).[10-14] It is important to recognize physiological changes associated with ageing in order to address toxicity-related issues early (Table 1.2). Early palliative care intervention is encouraged along with standard oncology care in all patients, as shown in a randomized trial.[15]

How should this patient be optimized prior to starting cancer treatment?

Falls and syncope

Falls associated with syncope should be thoroughly investigated to determine whether syncope is neural, orthostatic or cardiac in origin. All patients should have baseline ECG and postural BPs. If the diagnosis is uncertain, further investigations include 24 h ambulatory ECG for arrhythmias, tilt table testing encompassing carotid sinus massage (for carotid sinus and baroreceptor hypersensitivity), or an electroencephalogram.

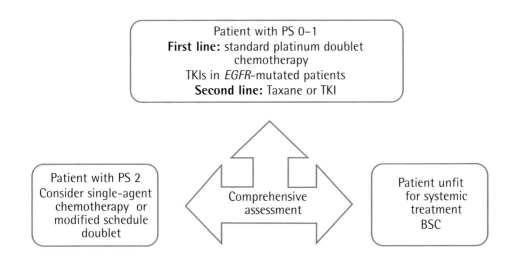

Figure 1.1 Recommendations for treatment in older patients with metastatic lung cancer.

Our patient was assessed in the falls clinic and found to have classical orthostatic hypotension (OH) with a systolic BP drop >20 mmHg.[16] His normal ECG ruled out a cardiac cause. His OH was most likely drug-induced and his amlodipine and ramipril were stopped with good effect. He was advised to drink plenty of fluids. If these measures had not been successful, cessation of his beta-blocker, full-leg compression stockings, and pharmacological interventions with fludrocortisone or midodrine would be the next steps.

In view of the Barthel screening showing difficulty with ADL, an occupational therapist performed a home visit. Grab rails for the bath and handrails for the stairs (leading to the flat) were fitted, and decluttering of the property and removal of loose rugs to reduce the risk of falls were advised.

Although treatment of hypertension improves cardiovascular and cerebrovascular outcomes, it must be weighed against the side effects of medications and the life-limiting nature of the patient's cancer. Preventing further falls was the most important factor in this patient.

COPD, smoking and shortness of breath
Lung function tests 1 year previously were consistent with moderate COPD (Global Initiative for Chronic Obstructive Lung Disease, stage II [GOLD-2]), with an FEV_1 at 65% of predicted. His MRC dyspnoea scale was grade 4, having a significant impact on his walking ability.

A tiotropium inhaler (long-acting muscarinic antagonist) was added to salbutamol, as he was undertreated according to NICE guidelines[17] (Figure 1.2). Tiotropium improves quality of life and reduces the number of chest infections. On assessment, the patient's inhaler technique was poor and was corrected. He was referred to the integrated respiratory team for follow-up.

Smoking cessation advice was given and nicotine replacement therapy offered, but he refused. There is no robust evidence to support smoking cessation in metastatic NSCLC. However, smoking after diagnosis of cancer increases the risk of a second primary tumour, cancer recurrence and treatment complications.[18]

Table 1.2 Physiological changes associated with ageing and how they should be addressed.

Reduced glomerular filtration rate	• Ensure hydration • Caution with diuretics • Avoid nephrotoxic drugs • Choose carboplatin over cisplatin and base dose on EDTA • Monitor renal function with nephrotoxic agents (platinum, pemetrexed)
Impaired fluid/electrolyte haemostasis	• Risk of fluid overload • Monitor prehydration • Monitor electrolytes in gastrointestinal toxicity
Impaired gastrointestinal function	• Supply mouthwashes • Caution with TKI-related diarrhoea • Constipation: consider early introduction of laxatives • Caution with antiemetics
Decrease in the activity of the cytochrome P450 system	• TKIs/taxanes may present increased toxicity • Ensure no drug interaction
Polypharmacy	• Review indication for medications
Warfarin	• Change to low-molecular-weight heparin
Coexisting peripheral neuropathy	• Monitor carefully with neurotoxic chemotherapy (taxanes, vinca alkaloids, platinum) and apply dose reduction if needed
Decreased cellularity in bone marrow	• Consider prophylactic growth colony-stimulating factor • Mid-cycle nadir blood counts • Anaemia should be treated aggressively • Folic acid and vitamin B_{12} should be administered with pemetrexed • Prophylactic antibiotics
Use of indwelling catheter	• Remove if possible (if needed discuss with urology or continence adviser) • Consider prophylactic antibiotics
Impaired memory	• Consider written instructions and contact numbers

Other considerations

Renal function. This is likely to be affected by chemotherapy. Nausea and vomiting may lead to dehydration and acute kidney injury. Discontinuation of ACE inhibitors (in this case, ramipril) should be considered during chemotherapy to reduce the risk of acute kidney injury. Dehydration will worsen OH.

B vitamins. This patient drinks more alcohol than the recommended limit, which can also increase OH. He is at risk of vitamin deficiencies (B_{12}, thiamine and folate), which can lead to neurological complications. Levels should be measured and corrected. He should be advised to reduce his alcohol intake. Certain chemotherapy agents can cause peripheral neuropathies and worsen symptoms.

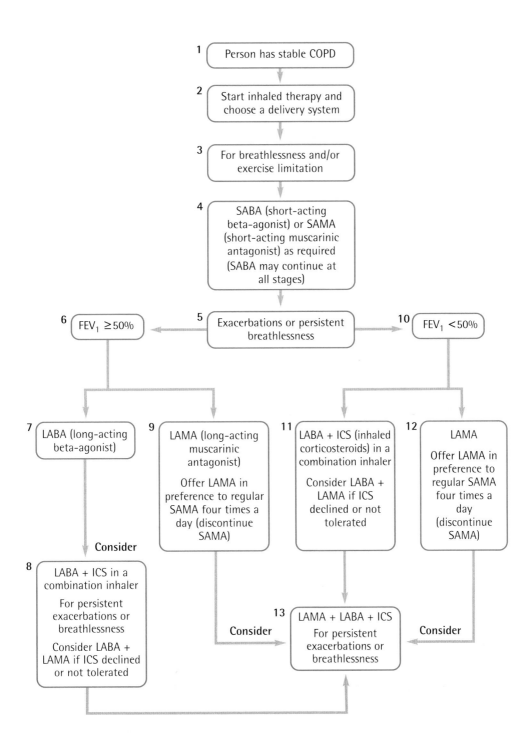

Figure 1.2 NICE pathway for inhaled therapy in COPD.[19]

Conclusion and learning points

- Older patients with metastatic lung cancer should not be excluded from palliative systemic therapy options on the basis of age alone.
- Treatment decisions should be based on a comprehensive assessment.
- Extra care should be applied to toxicity monitoring, and treatment modifications may be required.
- Falls associated with syncope must be investigated and managed in a multidisciplinary falls clinic.
- ECG and lying and standing BP can be measured in oncology clinics, and if OH is present with an unremarkable ECG first-line treatment of stopping antihypertensives and increasing fluid intake may be instituted.
- Symptomatic COPD can be optimized with additional inhalers and checking inhaler technique.

References

1 Reck M, Popat S, Reinmuth N, *et al.*; ESMO Guidelines Working Group. Metastatic non-small-cell lung cancer (NSCLC): ESMO clinical practice guidelines for diagnosis, treatment and follow-up. *Ann Oncol* 2014; 25 (suppl 3): iii27–39.

2 Gridelli C. The ELVIS trial: a phase III study of single-agent vinorelbine as first-line treatment in elderly patients with advanced non-small-cell lung cancer. Elderly Lung Cancer Vinorelbine Italian Study. *Oncologist* 2001; 6: 4–7.

3 Kudoh S, Takeda K, Nakagawa K, *et al.* Phase III study of docetaxel compared with vinorelbine in elderly patients with advanced non-small-cell lung cancer: results of the West Japan Thoracic Oncology Group Trial (WJTOG 9904). *J Clin Oncol* 2006; 24: 3657–63.

4 Gridelli C, Perrone F, Gallo C, *et al.* Chemotherapy for elderly patients with advanced non-small-cell lung cancer: the Multicenter Italian Lung Cancer in the Elderly Study (MILES). *J Natl Cancer Inst* 2003; 95: 362–72.

5 Frasci G, Lorusso V, Panza N, *et al.* Gemcitabine plus vinorelbine yields better survival outcome than vinorelbine alone in elderly patients with advanced non small cell lung cancer. A Southern Italy Cooperative Oncology Group (SICOG) phase III trial. *Lung Cancer* 2001; 34 (suppl 4): S65–9.

6 Comella P, Frasci G, Carnicelli P, *et al.* Gemcitabine with either paclitaxel or vinorelbine vs paclitaxel or gemcitabine alone for elderly or unfit advanced non-small-cell lung cancer patients. *Br J Cancer* 2004; 91: 489–97.

7 Quoix E, Zalcman G, Oster J-P. Carboplatin and weekly paclitaxel doublet chemotherapy compared with monotherapy in elderly patients with advanced non-small-cell lung cancer: IFCT-0501 randomized, phase 3 trial. *Lancet* 2011; 378: 1079–88.

8 Abe T, Takeda K, Ohe Y, *et al.* Randomized phase III trial comparing weekly docetaxel plus cisplatin versus docetaxel monotherapy every 3 weeks in elderly patients with advanced non-small-cell lung cancer: the intergroup trial JCOG0803/WJOG4307L. *J Clin Oncol* 2015; 33: 575–81.

9 Qi W-X, Tang L-N, He A-N. Doublet versus single cytotoxic agent as first-line treatment for elderly patients with advanced non-small-cell lung cancer: a systematic review and meta-analysis. *Lung* 2012; 190: 477–85.

10 Blanco R, Maestu I, de la Torre MG, *et al.* A review of the management of elderly patients with non-small-cell lung cancer. *Ann Oncol* 2014; 26: 1–13.

11 Pallis AG, Gridelli C, van Meerbeeck JP, *et al.* EORTC Elderly Task Force and Lung Cancer Group and International Society for Geriatric Oncology (SIOG) experts' opinion for the treatment of non-small-cell lung cancer in an elderly population. *Ann Oncol* 2010; 21: 692–706.

12 Wedding U, Ködding D, Pientka L, *et al.* Physicians' judgement and comprehensive geriatric assessment (CGA) select different patients as fit for chemotherapy. *Crit Rev Oncol Hematol* 2007; 64: 1–9.

13 Gajra A, Jatoi A. Non-small-cell lung cancer in elderly patients: a discussion of treatment options. *J Clin Oncol* 2014; 32: 2562–9.

14 Dawe D, Ellis PM. The treatment of metastatic non-small cell lung cancer in the elderly: an evidence-based approach. *Front Oncol* 2014; 4: 178.

15 Temel JS, Greer JA, Muzikansky A, *et al.* Early palliative care for patients with metastatic non-small-cell lung cancer. *N Engl J Med* 2010; 363: 733–42.

16 Moya A, Sutton R, Ammirati F, *et al.*; Task Force for the Diagnosis and Management of Syncope; European Society of Cardiology (ESC); European Heart Rhythm Association (EHRA); Heart Failure Association (HFA); Heart Rhythm Society (HRS). Guidelines for the diagnosis and management of syncope (version 2009). *Eur Heart J* 2009; 30: 2631–71.

17 National Institute for Health and Care Excellence (2010). *Chronic obstructive pulmonary disease. Management of chronic obstructive pulmonary disease in adults in primary and secondary care. NICE clinical guideline 101.* Available from: www.nice.org.uk/guidance/cg101 (accessed 27 March 2015).

18 Sitas F. Smoking cessation after cancer. *J Clin Oncol* 2014; 32: 3593–5.

19 National Institute for Health and Care Excellence (2010). *Chronic obstructive pulmonary disease pathway. Inhaled therapy in COPD.* Available from: pathways.nice.org.uk/pathways/chronic-obstructive-pulmonary-disease/inhaled-therapy-in-copd (accessed 27 March 2015).

02 Colorectal Cancer in a Patient with an Aortic Abdominal Aneurysm, Peripheral Vascular Disease and Poor Nutritional Status

Dimitra Repana, David Shipway, Paul Ross

Case history

A 75-year-old man presented to his GP complaining of fatigue, progressive weight loss of 12 kg and low mood. His past medical history consisted of peripheral vascular disease (PVD) presenting with calf claudication and hypertension diagnosed 20 years previously. He was an ex-smoker with a history of 40 pack-years and drank 4–6 units of alcohol per week. He was a retired librarian who lived alone after his wife died 2 years previously.

His medications included aspirin 75 mg/day, ramipril 10 mg/day, amlodipine 10 mg/day, bendroflumethiazide 2.5 mg/day, simvastatin 20 mg/day and naftidrofuryl oxalate 200 mg three times daily.

His performance status was 2 and his BMI was 21.2 kg/m^2 (height 175 cm, weight 65 kg). Physical examination revealed a palpable mass in the left lower abdomen. His score on the Patient Health Questionnaire (PHQ-9) was 10 (moderate depression).

Further investigations revealed microcytic anaemia with haemoglobulin 94 g/l and low iron levels 6 µmol/l. A colonoscopy was organized and a partially obstructing tumour was seen in the sigmoid. Biopsies confirmed a moderately differentiated adenocarcinoma of the colon. Staging was completed with a CT scan of chest, abdomen and pelvis, which showed, apart from the colonic tumour, pericolonic lymphadenopathy and a 7.5 cm abdominal aortic aneurysm (AAA).

The patient was started on mirtazapine for his depression and was assessed by a dietitian for his weight loss. Nutritional supplements were initiated in addition to carer support at home with meal preparation. After discussion with the vascular team it was decided that AAA repair with endoscopic repair of abdominal aortic aneurysm (EVAR) should proceed. A colonic stent was inserted and preoperative intravenous iron was given to optimize his haemoglobulin. EVAR was performed without complications. During admission, sodium was found to be low at 124 mmol/l and bendroflumethiazide was stopped. A laparoscopic anterior resection of his sigmoid tumour was performed 6 weeks afterwards. Histology showed a pT3N2 (6/18 lymph nodes) M0 adenocarcinoma of the sigmoid colon with lymphovascular invasion.

The patient was referred to the oncology team to discuss adjuvant chemotherapy after his surgery. Both options of single-agent capecitabine and doublet chemotherapy with fluoropyrimidine and oxaliplatin were discussed. After considering potential benefit and side effects, single-agent capecitabine was considered more appropriate.

What is the optimal management of his anaemia, weight loss and depression?

What are the usual causes of hyponatraemia in older people?

How do AAA and PVD affect his management?

What are the evidence-based data regarding surgical options in this population and what is the role of stenting used as a bridge to surgery?

What is the evidence for adjuvant chemotherapy?

What is the optimal management of his anaemia, weight loss and depression?

Preoperative anaemia has been associated with increased 30 day mortality and morbidity in patients undergoing major surgery.[1] Iron deficiency anaemia in patients with colorectal cancer is common, but further causes of anaemia in the older population should also be excluded[2] (Figure 2.1). Iron replacement with intravenous iron is safe and effective in the perioperative setting. It results in more rapid optimization of body iron stores, compared with enteric replacement, and may be better tolerated than oral preparations especially in patients vulnerable to constipation or obstructive symptoms[3] (Figure 2.2).

Pre-existing depression has been found to be a significant risk factor for complications and prolonged recovery from colorectal cancer surgery.[4] Antidepressants are chosen based on patient characteristics and toxicity profile.[5] Selective serotonin reuptake inhibitors (SSRIs) have been associated with increased bleeding risk.[6,7] Mirtazapine has been shown to be safer in this context and has a faster result in 2 weeks compared with SSRIs (OR 1.57, 95% CI 1.30–1.88; $p<0.00001$). It is also associated with improved appetite and weight gain.[8,9]

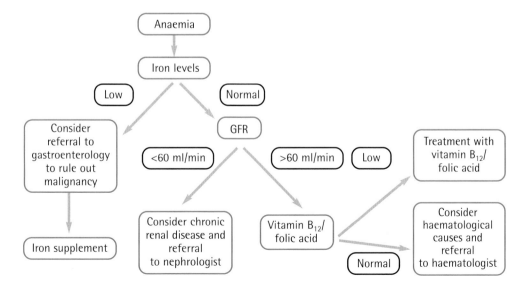

Figure 2.1 Algorithm for evaluation of anaemia in older patients (adapted from Goodnough and Schrier[2]). GFR, glomerular filtration rate.

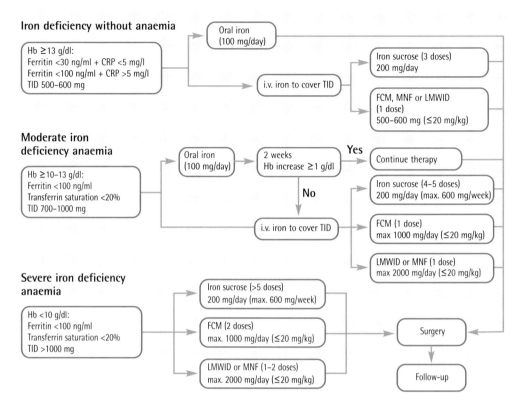

Figure 2.2 Algorithm for correction of anaemia (adapted from Muñoz *et al.*[3]). CRP, C-reactive protein; FCM, ferric caboxymaltose; LMWID, low molecular weight iron dextran; MNF, iron isomatolside-100; TID, total iron deficiency.

Weight loss in older people can be multifactorial and in this case, apart from cancer, depression and isolation contribute. Poor nutrition has been associated with worse outcomes for patients undergoing cancer surgery.[10] Various screening tools are used for initial assessment. Further management is determined according to severity of weight loss and circumstances. This includes assistance with feeding or shopping, especially for isolated patients, nutritional supplements, appetite stimulants, and enteral and parenteral feeding. For surgical candidates who are at risk of malnutrition (Table 2.1), or who are already malnourished and oral intake is inadequate or unsafe, an enteral tube should be considered if they have a functional and accessible gastrointestinal tract. In case of a non-functional, perforated or inaccessible gastrointestinal tract, parenteral nutrition is indicated.[11]

Table 2.1 Definitions of malnutrition and risk of malnutrition.[11]

Malnutrition	• BMI <18.5 kg/m²
	• Unintentional weight loss >10% within last 3–6 months
	• BMI <20 kg/m² and unintentional weight loss >5% within last 3–6 months
Risk of malnutrition	• Has eaten little or nothing in last 5 days and/or is likely to eat little or nothing in the next 5 days or longer
	• Poor absorption and/or high nutritional losses and/or high nutritional needs

What are the usual causes of hyponatraemia in older people?

Hyponatraemia is the most common electrolyte disorder in older patients and is observed in more than 20% of geriatric inpatients.[12] It is associated with impaired cognition, higher risk of osteoporosis, falls and fractures, prolonged admission and readmission to hospital and increased mortality.[13] Mild hyponatraemia is usually asymptomatic; neurological symptoms develop depending on severity and onset and include headaches, malaise, nausea and vomiting, confusion, cramps, seizures, delirium, coma, neurogenic pulmonary oedema and brain oedema with fatal herniation.[14]

Hyponatraemia can often be multifactorial: the usual causes are shown in Table 2.2.[15] Several medications can cause low sodium levels, and a thorough medication history should be obtained. In our patient, hyponatraemia was attributed to the combination of a thiazide diuretic with an antidepressant.

Table 2.2 Major causes of hyponatraemia (adapted from Sterns[15]).

Disorders in which ADH levels are elevated

Effective circulating volume depletion
- True volume depletion
- Heart failure
- Cirrhosis
- Thiazide diuretics

Syndrome of inappropriate ADH secretion, including reset osmostat pattern

Hormonal changes
- Adrenal insufficiency
- Hypothyroidism
- Pregnancy

Disorders in which ADH levels may be appropriately suppressed

Advanced renal failure
Primary polydipsia
Beer drinker's potomania

Hyponatraemia with normal or elevated plasma osmolality

High plasma osmolality (effective osmols)
- Hyperglycaemia
- Mannitol

High plasma osmolality (ineffective osmols)
- Renal failure
- Alcohol intoxication with an elevated serum alcohol concentration

Normal plasma osmolality
- Pseudohyponatraemia (laboratory artefact)
  - High triglycerides
  - Cholestatic and obstructive jaundice (lipoprotein X)
  - Multiple myeloma
- Absorption of irrigant solutions
  - Glycine
  - Sorbitol
  - Mannitol

ADH, antidiuretic hormone.

How do AAA and PVD affect his management?

For AAA greater than 5.5 cm there is at least a 20% risk of rupture at 1 year, which increases exponentially with diameter; thus, surgical intervention should be considered[16] (Figure 2.3). EVAR is a major advance in vascular surgery, since it is associated with reduced perioperative mortality.[17] Data support the use of EVAR in older patients who meet the anatomical criteria for the procedure.[18]

Age, smoking, diabetes, hypertension and hypercholesterolaemia are well-established risk factors for PVD. Undiagnosed ischaemic heart disease is an underlying factor in 40–60% of patients with PVD,[19] and a meticulous history of cardiac and respiratory symptoms should be sought, along with routine preoperative ECG. Patients with vascular disease have a high prevalence of undiagnosed cognitive impairment that can affect up to 60% of those presenting for vascular surgery; these patients are at high risk of perioperative delirium, which may influence the choice of anaesthetic technique.[20]

PVD is graded according to severity, and mild claudication improves with medical treatment and increased exercise. In this case it should not influence decisions regarding further management.[21] Secondary prevention medications are likely to be in use, and ACE inhibitors should be withheld on the morning of surgery. Antiplatelet agents may also need to be discontinued depending on the nature of the surgery undertaken, although in the context of coexisting ischaemic heart disease this may need to be with caution.

What are the evidence–based data regarding surgical options in this population and what is the role of stenting used as a bridge to surgery?

Comprehensive Geriatric Assessment (CGA) in the perioperative setting can identify risks that may increase mortality and help the multidisciplinary team of surgeons and oncologists towards better and safer treatment decisions for older patients with cancer.[22]

Data support a laparoscopic approach over open surgery in this age group.[23] A recently published meta-analysis including more than 70,000 older patients showed no difference in survival outcomes (OR 0.89, 95% CI 0.45–0.68; $p<0.01$) but improved postoperative complications (OR 0.55, 95% CI 0.48–0.63; $p<0.01$) and mortality (OR 0.55, 95% CI 0.45–0.68; $p<0.01$).[23]

Colonic stenting versus emergency surgery for obstructing left-sided tumours has been

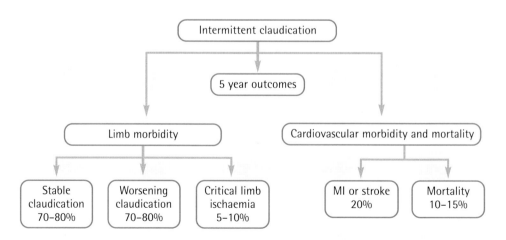

Figure 2.3 Natural history of PVD (adapted from Conte *et al.*[21]). MI, myocardial infarction.

associated with reduced stoma formation and higher primary anastomosis.[24] Owing to lack of randomized trials, few data are available for the use of colonic stents as a bridge to elective surgery. It may be reasonable to use stenting whilst medical optimization is achieved.[25]

What is the evidence for adjuvant chemotherapy?

Between 2009 and 2011, 43% of all patients diagnosed with colorectal cancer in the UK were >75 years old.[26] Management of older patients demands an individualized approach due to significant heterogeneity in this group. Holistic assessment allows consideration of physiological rather than chronological age, comorbidities and social issues.[27]

There are concerns about oncological undertreatment of older patients,[27] and age has been observed as a major reason for not offering adjuvant treatment.[28]

Adjuvant chemotherapy following colorectal cancer surgery improves disease-free survival and overall survival (OS); therefore, it should be discussed with patients with node-positive tumours and selected patients with node-negative tumours with other adverse prognostic features.[29] The discussion will need to consider recurrence risk, potential survival advantage and risks of chemotherapy. Subgroup analyses of both the Multicenter International Study of Oxaliplatin/5-Fluorouracil/Leucovorin in the Adjuvant Treatment of Colon Cancer Trial (MOSAIC)[30] and the National Surgical Adjuvant Breast and Bowel Project (NSABP C-07)[31] questioned the benefit of adding oxaliplatin to fluorouracil-based chemotherapy for patients above 70 years of age. Conflicting results were reported in the Study of Bevacizumab Alone or Combined with Capecitabine and Oxaliplatin as Support Therapy in Metastatic Colorectal Cancer Patients (XELOXA), where adding oxaliplatin to capecitabine chemotherapy in patients with colon cancer was found to be beneficial for all age groups compared with fluoropyrimidines.[32] The ACCENT database, which used individual patient data and included all previous studies plus four further trials, suggested that there may be a disease-free survival benefit for patients >70 years but not an OS benefit.[33] Another recently published pooled analysis supported the benefit of oxaliplatin in patients over 70, which was maintained even after adjustment for comorbidities.[34] As randomized controlled trials are lacking in this specific age group, and data from subgroup analyses from previous studies are conflicting, adding oxaliplatin appears reasonable for fit patients between 70 and 75 years of age. Online tools such as Adjuvant! Online (www.adjuvantonline.com) can help shared decision making and estimate the risk of recurrence, life expectancy and potential benefit of chemotherapy.

Conclusion and learning points

- Optimization of haemoglobulin prior to surgery with intravenous iron is both safe and effective. It may be better tolerated in patients with colorectal cancer, who are vulnerable to symptoms of gastrointestinal upset associated with oral iron preparation. Other contributing causes of anaemia should also be excluded.

- Antidepressant treatment with SSRIs has been associated with increased bleeding risk and should be avoided. Mirtazapine is an excellent alternative, as it offers appetite stimulation, which may promote secondary nutritional optimization.

- Dietetic review should be carried out to assess nutritional status and habits, with further management according to severity of weight loss.

- Older patients often have chronic low sodium levels associated with complications and mortality.

- CGA and optimization throughout the surgical pathway reduce complications and inpatient length of stay.
- EVAR is safe and provides advantages compared with open surgery for AAA.
- Laparoscopic surgery is preferred in older patients, since it is associated with fewer complications and mortality.
- Referral to the oncology team for discussion of risks and benefits of adjuvant chemotherapy for all patients who are fit for treatment should always be considered.

References

1 Musallam K, Tanim H, Richards T, *et al.* Perioperative anaemia and postoperative outcomes in non-cardiac surgery: a retrospective cohort study. *Lancet* 2011; 378: 1396–407.

2 Goodnough LT, Schrier SL. Evaluation and management of anaemia in the elderly. *Am J Hematol* 2014; 89: 88–96.

3 Muñoz M, Gómez-Ramirez S, Martin-Mortañez E, Auerbach M. Perioperative management in colorectal cancer patients: a pragmatic approach. *World J Gastroenterol* 2014; 20: 1972–85.

4 Balentine C, Hermosillo-Rodriguez J, Robinson C, *et al.* Depression is associated with prolonged and complicated recovery following colorectal surgery. *J Gastrointest Surg* 2011; 15: 1712–17.

5 Bottino C, Barcelos-Ferreira R, Ribeiz S. Treatment of depression in older adults. *Curr Psychiatry Rep* 2012; 14: 289–97.

6 Mahdanian A, Rej S, Bacon S, *et al.* Serotonergic antidepressants and perioperative bleeding risk: a systematic review. *Exp Opin Drug Saf* 2014; 13: 695–704.

7 Auerbach AD, Vittnghoff E, Maselli J, *et al.* Perioperative use of selective serotonin reuptake inhibitors and risks for adverse outcomes of surgery. *JAMA Intern Med* 2013; 173: 1075–81.

8 Watanabe N, Omori MI, Nakagawa A, *et al.*; MANGA (Meta-Analysis of New Generation Antidepressants) Study Group. Safety reporting and adverse-event profile of mirtazapine described in randomized controlled trials in comparison with other classes of antidepressants in the acute-phase treatments of adults with depression. *CNS Drugs* 2010; 24: 35–53.

9 Serretti A, Mandelli L. Antidepressants and body weight: a comprehensive review and meta-analysis. *J Clin Psychiatry* 2010; 71: 1259–72.

10 Sun K, Chen S, Xu J, *et al.* The prognostic significance of the prognostic nutritional index in cancer: a systematic review and meta-analysis. *J Cancer Res Clin Oncol* 2014; 140: 1537–49.

11 National Institute of Health and Care Excellence (2006). *Nutrition support in adults. Oral nutrition support, enteral tube feeding and parenteral nutrition. NICE clinical guideline 32.* Available from: www.nice.org.uk/guidance/cg32/resources/guidance-nutrition-support-in-adults-pdf (accessed 27 June 2015).

12 Gosch M, Joosten-Gstrein B, Heppner HJ, *et al.* Hyponatraemia in geriatric inhospital patients: effects on results of a comprehensive geriatric assessment. *Gerontology* 2012; 58: 430–40.

13 Cowen L, Hodak S, Verbalis J. Age-associated abnormalities of water homeostasis. *Endocrinol Metab Clin North Am* 2013; 42: 349–70.

14 Sterns R. Disorders of plasma sodium – causes, consequences, and correction. *N Engl J Med* 2015; 372: 55–65.

15 Sterns R. Causes of hyponatraemia in adults. *UptoDate* 2015; May.

16 Davis M, Harris M, Earnshaw J. Implementation of the National Health Service Abdominal Aortic Aneurysm Screening Program in England. *J Vasc Surg* 2013: 57: 1440–5.

17 Giles KA, Pomposelli F, Hamdan A. Decrease in total aneurysm related deaths in the era of endovascular aneurysm repair. *J Vasc Surg* 2009; 49: 543–51.

18 Saratzis A, Mohamed S. Endovascular abdominal aortic aneurysm repair in the geriatric population. *J Geriatr Cardiol* 2012; 9: 285–91.

19 Norgren L, Hiatt WR, Dormandy JA, *et al.*; TASC II Working Group. Inter-society consensus for the management of peripheral arterial disease (TASC II). *J Vasc Surg* 2007; 45 (suppl S): 45–67.

20 Partridge J, Dhesi J, Cross J, *et al.* The prevalence and impact of undiagnosed cognitive impairment in older vascular surgical patients. *J Vasc Surg* 2014; 60: 1002–11.

21 Conte M, Pomposelli F, Clair D, *et al.*; Society for Vascular Surgery Lower Extremity Guidelines Writing Group. Society for Vascular Surgery practice guidelines for atherosclerotic occlusive disease of the lower extremities: management of asymptomatic disease and claudication. *J Vasc Surg* 2015; 61 (3 suppl): 2–41S.

22 Shipway DJH, Harari D, Dhesi JK. Peri-operative management of older people undergoing surgery. *Rev Gerontol* 2013; 24: 78–92.

23 Ugolini G, Ghignone F, Zattoni D, *et al.* Personalized surgical management of colorectal cancer in elderly population. *World J Gastroenterol* 2014; 20: 3762–77.

24 Cirocchi R, Farinella E, Trastulli S, *et al.* Safety and efficacy of endoscopic colonic stenting as a bridge to surgery in the management of intestinal obstruction due to left colon and rectal cancer: a systematic review and meta-analysis. *Surg Oncol* 2013; 22: 14e21.

25 Ansaloni L, Andersson R, Bazzoli F, *et al.* Guidelines in the management of obstructing cancer of the left colon: consensus conference of the World Society of Emergency Surgery (WSES) and Peritoneum and Surgery (PnS) Society. *World J Emerg Surg* 2010; 5: 29.

26 Cancer Research UK. *Cancer statistics explained.* Available from: www.cancerresearchuk.org/health-professional/cancer-statistics/cancer-stats-explained (accessed 27 June 2015).

27 Papamichael D, Audisio RA, Glimelius B, *et al.* Treatment of colorectal cancer in older patients: International Society of Geriatric Oncology (SIOG) consensus recommendations 2013. *Ann Oncol* 2015; 26: 463–76.

28 Chagpar R, Xing Y, Chiang YJ, *et al.* Adherence to stage-specific treatment guidelines for patients with colon cancer. *J Clin Oncol* 2012; 30: 972–9.

29 Labianca R, Nordlinger B, Beretta GD, *et al.*; ESMO Guidelines Working Group. Early colon cancer: ESMO clinical practice guidelines for diagnosis, treatment and follow up. *Ann Oncol* 2013; 24 (suppl 6): vi64–72.

30 Tournigand C, Andre T, Bonnetain F, *et al.* Adjuvant therapy with fluorouracil and oxaliplatin in stage II and elderly patients (between ages 70 and 75 years) with colon cancer: subgroup analyses of the Multicenter International Study of Oxaliplatin, Fluorouracil, and Leucovorin in the Adjuvant Treatment of Colon Cancer Trial. *J Clin Oncol* 2012; 30: 3353–60.

31 Yothers G, O'Connell M, Allegra C, *et al.* Oxaliplatin as adjuvant therapy for colon cancer: updated results of NSABP C-07 Trial, including survival and subset analyses. *J Clin Oncol* 2011; 29: 3768–74.

32 Haller D, Tabernero J, Maroun J, *et al.* Capecitabine plus oxaliplatin compared with fluorouracil and folinic acid as adjuvant therapy for stage III colon cancer. *J Clin Oncol* 2011; 20: 1465–71.

33 McCleary N, Meyerhardt J, Green E, *et al.* Impact of age on the efficacy of newer adjuvant therapies in patients with stage II/III colon cancer: findings from the ACCENT database. *J Clin Oncol* 2013; 31: 2600–6.

34 Haller DG, Connell MJ, Cartwright TH, *et al.* Impact of age and medical comorbidity on adjuvant treatment outcomes for stage III colon cancer: a pooled analysis of individual patient data from four randomized controlled trials. *Ann Oncol* 2015; 26: 1715–24.

03 A Patient with Early-Stage Lung Cancer and Heart Disease

Adam P. Januszewski, Danielle Harari, Mary E.R. O'Brien

Case history

An 84-year-old woman with a persistent cough was referred to the respiratory physicians by her GP. A CT scan identified a 3.5×2.6 cm mass in the left upper lobe, and a subsequent biopsy demonstrated a poorly differentiated adenocarcinoma (cytokeratin 7- and thyroid transcription factor-1-positive). Full staging (CT-PET and MR brain scans) confirmed a T2aN1M0 (stage IIA) lung adenocarcinoma. Her past medical history included a myocardial infarction in 2009 (managed medically) and atrial fibrillation (AF). Examination was unremarkable with adequate pulmonary function (>80% predicted FEV_1 and diffusion factor). The patient was taking omeprazole, digoxin, warfarin and simvastatin. She was a widow with two daughters and an ex-smoker of 38 years with a 20 pack-year history. She was fully independent.

The lung multidisciplinary team (MDT) recommended primary resection and she proceeded to have a video-assisted left upper lobectomy. She recovered well postoperatively and the pathological stage was pT2pN1M0. After a further MDT discussion, the benefits and toxicities of vinorelbine/carboplatin were outlined to the patient and her family and she elected to receive chemotherapy. This was preferred over vinorelbine/cisplatin because of the potential cardiac and renal toxicities associated with cisplatin. Given her past medical history, early referral was made to the cardiologists, who converted her warfarin to rivaroxaban and continued her digoxin.

Cycle 1 of chemotherapy was complicated by grade 1 sensory neuropathy and cycle 2 by a urinary tract infection. The vinorelbine dose was reduced for cycle 3. The patient had ongoing difficulties with urinary symptoms, weight loss and worsening paraesthesia; therefore, cycle 4 was omitted.

What is the goal of treatment in this patient?

What preoperative assessments should be performed to risk-stratify older patients?

What is the evidence base for adjuvant treatment in older patients with lung cancer?

What considerations for heart disease need to be made in the older oncology patient?

What is the goal of treatment in this patient?

Limited-stage lung cancer is treated by surgery with curative intent. There are numerous series of surgical cases describing well-selected patients who tolerated the procedure as well as younger patients. However, population data in the 2014 UK National Clinical Lung Cancer Audit show that age is an independent prognostic factor and that patients aged over 80 have significantly worse outcome. If patients have adequate respiratory and cardiac function, regardless of age, they are offered surgery for early-stage non-small-cell lung carcinoma (NSCLC). Adjuvant chemotherapy trials have demonstrated consistently that the benefits at 5 years are a gain in overall survival (OS) of 5–10% and a 30% decrease in the rate of recurrence.[1] In general, however, patients over the age of 70 were not included in these trials, although subsequent series suggest that older patients tolerate chemotherapy and therefore have the potential to benefit to the same extent as those under the age of 70.

What preoperative assessments should be performed to risk–stratify older patients?

Surgery remains the cornerstone for the radical treatment of stage I–II NSCLC. Preoperative risk assessment is paramount to enable informed decision making. Regardless of age, baseline pulmonary function tests need to be performed to ensure that their predicted FEV_1 and DLCO are greater than 80%. Anything below normal values would require further functional pulmonary assessment to predict postoperative complications, mortality and morbidity. Some centres perform a ventilation/perfusion scan to identify mismatches in preoperative planning.

The risk of in-hospital death can be predicted using validated models such as the thoracic surgery scoring system Thoracoscore, which uses, amongst others, age, performance status and comorbidities to predict the chance of in-hospital death.[2] Preoperative geriatric-specific models for risk scoring have been developed but not widely used or validated. When using markers such as impaired cognition, recent falls, functional dependence and comorbidities in a predictive scoring model, one study was able to predict postoperative mortality and institutionalization.[3]

To estimate the risk of operative mortality there has been a move towards cardiac risk scoring and functional assessment. The Revised Cardiac Risk Index (recommended by the European Society for Medical Oncology) assigns a risk score to help guide which patients require further investigations. Coronary heart disease, history of cerebrovascular disease, creatinine >2 mg/dl and planned pneumonectomy are scored, although age is not.[4] This externally validated model is used to determine which patients should have further cardiac investigation. Recent guidelines, however, advise that all patients over 70 should have cardiopulmonary functional assessment prior to radical surgery.[5]

Postoperative quality of life has only been assessed in a small number of trials. Findings suggest that older patients have a lower preoperative quality of life compared with their younger counterparts and that postoperative recovery is similar (after an initial decrement).[6]

What is the evidence base for adjuvant treatment in older patients with lung cancer?

The standard of care for stage IB–IIIA NSCLC is postoperative cisplatin-based chemotherapy based on randomized phase III studies summarized in the Lung Adjuvant Cisplatin Evaluation (LACE) meta-analysis, which reported an OS benefit of 5.4% at 5 years.[7] There are, however, no prospective studies in the older population.

JBR-10 trial

This prospective phase III trial randomized 482 patients with completely resected stage IB–II NSCLC to vinorelbine/cisplatin or observation. In this landmark study, chemotherapy improved median OS from 73 to 97 months (HR 0.69; $p=0.04$) and 5 year survival (69% vs 54%; $p=0.04$).[8] A subgroup analysis by Pepe et al.[9] compared patients over and under 65 years. There were no differences in adverse events, and chemotherapy had an ongoing benefit in OS (HR 0.61; 95% CI 0.38–0.98; $p=0.04$). The analysis demonstrated that fewer doses of cisplatin were given to older patients, with an ongoing benefit in OS during up to 10 years' median follow-up (although this appears to have been confined to the patients with stage N1 disease).[10]

LACE

This meta-analysis comprising data of 4584 patients across five cisplatin-based prospective adjuvant chemotherapy trials demonstrated an absolute OS benefit of 5.4% at 5 years with treatment (HR 0.89, 95% CI 0.82–0.96; $p=0.005$).[1] Subgroup analysis by Früh et al.[7] categorized patients into age categories of young (<65 years), middle and older (>70 years) and found no age-based differences in HR ($p_{trend}=0.29$). Rates of severe toxicities were similar between groups, although there was a significant reduction in the first and total dose of cisplatin given to the older patients (X^2 test, $p<0.0001$).

Other studies have investigated retrospective data regarding adjuvant chemotherapy in older versus younger populations. In these retrospective database analyses the non-cancer-related deaths and chemotherapy toxicities were increased in older patients. However, there was no survival advantage for patients aged over 80 (supported by two further retrospective studies). This suggests that, although age should not be a definitive cut-off, caution should be used when using adjuvant chemotherapy in the over-80s.[11,12] Predictive models estimating the degree of benefit from adjuvant treatments are based on studies with small numbers of older patients; therefore, their validity is questionable and should be interpreted with caution.

What considerations for heart disease need to be made in the older oncology patient?

Heart disease remains the leading cause of death in the over-65s. It is important to optimize patients prior to oncological treatments and subsequently manage long-term survivors of cancer.

AF is the most common arrhythmia in older patients and increases in prevalence with age. Poorly controlled AF results in palpitations, shortness of breath and reduced exercise tolerance, and if left untreated leads to heart failure and embolic events. It can be managed by rate or rhythm control; however, evidence suggests that the risk of death is higher in patients aged over 65 undergoing rhythm compared with rate control.[13] The recommendation would be to ensure that AF is rate-controlled.

In the present case the patient is not symptomatic from AF and has been on digoxin for many years. However, as previously discussed, she would require baseline pulmonary and cardiac investigations: ECG and echocardiogram. If she had cardiac symptoms they may warrant referral to a cardiologist for functional assessments (stress echocardiogram or perfusion scans). The thoracic team needs to work closely with the cardiologists, as revascularization would require dual antiplatelet therapy, which may delay surgical intervention. Should the patient have impaired left ventricular function, a beta-blocker and ACE inhibitor may be commenced to preserve and optimize cardiac function.

Anticoagulation should be considered in all patients with AF to reduce the risk of embolic events. This would be based on a risk stratification model of embolic/bleeding events such as the CHA_2DS_2-VASc score. Providers are sometimes reluctant to prescribe anticoagulation in older people with AF despite well-documented evidence of benefit. In frailer patients, however, the risk–benefit decision may be complicated by individual patient factors (e.g. risk of falls) and should be taken on an individual basis. There is no longer a place for aspirin in the prevention of thromboembolic events. New anticoagulants, like rivaroxaban, are being used increasingly in patients with cancer because of their predictable pharmacological profiles.

Regardless of age, chemotherapy in patients with heart disease needs to be used with caution. This is important in platinum regimens, as they induce thrombosis and platelet aggregation, and administration of chemotherapy requires significant intravenous hydration that can be difficult to manage with impaired cardiac function. Some physicians use carboplatin instead of cisplatin in patients where there is concern about renal or cardiac function. The small retrospective studies in older patients do not suggest significant differences in outcomes. However, the use of carboplatin should be with the caveat that its efficacy is not proven and it carries the risk of increased myelosuppression.

Conclusion and learning points

- Older patients derive significant benefit from radical approaches to early-stage lung cancer, which includes adjuvant chemotherapy. However, caution should be used with adjuvant treatment in those aged over 80, as there is a lack of evidence of benefit, and toxicities are more significant.

- Comorbidities (including heart disease) are common in older patients but should not be a reason not to proceed with radical treatment. Pretreatment investigation of cardiac function should be considered in any patient with a past history or symptoms of cardiac disease, with early referral to cardiology.

- Risk assessment prior to surgery allows informed decision making, and, although recovery from surgery for lung cancer is similar to that in younger patients, older patients do exhibit an initial detriment in function.

- Optimization of cardiac function for patients with AF and coronary heart disease is desirable to reduce the risk of decompensating during stressors. Addressing secondary risk factors is important for improving long-term survival.

References

1 Pignon J-P, Tribodet H, Scagliotti GV, et al. Lung adjuvant cisplatin evaluation: a pooled analysis by the LACE Collaborative Group. J Clin Oncol 2008; 26: 3552–9.

2 Falcoz PE, Conti M, Brouchet L, et al. The thoracic surgery scoring system (Thoracoscore): risk model for in-hospital death in 15,183 patients requiring thoracic surgery. J Thorac Cardiovasc Surg 2007; 133: 325–32.

3 Robinson TN, Eiseman B, Wallace JI, et al. Redefining geriatric preoperative assessment using frailty, disability and co-morbidity. Ann Surg 2009; 250: 449–55.

4 Brunelli A, Cassivi SD, Fibla J, et al. External validation of the recalibrated thoracic revised cardiac risk index for predicting the risk of major cardiac complications after lung resection. Ann Thorac Surg 2011; 92: 445–8.

5 Brunelli A, Charloux A, Bolliger CT, et al. ERS/ESTS clinical guidelines on fitness for radical therapy in lung cancer patients (surgery and chemo-radiotherapy). Eur Respir J 2009; 34: 17–41.

6 Brunelli A, Socci L, Refai M, et al. Quality of life before and after major lung resection for lung cancer: a prospective follow-up analysis. Ann Thorac Surg 2007; 84: 410–16.

7 Früh M, Rolland E, Pignon J-P, *et al.* Pooled analysis of the effect of age on adjuvant cisplatin-based chemotherapy for completely resected non-small-cell lung cancer. *J Clin Oncol* 2008; 26: 3573–81.

8 Winton T, Livingston R, Johnson D, *et al.* Vinorelbine plus cisplatin vs. observation in resected non-small-cell lung cancer. *N Engl J Med* 2005; 352: 2589–97.

9 Pepe C, Hasan B, Winton TL, *et al.* Adjuvant vinorelbine and cisplatin in elderly patients: National Cancer Institute of Canada and Intergroup Study JBR.10. *J Clin Oncol* 2007; 25: 1553–61.

10 Butts CA, Ding K, Seymour L, *et al.* Randomized phase III trial of vinorelbine plus cisplatin compared with observation in completely resected stage IB and II non-small-cell lung cancer: updated survival analysis of JBR-10. *J Clin Oncol* 2010; 28: 29–34.

11 Cuffe S, Booth CM, Peng Y, *et al.* Adjuvant chemotherapy for non-small-cell lung cancer in the elderly: a population-based study in Ontario, Canada. *J Clin Oncol* 2012; 30: 1813–21.

12 Wisnivesky JP, Smith CB, Packer S, *et al.* Survival and risk of adverse events in older patients receiving postoperative adjuvant chemotherapy for resected stages II–IIIA lung cancer: observational cohort study. *BMJ* 2011; 343: d4013.

13 Wyse DG, Waldo AL, DiMarco JP, *et al.* A comparison of rate control and rhythm control in patients with atrial fibrillation. *N Engl J Med* 2002; 347: 1825–33.

Further reading

• Gajra A, Jatoi A. Non-small-cell lung cancer in elderly patients: a discussion of treatment options. *J Clin Oncol* 2014; 32: 2562–9.

• Vedovati MC, Germini F, Agnelli G, Becattini C. Direct oral anticoagulants in patients with VTE and cancer: a systematic review and meta-analysis. *Chest* 2015; 147: 475–83.

• National Institute for Health and Care Excellence (2014). *Atrial fibrillation: the management of atrial fibrillation. NICE guidelines CG180.* Available from: www.nice.org.uk/guidance/cg180 (accessed 12 June 2015).

• Lichtman SM, Wildiers H, Chatelut E, *et al.* International Society of Geriatric Oncology Chemotherapy Taskforce: evaluation of chemotherapy in older patients – an analysis of the medical literature. *J Clin Oncol* 2007; 25: 1832–43.

04 A Patient with Colorectal Cancer, Liver Metastases and Falls

Sarah J.L. Payne, Margot Gosney, Matthew Seymour

Case history

A 79-year-old woman had a 2 week history of rectal bleeding. Her past medical history included hypertension, osteoarthritis, type 2 diabetes and myocardial infarction. Clinically she was assessed as having Eastern Cooperative Oncology Group performance status 1 at baseline. Investigations showed a non-obstructing, non-bleeding lesion of the sigmoid colon, with bilobar liver metastases and a pulmonary embolus. Biopsies confirmed a *RAS*-mutant moderately differentiated adenocarcinoma. Blood tests revealed iron deficiency anaemia (Hb 102 g/l). Dalteparin was started for the pulmonary embolus, and the patient's case was discussed by the hepatobiliary multidisciplinary team (MDT), who recommended primary chemotherapy.

At the initial oncology appointment, the oncologist recommended fluorouracil (5-FU)/oxaliplatin chemotherapy. A screening Comprehensive Geriatric Assessment revealed a history of falls, which prompted an urgent referral to the falls clinic. The review identified two recent falls due to multifactorial causes:

- Postural hypotension attributed to antihypertensive drugs.
- Grade 2 peripheral neuropathy (touch and pinprick) attributable to diabetes and vitamin B_{12} deficiency.
- Poor strength, especially in the proximal lower limbs, and poor balance.

In light of the peripheral neuropathy, the oncologist changed the chemotherapy to full-dose 5-FU/irinotecan. A dose reduction was required at cycle 4 due to grade 2 anaemia and fatigue. The patient completed 12 cycles of doublet chemotherapy, with stable disease on an outcome CT. The hepatobiliary MDT recommended a two-stage (bowel, then liver) operation. Radiofrequency liver ablation was not an option, given the tumour location. Following discussion of the options, the patient declined surgery and was therefore put on surveillance.

What is the goal of cancer treatment for this patient?

What could be done to reduce her risk of falls as she undergoes cancer treatment?

What is the evidence base for her treatment options?

How did her comorbidities affect the cancer treatment decisions?

How can falls be identified and managed in cancer services?

What is the goal of cancer treatment for this patient?

It is important to be clear about the long-term goal of therapy at the outset, carefully considering the priorities and goals of the patient. In this case there were two options: a potentially curative approach involving intensive chemotherapy and multiple operations, or a palliative approach that would involve less intensive chemotherapy. Clear discussion of these options with the patient at the outset might have avoided the apparent mismatch between the priorities and goals of the doctors and those of the patient.

What could be done to reduce her risk of falls as she undergoes cancer treatment?

The management of comorbidities should always be reviewed at the time of starting cancer treatment: long-standing medical conditions might have changed; pharmacology might have altered; and the cost–benefit balance of preventive medications might have shifted.[1]

In this patient, antihypertensives were discontinued and her GP was asked to monitor her BP. Vitamin B_{12} level should be checked, and supplemented if necessary, in patients with falls and/or peripheral neuropathy and/or anaemia. Similarly, this patient received intravenous iron for her baseline iron deficiency anaemia. She was started on calcium and vitamin D tablets to reduce the risk of fracture should she have another fall.

Diabetic control should be optimized, but prevention of long-term diabetic complications may now be less relevant. This patient's HbA_{1c} level was raised and the GP was asked to increase medication whilst avoiding long-acting drugs which may risk early morning hypoglycaemia. Plans were made for extra diabetic monitoring in the community during chemotherapy, and pre-emptive plans were made should her oral intake decline. She was referred to a community physiotherapist, who started home-based therapy for strength and balance. An occupational therapist assessed her home and advised her to dispose of loose rugs and increased the wattage on her light bulbs, and installed grab rails and a bath stool.

What is the evidence base for her treatment options?

Chemotherapy is used in both the curative (neoadjuvant, adjuvant) and the palliative setting, and for both there is rather limited evidence relating to patients whose advanced age, frailty or comorbidity may affect treatment decisions.

5-FU, given with folinic acid, improves survival compared with supportive care alone, with benefits seen in both younger and older patients.[2] Cytotoxic doublets (5-FU/oxaliplatin, capecitabine/oxaliplatin, 5-FU/irinotecan) substantially improve the rate of response and progression-free interval over that of 5-FU alone, and their efficacy may be further increased by adding a targeted drug or a third cytotoxic agent.[3,4] When interval curative surgery is an aim or possibility, the higher response rate of these more intensive therapies improves the probability of cure; however, when the aim is purely palliative, evidence from several large sequencing trials suggests that side effects may be reduced and survival is not compromised by sequenced therapy, starting with 5-FU and keeping other options in reserve.[5]

To date there have been three prospective trials that have specifically considered the choice of chemotherapy for inoperable metastatic colorectal cancer in older patients: Fluorouracil, Oxaliplatin, Irinotecan: Use and Sequencing (FOCUS)2;[6] Fédération Francophone de Cancérologie Digestive (FFCD) 2001–02;[7] and A Study of Bevacizumab in Combination with Capecitabine in Elderly Patients with Metastatic Colorectal Cancer (AVEX).[8]

FOCUS2[6]

This UK phase III trial recruited 459 patients with inoperable colorectal cancer who were considered unsuitable for full-dose chemotherapy because of advanced age or frailty: 78% were aged over 70 years, 43% over 75 years. Randomization was to 5-FU/levofolinic acid, 5-

FU/oxaliplatin, capecitabine, or capecitabine/oxaliplatin in a 2×2 design, in each case starting at 80% standard dose with an optional escalation after 6 weeks. Oxaliplatin produced only borderline significant improvement in progression-free survival (PFS) and no difference in overall survival (OS). There were no efficacy differences between capecitabine and 5-FU, although 5-FU was better tolerated. Interestingly, the rates of toxicity with each of the 80% regimens in FOCUS2 were very similar to those seen with full-dose regimens in standard trials of young, fit patients.

FFCD 2001–02[7]

This French phase III trial randomly assigned 282 untreated patients with metastatic colorectal cancer age >75 years to 5-FU versus 5-FU/irinotecan. Irinotecan produced an improved response rate (46.3% vs 27.4%; OR 2.3, 95% CI 1.4–3.8, $p=0.001$), a non-significant improvement in PFS (7.3 months vs 5.2 months; HR 0.84, 95% CI 0.66–1.07, $p=0.15$), but no OS benefit. A substudy performed geriatric evaluations on approximately half of the patients recruited to the study and demonstrated a 58% rate of grade 3–4 toxicity, a 54% rate of unexpected hospitalization and a 33% rate of dose reduction. The strongest predictors of toxicity were dependence in the instrumental activities of daily living scale and decreased cognitive function assessed using the Mini-Mental State Examination. These factors perhaps warrant a particular focus in pretreatment assessment to identify modifiable aspects and support needs.

AVEX[8]

This phase III randomized trial compared capecitabine versus capecitabine/ bevacizumab in an older population deemed unfit for combination chemotherapy treatment. The response rate and PFS were significantly increased with bevacizumab (RR 19% vs 10%, $p=0.04$; PFS 9.1 months vs 5.1 months, $p<0.0001$), but OS was not. The frequency of grade 3–4 toxicities was greater in the combination arm, mainly hand-foot syndrome and venous thromboembolism; overall, however, capecitabine/ bevacizumab was felt to be a safe therapeutic option in this population.

How did her comorbidities affect the cancer treatment decisions?

This patient's treatment was initiated with potentially curative intent, with 5-FU/oxaliplatin prior to possible surgical resection of bowel and liver. This was modified to 5-FU/irinotecan when the history of peripheral neuropathy and falls became apparent. The patient was able to complete all chemotherapy cycles, albeit after a dose reduction. Her diabetic control was monitored, but no problems arose despite the use of dexamethasone as an antiemetic.

How can falls be identified and managed in cancer services?

Falls occur in approximately 30% of people aged ≥65 years. They are more common in patients with cancer, notably affecting up to 50% of those with advanced cancer.[9] Falls are often not mentioned by patients; therefore, a falls screening question is useful.

Falls can be divided into two broad categories, which are managed differently:

- Falls with syncope are usually cardiogenic/neurogenic and require medical investigations (e.g. 24 h tape) and treatment following specialist assessment.
- Falls without syncope are more common, usually multifactorial and often associated with postural instability. Watching gait as patients walk into the clinic room may help to identify these cases (e.g. slow/unsteady/shuffling), or watching patients get up from the clinic room chair (slow/using arms to push up from chair). Several major falls risk factors are potentially

modifiable (e.g. muscle weakness, vision, polypharmacy and environmental hazards).[10] There are numerous simple interventions that can be initiated by an oncologist (e.g. reviewing medications, measuring BP and stopping antihypertensives if BP is low, referring to physiotherapy if gait is unsteady, referring for cataract surgery/new glasses). Complex cases should be referred for further assessment.

Most UK hospitals/GPs have access to multidisciplinary falls clinics run either in hospital or in the community. Where there is uncertainty about what services are available, local geriatrics departments will be able to direct.

Conclusion and learning points

- Treatment aims and choices should be discussed with patients at the outset.
- For patients with significant age- or comorbidity-related frailty, less intensive chemotherapy treatments may be preferable to achieve palliation.
- A thorough comorbidity assessment will inform decision making.
- Assess for peripheral neuropathy prior to chemotherapy such as oxaliplatin (pinprick and light touch), especially if there is a history of falls, diabetes or alcohol excess, and review modifiable causes.
- Falls should be assessed as part of the oncology consultation.
- Refer complex cases (recurrent falls or unclear aetiology) for further specialist assessment.

References

1   Hall PS, Lord SR, El-Laboudi A, Seymour MT. Non-cancer medications for patients with incurable cancer: time to stop and think? *Br J Gen Pract* 2010; 60: 243–4.

2   Folprecht G, Cunningham D, Ross P, *et al.* Efficacy of 5-fluorouracil-based chemotherapy in elderly patients with metastatic colorectal cancer: a pooled analysis of clinical trials. *Ann Oncol* 2004; 15: 1330–8.

3   Folprecht G, Seymour MT, Saltz L, *et al.* Irinotecan/fluorouracil combination in first-line therapy of older and younger patients with metastatic colorectal cancer: combined analysis of 2,691 patients in randomized controlled trials. *J Clin Oncol* 2008; 26: 1443–51.

4   Goldberg RM, Tabah-Fisch I, Bleiberg H, *et al.* Pooled analysis of safety and efficacy of oxaliplatin plus fluorouracil/leucovorin administered bimonthly in elderly patients with colorectal cancer. *J Clin Oncol* 2006; 24: 4085–91.

5   Seymour MT, Punt CJA. Sequential chemotherapy for advanced colorectal cancer: should we ever start with a single cytotoxic agent? *Curr Colorectal Cancer Rep* 2008; 4: 130–8.

6   Seymour MT, Thompson LC, Wasan HS, *et al.* Chemotherapy options in elderly and frail patients with metastatic colorectal cancer (MRC FOCUS2): an open-label, randomised factorial trial. *Lancet* 2011; 377: 1749–59.

7   Aparicio T, Jouve JL, Teillet L, *et al.* Geriatric factors predict chemotherapy feasibility: ancillary results of FFCD 2001–02 phase III study in first-line chemotherapy for metastatic colorectal cancer in elderly patients. *J Clin Oncol* 2013; 31: 1464–70.

8   Cunningham D, Lang I, Marcuello E, *et al.* Bevacizumab plus capecitabine versus capecitabine alone in elderly patients with previously untreated metastatic colorectal cancer (AVEX): an open-label, randomised phase 3 trial. *Lancet Oncol* 2013; 14: 1077–85.

9   Stone CA, Lawlor PG, Savva GM, *et al.* Prospective study of falls and risk factors for falls in adults with advanced cancer. *J Clin Oncol* 2012; 30: 2128–33.

10 Rubenstein LZ. Falls in older people: epidemiology, risk factors and strategies for prevention. *Age Ageing* 2006; 35 (suppl 2): ii37–41.

Further reading

· Papmichael D, Audisio RA, Glimelius B, *et al.* Treatment of colorectal cancer in older patients: International Society of Geriatric Oncology (SIOG) consensus recommendations. *Ann Oncol* 2013; 26: 463–76.

· McCleary NJ, Dotan E, Browner I. Refining the chemotherapy approach for older patients with colon cancer. *J Clin Oncol* 2014; 32: 2570–80.

· Wildes TM, Dua P, Fowler SA, *et al.* Systematic review of falls in older adults with cancer. *J Geriatr Oncol* 2015; 6: 70–83.

· Chang JT, Morton SC, Rubenstein LZ, *et al.* Interventions for the prevention of falls in older adults: a systematic review and meta-analysis of randomized clinical trials. *BMJ* 2004; 328: 680–4.

· National Institute for Health and Care Excellence (2013). *Falls: assessment and prevention of falls in older people. NICE clinical guideline 161.* Available from: www.nice.org.uk/guidance/cg161 (accessed 14 June 2015).

05 Adjuvant Chemotherapy in a Patient with Breast Cancer

Jenny Seligmann, Margot Gosney, Bob Leonard

Case history

A 74-year-old woman attended for adjuvant chemotherapy 8 weeks after surgery for a T1G3N0, oestrogen receptor (ER)-negative, progesterone receptor-negative, human epidermal growth factor receptor 2 (HER2)-positive breast cancer, with clear surgical margins. She had returned to preoperative functioning.

Her past medical history included angina, hypertension, and urinary incontinence on coughing with occasional urgency. She was Afro-Caribbean and lived with her husband. None of her four children lived nearby. She was self-caring, had normal cognitive function, occasional breathlessness and intermittent headaches.

Her medications included bisoprolol, co-amilofruse, aspirin, pravastatin, isosorbide mononitrate and glyceryl trinitrate (GTN) spray.

On examination, her performance status was 1, BMI 32 kg/m² and BP 178/90 mmHg. An adenosine stress test demonstrated normal left ventricular function, perfusion and no inducible ischaemia. Blood tests were normal and urine culture was negative.

The patient wanted the most effective adjuvant treatment but was concerned about the impact of chemotherapy on her symptoms. She reported that she omitted her medication at times, as it worsened her urinary incontinence.

What is the evidence for the use of adjuvant chemotherapy in older patients with breast cancer?

What potential risks and toxicities should the patient be made aware of?

How can we best select older patients for adjuvant chemotherapy?

How should the hypertension and headaches be managed?

How can urinary incontinence be identified and managed in cancer services?

Patient outcome

Recent developments

What is the evidence for the use of adjuvant chemotherapy in older patients with breast cancer?

Breast cancer in the over-70s is associated with increased tumour size, nodal involvement, biological differences (more ER-positive and fewer HER2-positive cancers)[1,2] and inferior outcomes.[3] The incidence of male breast cancer increases with age.[4] Therefore, adjuvant systemic therapy is important for some older patients.

Few adjuvant chemotherapy randomized controlled trial (RCT) data are available for breast cancer in the over-70s.[5] Trials comparing adjuvant chemotherapy with no chemotherapy were closed early due to insufficient accrual (Chemotherapy Adjuvant Studies for Women at Advanced Age [CASA] and Adjuvant Cytotoxic Chemotherapy in Older Women [ACTION]). RCT data have not supported less intensive adjuvant chemotherapy: a trial of combination therapy (cyclophosphamide, methotrexate and fluorouracil [CMF] or cyclophosphamide and doxorubicin) versus less intensive capecitabine monotherapy reported decreased relapse-free survival and worse overall survival for capecitabine.[6] Furthermore, inferior breast cancer outcomes were seen with weekly docetaxel compared with CMF, accompanied by poorer quality of life.[7] Conversely, others support the use of docetaxel with cyclophosphamide.[8] Current evidence is insufficient to recommend an optimal chemotherapy regimen, but less intensive treatment is associated with poorer outcomes. Patients with HER2-positive breast cancer, without significant cardiac disease, should also receive trastuzumab.[9] Single-agent trastuzumab may be indicated in unfit patients,[10] although it is not recommended in NICE guidelines.

What potential risks and toxicities should the patient be made aware of?

Increasing age, poorer function and comorbidity may necessitate dose reductions.[11] Notable toxicities include mucositis with CMF,[12] congestive cardiac failure with anthracyclines,[13] and myelodysplastic syndromes.[14]

A large study found hearing deficits, recent falls and difficulty 'walking a block' were independently predictive of toxicity during adjuvant chemotherapy.[15] Another study found that 41% of older patients starting adjuvant chemotherapy had objective cognitive deficits.[16]

How can we best select older patients for adjuvant chemotherapy?

Given the lack of guidelines, a personalized approach is required for individual patients. Guidelines issued by the International Society of Geriatric Oncology and the European Society of Breast Cancer Specialists state that: 'Age alone should not influence any aspect of management of older patients with breast cancer; however, careful assessment of biological age, estimated life expectancy, risks, benefits, anticipated treatment tolerance, patient preference and potential barriers to treatment should be considered.'[9]

In the setting of adjuvant treatment, estimation of life expectancy and non-cancer-related causes of death are important. Scores such as the Charlson Comorbidity Index, which combines age with comorbidity, Adjuvant! Online (www.adjuvantonline.com) and Predict (www.predict.nhs.uk) may be helpful. An overall comorbidity score does not lead to optimization, but identifying specific comorbidities that can be optimized is helpful.

Considering chemotherapy regimens, a number of patient-specific factors must be taken into account, including the impact of specific comorbidities and choice of regimen (for instance, avoiding anthracyclines in patients with cardiac disease); polypharmacy issues; and potential barriers to treatment, such as social circumstances, carer responsibilities and transport difficulties. Some patients may benefit from referral to a geriatrician to optimize their condition prior to treatment.

A clear and detailed discussion must be had with the patient concerning the risks and benefits of chemotherapy and potential toxicity. Emergency contact details need to be provided and communication with the patient's GP is essential.

How should the hypertension and headaches be managed?

Whilst an isolated BP reading of 178/90 mmHg may reflect white coat hypertension (twice as common in older patients), it is essential that further estimates of BP are recorded. The difference between daytime ambulatory BP monitoring readings and clinic BP may be as much as 20 mmHg. In sustained hypertension it is important to obtain a target BP with a drug or combination that works and is tolerated. The National British Hypertension Society and WHO guidelines recommend those aged over 55 or Afro-Caribbean of any age be initially treated with a calcium channel blocker, with an angiotensin receptor blocker added as second line and a diuretic added as third line. Two drugs at a lower dose with no adverse effects are preferred to one at a higher dose that is poorly tolerated.

Whilst headaches may be the result of uncontrolled hypertension it is important in this age group to exclude temporal arteritis (mandatory determination of erythrocyte sedimentation rate); migraine, which rarely presents at this age, or in this particular patient; and a space-occupying lesion (mandatory CT brain scan). A targeted history is essential to ensure that the intermittent headaches are not associated with the GTN spray and to consider whether a calcium channel blocker may worsen pre-existing headaches.

How can urinary incontinence be identified and managed in cancer services?

Urinary incontinence is an important concern and is often under-assessed and undertreated in cancer patients. It often occurs as a complication of tumours of the prostate, bladder, cervix, lung, spine, vagina and urethra. All forms of cancer treatment can lead to incontinence, as the peripheral nerves and blood supply controlling the bladder may be damaged during surgery. Pelvic radiotherapy may cause nerve damage or lead to dryness and thinning of the urethra. Chemotherapeutic agents may also lead to peripheral neuropathy, and hormone therapies may cause vaginal and urethral dryness, and, hence, incontinence.

The risks of incontinence are magnified when cancer treatments are combined, and other medications (e.g. antidepressants and sedatives) may cause or exacerbate it. Many older patients have pre-existing urinary incontinence, the causes of which may be multifactorial. Causes include anatomical changes with ageing, functional ability, environmental factors, cognitive deficits and psychological problems, medications, infections, constipation, faecal loading and excess urine output (e.g. with hyperglycaemia or hypercalcaemia).

Urge incontinence (involuntary loss of urine associated with a strong desire to micturate) accounts for 50–70% of incontinence and is secondary to detrusor overactivity. Patients should be asked whether they suddenly feel the urge to go and have less than 10 min to make it to the toilet. Patients may be woken up with symptoms. Stress incontinence is the involuntary loss of urine when coughing or laughing, which is usually due to lax pelvic floor musculature.

Clinical assessment should focus on reversible factors: review of medication, constipation, environmental and psychological factors. Examination should include identifying atrophic vaginitis (treatable with vaginal oestrogen, requiring caution in breast cancer), a contributor to urgency and discomfort; prolapse or stress leak on coughing; and bladder palpation or hand-held bladder scan to rule out retention and overflow. Pelvic floor exercises should be explained and handouts given (see Bladder and Bowel Foundation at www.bladderandbowelfoundation.org), together with encouragement to 'hold on' in order to retrain the bladder. Investigations should include urinalysis, which includes analysis of urine culture, urea and electrolytes, serum glucose and calcium. Initial treatment as above should be given, but if the problem persists, specialist referral to local continence services should be considered.

Any potential impact on urinary symptoms should be considered when planning cancer treatment, such as lesser volume of fluid (e.g. avoiding cisplatin), and practical issues such as proximity of toilets.

Patient outcome

This patient had a 44% chance of developing recurrent disease and a 26% chance of death from breast cancer over 10 years (using Adjuvant! Online). Using the Charlson Comorbidity Index she had a predicted 1 and 10 year survival of 81% and 53%, respectively. Following discussion she was keen to proceed with adjuvant chemotherapy with paclitaxel, trastuzumab and radiotherapy. The suggested regimen was attractive given the short infusion duration and volume. Prior to commencing treatment she attended her GP for a medication review. Following cessation of the diuretic and commencement of pelvic floor exercises her symptoms improved. Her hypertension responded well to amlodipine and it did not worsen her headaches, which were attributed to stress when other pathology was excluded.

She stopped paclitaxel after 6 weeks due to toxicity (lethargy and neuropathy); however, she completed trastuzumab (18 cycles) and radiotherapy. She had no evidence of disease recurrence 2 years later. She had no cardiac events and no worsening of symptoms of incontinence.

Recent developments

Whilst there have been improvements in survival outcomes in older patients with breast cancer, it remains less than that observed among younger patients.[3] Older patients therefore comprise an underserved population and a better evidence base is needed. Several trials currently recruiting or awaiting reporting may contribute to evidence-based knowledge. Several RCTs will provide information on optimal adjuvant regimens in high-risk older patients (NCT00196859, NCT01204437, NCT01564056, NCT00284336). Further trials will investigate adjuvant treatment in HER2-positive cancer (NCT02102438), including single-agent trastuzumab (NCT01104935). However, older breast cancer patients included in RCTs tend to have less comorbid disease, higher socioeconomic status and lower overall mortality than an unselected population of a corresponding age.[17] Caution is therefore needed when applying RCT evidence to clinical practice.

Further studies will report on the impact of cognitive side effects of breast cancer treatment (NCT00550134) and the effect of age-related changes in the immune system on breast cancer biology (NCT02327572).

More work is urgently needed to aid selection of older patients for adjuvant systemic therapy, particularly assessing risk, both in terms of risk of breast cancer recurrence and of treatment complications. Further work to establish the gold standard of Comprehensive Geriatric Assessment within oncology is also essential.

Conclusion and learning points

- Age alone should not impede use of adjuvant chemotherapy in older breast cancer patients.

- Careful evaluation of potential benefit is crucial, particularly in terms of relative survival.

- Careful assessment of toxicity risk is important.

- Patient and family views must prevail: barriers to treatment must be identified and resolved prior to starting treatment.

- Optimization of patient condition prior to starting treatment is important, particularly a review of medication and comorbidities.

- RCT evidence is limited. Currently there is no strong evidence to support use of a specific regimen. RCT evidence suggests that less intensive chemotherapy results in inferior survival but does not ameliorate toxicity. Patient-directed regimens may be selected based on side effect profile.

- Each patient requires individual assessment and a tailored management plan.

- Urinary incontinence in older cancer patients is under-assessed and undertreated.

- A careful history and understanding of the causes of incontinence will aid diagnosis and treatment.

- It should be established whether hypertension is a real phenomenon; if so, it should be treated according to WHO guidelines.

- Headaches are often benign in nature but can indicate serious underlying pathology. Frequently used cardiac drugs may cause or worsen headaches.

References

1 Schonberg MA, Marcantonio ER, Li D, *et al.* Breast cancer among the oldest old: tumor characteristics, treatment choices, and survival. *J Clin Oncol* 2010; 28: 2038–45.

2 Wildiers H, Van Calster B, van de Poll-Franse LV, *et al.* Relationship between age and axillary lymph node involvement in women with breast cancer. *J Clin Oncol* 2009; 27: 2931–7.

3 Rosso S, Gondos A, Zanetti R, *et al.* Up-to-date estimates of breast cancer survival for the years 2000–2004 in 11 European countries: the role of screening and a comparison with data from the United States. *Eur J Cancer* 2010; 46: 3351–7.

4 Giordano SH, Cohen DS, Buzdar AU, *et al.* Breast carcinoma in men: a population-based study. *Cancer* 2004; 101: 51–7.

5 Early Breast Cancer Trialists' Collaborative (EBCTG). Effects of chemotherapy and hormonal therapy for early breast cancer on recurrence and 15-year survival: an overview of the randomised trials. *Lancet* 2005; 365: 1687–717.

6 Muss HB, Berry DA, Cirrincione CT, *et al.* Adjuvant chemotherapy in older women with early-stage breast cancer. *New Engl J Med* 2009; 360: 2055–65.

7 Perrone F, Nuzzo F, Di Rella F, *et al.* Weekly docetaxel versus CMF as adjuvant chemotherapy for older women with early breast cancer: final results of the randomized phase III ELDA trial. *Ann Oncol* 2015; 26: 675–82.

8 Jones S, Holmes FA, O'Shaughnessy J, *et al.* Docetaxel with cyclophosphamide is associated with an overall survival benefit compared with doxorubicin and cyclophosphamide: 7-year follow-up of US Oncology Research Trial 9735. *J Clin Oncol* 2009; 27: 1177–83.

9 Biganzoli L, Wildiers H, Oakman C, *et al.* Management of elderly patients with breast cancer: updated recommendations of the International Society of Geriatric Oncology (SIOG) and European Society of Breast Cancer Specialists (EUSOMA). *Lancet Oncol* 2012; 13: e148–60.

10 Goldhirsch A, Wood WC, Coates AS, *et al.* Strategies for subtypes – dealing with the diversity of breast cancer: highlights of the St. Gallen International Expert Consensus on the Primary Therapy of Early Breast Cancer 2011. *Ann Oncol* 2011; 22: 1736–47.

11 Garg P, Rana F, Gupta R, *et al.* Predictors of toxicity and toxicity profile of adjuvant chemotherapy in elderly breast cancer patients. *Breast J* 2009; 15: 404–8.

12 Crivellari D, Bonetti M, Castiglione-Gertsch M, *et al.* Burdens and benefits of adjuvant cyclophosphamide, methotrexate, and fluorouracil and tamoxifen for elderly patients with breast cancer: the International Breast Cancer Study Group Trial VII. *J Clin Oncol* 2000; 18: 1412–22.

13 Pinder MC, Duan Z, Goodwin JS, *et al.* Congestive heart failure in older women treated with adjuvant anthracycline chemotherapy for breast cancer. *J Clin Oncol* 2007; 25: 3808–15.

14 Patt DA, Duan Z, Fang S, *et al.* Acute myeloid leukemia after adjuvant breast cancer therapy in older women: understanding risk. *J Clin Oncol* 2007; 25: 3871–6.

15 Hurria A, Togawa K, Mohile SG, *et al.* Predicting chemotherapy toxicity in older adults with cancer: a prospective multicenter study. *J Clin Oncol* 2011; 29: 3457–65.

16 Lange M, Giffard B, Noal S, *et al.* Baseline cognitive functions among elderly patients with localised breast cancer. *Eur J Cancer* 2014; 50: 2181–9.

17 van de Water W, Kiderlen M, Bastiaannet E, *et al.* External validity of a trial comprised of elderly patients with hormone receptor-positive breast cancer. *J Natl Cancer Inst* 2014; 106: dju051.

Further reading

- Muss HB. Adjuvant chemotherapy in older women with breast cancer: who and what? *J Clin Oncol* 2014; 32: 1996–2000.

06 A Patient with Intermediate-Risk Prostate Cancer, Transient Ischaemic Attack and Impotence

Kathryn Mitchell, Hannah Taylor, Danielle Harari, Malcolm Mason

Case history

A 79-year-old man was referred to the urology department following a routine blood test in primary care which revealed a prostate-specific antigen (PSA) level of 17 ng/ml. He did not have any lower urinary tract symptoms. His past medical history included hypertension, type 2 diabetes, and a history of transient ischaemic attack (TIA).

In the one-stop urology clinic, digital rectal examination revealed a hard nodule in the prostate, and a biopsy confirmed adenocarcinoma of the prostate with a Gleason score of 3+4=7. An MRI revealed a large tumour in the right lobe of the prostate; however, it had not breached the capsule. He had a staging bone scan which was normal. He was therefore staged at T2bN0M0. The urology multidisciplinary team recommended consideration and discussion of radical treatment options.

At the initial oncology clinic, the patient's general fitness for treatment was assessed by taking a medical history and doing baseline tests. He was on aspirin 75 mg for a previous TIA with no neurological consequences; his BP and blood glucose were well controlled on medication. These comorbidities did not preclude his having surgery (radical prostatectomy), but other options were discussed particularly in the context of increased postoperative risk of incontinence with advancing age. Detailed discussions were had with the patient regarding the practicalities, risks and benefits of radical radiotherapy with concurrent androgen deprivation therapy (ADT) versus watchful waiting.

The patient decided to proceed with radical radiotherapy. The oncologist liaised with the GP to ensure that cardiac risk factors were optimized to reduce the increased risk of cardiovascular morbidity associated with ADT. The patient completed a treatment course of 3 months of neoadjuvant ADT (goserelin 3.6 mg monthly), followed by 74 Gy in 37 fractions of external beam radiation therapy (EBRT) to the prostate with concurrent ADT.

The patient developed grade 1 acute bowel and urinary toxicities during treatment but otherwise had no significant short-term side effects. He was put on surveillance after treatment with 3 monthly PSA blood tests to monitor for evidence of biochemical relapse. At the 3 month follow-up visit he reported having experienced a transient weakness and tingling in his left hand and the oncologist referred him to the stroke physician for assessment of TIA (Table 6.1). At the 6 month follow-up he mentioned that he had persistent problems with impotence that were affecting his quality of life.

What was the goal of the cancer treatment for this patient?

How can health status be evaluated and optimized in this older patient particularly in relation to history of TIA and increased risk associated with ADT?

How can the longer term consequence of impotence be managed?

What is the evidence base for the cancer treatment options?

What was the goal of the cancer treatment for this patient?

The goals of cancer treatment should be driven by a balance of risk. The main concern is that there may be future complications of the disease that result in significant morbidity to the patient, or indeed cancer-related mortality. The patient's age and comorbidities have to be

Table 6.1 Evidence-based diagnosis and management of TIA (adapted from NICE[9] and Royal College of Physicians[10] guidelines).

Symptoms of likely TIA: focal symptoms with complete resolution of focal neurology
Sudden onset of:
- Loss of power (weakness or clumsiness on one side)
- Loss of speech (dysphasia/dyslexia/dysgraphia)
- Loss of sensation
- Loss of vision

Unlikely TIA symptoms
- Faintness, syncope
- Non-specific dizziness, light-headedness
- Confusion, mental disorientation
- Spreading sensory disturbance to adjacent body parts over several minutes (consider migraine or focal sensory seizure)

Risk assessment
People who have had a suspected TIA should be assessed as soon as possible for their risk of subsequent stroke using a validated scoring system, such as ABCD2:
A = age >60 (1 point)
B = BP >140/90 mmHg (1 point)
C = clinical feature: unilateral weakness (2 points), speech disturbance with no weakness (1 point)
D = duration of symptoms >60 min (2 points), 10–59 min (1 point)
D = diabetes (1 point)
High risk of stroke = ABCD2 score ≥4

Investigation
Patient at high risk of stroke (ABCD2 score ≥4) should have investigation within 24 h of onset of symptoms, and those at low risk within 1 week
- Urgent brain imaging (diffusion-weighted MRI)
- Carotid imaging to look for stenosis that may require surgical intervention (carotid endarterectomy)

Treatment
All patients should be prescribed aspirin 300 mg daily, initiated as soon as possible following TIA, and continued for up to 14 days after which clopidogrel monotherapy (75 mg daily) should be given indefinitely for secondary prevention

balanced with his estimated life expectancy and the potential side effects that may result from radical treatment. The patient's own goals and expectations should also be explored to aid with joint decision making. In this case, further assessment and management of the patient's comorbidities by a geriatrician (to comprehensively manage cardiac risk factors, TIA and diabetes) could have optimized him for anaesthesia and surgery, but his choice was to proceed with radiotherapy. The emphasis therefore needed to be on reducing toxicity both in the short and long term.

Patients should be assessed for pre-existing bowel problems: some conditions, such as active inflammatory bowel disease, are a contraindication to radiotherapy. Baseline information was taken regarding lower urinary tract symptoms and sexual function (e.g. using the King's Health Questionnaire), as well as bowel function. Radiotherapy will result in some degree of minor, long-term bowel dysfunction in nearly half of patients, but in a small percentage it can be significant. Radiotherapy is also associated with an increased risk of incontinence, especially in patients who have had a transurethral resection in the past.

How can health status be evaluated and optimized in this older patient particularly in relation to history of TIA and increased risk associated with ADT?

In localized prostate cancer, a life expectancy of greater than 10 years is considered mandatory to ensure that there is benefit from radical treatment. With increasing life expectancy a greater number of older men will be treated. At present in the UK, the average life expectancy for a man of 65 is 18.2 years (Office for National Statistics data). Comorbidity assessment is essential to inform mortality risk unrelated to cancer per individual. Comorbidity screening tools such as the Cumulative Illness Rating Scale–Geriatrics (CIRS-G) and the Charlson Comorbidity Index (CCI) can identify people with low risk and those who need further assessment and optimization for consideration of radical treatment. In a study assessing the impact of comorbidity on survival among men with localized prostate cancer, at 10 years most men with a CCI score >2 had died from non-cancer-related causes (regardless of the grade of tumour or patient age).[1] Comprehensive assessment will lead to optimization of comorbidities that may in turn impact life expectancy in individuals, e.g. diabetes, high BP, cardiac risk factors, poor nutritional status. The International Society of Geriatric Oncology Geriatric Screening Tool (G8) is a systematic evaluation of health status. It assesses age, nutrition, mobility, neuropsychological problems, polypharmacy, and patients' perception of their own health. A score >14 suggests that the patient should receive the same treatment as younger patients and those with a score ≤14 should undergo a full comprehensive geriatric review to assess for reversible pathology and potential for optimizing treatment of underlying problems.

This patient's primary comorbidity was a history of TIA a few years previously. He described it as a sudden but short-lived loss of speech. When he developed a transient weakness in the left side during ADT treatment he required further assessment (Table 6.1) and was urgently referred by oncology to the stroke service. Brain MRI showed small-vessel disease only and carotid Doppler ultrasonography showed <70% stenosis, so no surgical intervention was required. He was switched from aspirin to long-term clopidogrel.

ADT is unequivocally associated with an increased risk of all forms of cardiovascular disease, as well as an increased risk of developing diabetes or metabolic syndrome. It is recommended that patients should be informed about the increased risk of cardiovascular morbidity associated with ADT and advised to adopt relevant lifestyle changes to optimize their risk factors. Patients should be encouraged to take regular physical exercise, normalize their BMI, decrease alcohol intake and stop smoking. Optimization of cardiac risk factors should also be considered. BP, serum cholesterol and glycaemic control can all be addressed to reduce the risk of cardiovascular morbidity and mortality.

How can the longer term consequence of impotence be managed?

This patient developed erectile dysfunction following treatment: it is important to consider sexuality in older patients. Comorbidities may affect sexuality in complicated ways. Men who have had a heart attack may be anxious about having a further event during sex, which can reduce libido, but studies have shown that the risk of having a recurrent event during sex is in fact only 2 in 1 million. Medical causes of erectile dysfunction in older men that can be optimized include diabetes (tight glucose control may restore potency), untreated hypertension, and Parkinson's disease. Certain medications affect sexual functioning (e.g. certain types of antihypertensives, diuretics, alpha-blockers and antidepressants) and these can be reviewed.

All forms of ADT will cause impotence, which may improve once serum testosterone levels have recovered following ADT cessation. Typically, after 3 months of ADT, this can take as much as 1 year, and sometimes longer. There is some evidence that sildenafil improves ADT- and radiation-induced erectile dysfunction, but responses are seen only in a minority of patients. Long-term erectile dysfunction will occur in 30–80% of patients who were not impotent before radiotherapy.

What is the evidence base for the cancer treatment options?

Surveillance

A recent study evaluated the outcomes of surgery versus surveillance for low-risk prostate cancer. The study assessed the impact of patient age, baseline health status and patient preferences. Older patients with poor baseline health had a much smaller benefit from radical treatment and were likely to have a better quality-adjusted life expectancy with surveillance.[2]

Radical prostatectomy

The Scandinavian Prostate Cancer Group study number 4 (SPCG-4) randomized patients with localized prostate cancer to radical prostatectomy versus watchful waiting. Patients under the age of 65 treated by radical prostatectomy had significantly better overall survival (OS). In men over 65, however, surgery did not prolong OS but was associated with a reduced risk of metastasis (RR 0.68) and a reduction in the need for ADT (RR 0.6),[3] both of which might be considered to be beneficial in selected men, even in the absence of a survival benefit. It was also noted that postoperative complications were related more to the presence of comorbidities than to increasing age. Incontinence was present more frequently in older patients.[4,5]

EBRT with ADT

Regardless of age, EBRT (intensity-modulated radiation therapy at a dose of >72 Gy) and radical prostatectomy have comparable efficacy and result in similar treatment-related comorbidities.[6]

There is often concern with regard to neoadjuvant and concurrent ADT alongside EBRT in older patients, especially in those with pre-existing heart conditions. ADT increases the efficacy of EBRT;[7] however, in the presence of moderate to severe comorbidities the survival benefit may be less significant.[8]

Conclusion

- Older patients with localized prostate cancer should have a thorough assessment of their health status to ensure benefit from radical treatment.
- Patients with symptoms of TIA should be investigated promptly with review by the stroke service. ADT increases the risk of TIA and other vascular events.
- Sexual function should be considered in older men undergoing prostate cancer treatment, especially in those with medical comorbidities that may contribute to impotency.

References

1 Albertsen PC, Moore DF, Shih W, *et al.* Impact of comorbidity on survival among men with localised prostate cancer. *J Clin Oncol* 2011; 29: 1335–41.

2 Liu D, Lehmann HP, Frick KD, *et al.* Active surveillance versus surgery for low risk prostate cancer: a clinical decision analysis. *J Urol* 2012; 187: 1241–6.

3 Bill-Axelson A, Holmberg L, Garmo H, *et al.* Radical prostatectomy or watchful waiting in early prostate cancer. *N Engl J Med* 2014; 370: 932–42.

4 Begg CB, Riedel ER, Bach PB, *et al.* Variations in morbidity after radical prostatectomy. *N Engl J Med* 2002; 346: 1138–44.

5 Stanford JL, Feng Z, Hamilton AS, *et al.* Urinary and sexual function after radical prostatectomy for clinically localised prostate cancer: the Prostate Cancer Outcomes Study. *JAMA* 2000; 283: 354–60.

6 Kupelian PA, Elshaikh M, Reddy CA, *et al.* Comparison of the efficacy of local therapies for localised prostate cancer in the prostate-specific antigen era: a large single-institution experience with radical prostatectomy and external bean radiotherapy. *J Clin Oncol* 2002; 20: 3376–85.

7 Bolla M, Van Teinhoven G, Warde P, *et al.* External irradiation with or without long-term androgen suppression for prostate cancer with high metastatic risk: 10-year results of an EORTC randomised study. *Lancet Oncol* 2010; 11: 1066–73.

8 D'Amico A, Renshaw AA, Loffredo M, *et al.* Androgen suppression and radiation vs radiation alone for prostate cancer: a randomised controlled trial. *JAMA* 2008; 299: 289–95.

9 National Institute for Health and Clinical Excellence (2010). *Clopidogrel and modified-release dipyridamole for the prevention of occlusive vascular events. NICE technology appraisal guidance 210.* Available from: www.nice.org.uk/guidance/TA210 (accessed 14 August 2015).

10 Royal College of Physicians, Intercollegiate Stroke Working Party (2012). *National clinical guideline for stroke.* 4th ed. Available from: www.rcplondon.ac.uk/resources/stroke-guidelines (accessed 15 September 2015).

07 Surgery for Upper Gastrointestinal Cancer in a Morbidly Obese Patient with Diabetes and Renal Impairment

Doraid Alrifai, David Shipway, Sarah Ngan

Case history

An 81-year-old man presented with a 4 month history of nausea, epigastric discomfort and unintentional 6 kg weight loss. He was found to have mild anaemia (Hb 98 g/l, mean corpuscular volume 92 fl) and low iron indices. His baseline creatinine was 144 µmol/l and estimated glomerular filtration rate (eGFR) 47 ml/min. He underwent gastroscopy, during which an ulcer was detected at the gastro-oesophageal junction (GOJ). Histopathology confirmed an undifferentiated adenocarcinoma. CT staging demonstrated tumour invasion into the gastric subserosa and two enlarged perigastric lymph nodes. His tumour was clinically staged as T3N1M0.

His past medical history included type 2 diabetes mellitus, diabetic nephropathy (stage 3 chronic kidney disease) and obesity (BMI 35.2 kg/m^2). He suffered from painful osteoarthritis of the hips and knees and had an exercise tolerance of 100 m. He struggled to climb two flights of stairs without resting, mainly because of arthritic symptoms rather than because of dyspnoea or chest pain.

He was an ex-smoker who drank minimal alcohol. He lived in a first floor flat with his wife, who had had a stroke and suffered from reduced mobility. He was independent in his activities of daily living and required no support from social services. His medication at presentation included amlodipine, ramipril, metformin, gliclazide, and ibuprofen as and when required.

What are the current evidence-based treatment options for managing this tumour type?

What other information might influence treatment decisions?

What is the relevance of morbid obesity to perioperative management?

How will stage 3 chronic kidney disease affect his management?

What is important specifically about diabetes in this context?

Patient outcome

What are the current evidence-based treatment options for managing this tumour type?

The commonest locations for upper gastrointestinal malignancies include the oesophagus, stomach and GOJ. Ninety percent of gastric tumours are adenocarcinomas, which can be subdivided into diffuse (undifferentiated) and intestinal (well differentiated). Gastrointestinal stromal tumours, lymphoma and neuroendocrine tumours constitute the remaining 10%. Oesophageal tumours can consist of adenocarcinoma, squamous cell carcinoma or, rarely, small cell carcinoma.[1] The commonest risk factors and clinical features are shown in Tables 7.1 and 7.2, respectively.

Initial staging investigations for tumours of gastric and oesophageal origin should involve a CT scan including multiplanar reconstruction of the thorax, abdomen and pelvis to determine the presence of metastatic disease. Further staging with PET-CT, endoscopic ultrasound and staging laparoscopy may be considered in addition, depending on the location of the primary lesion.

Gold standard treatment for gastro-oesophageal tumours follows a complex pathway. Early tumours (T1a or less) may be treated with endoscopic mucosal resection.[2] Oesophageal tumours with no lymph node involvement (T2 or less) may proceed directly to radical resection.

More advanced gastric and oesophageal adenocarcinomas (including Siewert types I, II and III GOJ adenocarcinomas) should be considered for surgical resection. Proximal gastric tumours can be treated with total gastrectomy, and distal tumours with subtotal gastrectomy. Cardia, subcardia and type II GOJ tumours are treated with extended gastrectomy or oesophagogastrectomy. Lower oesophageal types I and II GOJ tumours are treated with oesophageal resection. The extent of lymphadenectomy is tailored to the location and stage of the tumour.

Table 7.1 Commonest risk factors for upper gastrointestinal tumours.

- Male
- Age
- Tobacco smoking
- Alcohol (>6 units/day)
- *Helicobacter pylori*
- Atrophic gastritis
- High BMI
- Rubber production
- Gamma radiation/x-ray
- Partial gastrectomy
- Blood group A
- Chronic gastro-oesophageal reflux disease
- Barrett's oesophagus
- Family history
- Familial (hereditary diffuse gastric cancer, hereditary non-polyposis colorectal cancer, familial adenomatous polyposis, Peutz–Jeghers syndrome)

Table 7.2 Clinical features of non-disseminated gastrointestinal tumours.

- Retrosternal or epigastric pain/dyspepsia
- Upper gastrointestinal bleeding
  - Haematemesis
  - Malaena
  - Anaemia
- Dysphagia/odynophagia
- Nausea/vomiting
- Weight loss
- Epigastric mass (also lower oesophageal tumours)

Perioperative combination chemotherapy (combined pre- and postoperative treatment) improves the survival of patients diagnosed with locally advanced tumours (T2+).[3] For oesophageal adenocarcinomas, preoperative chemoradiotherapy may also be considered, as it improves long-term survival over surgery alone.[4] Adjuvant chemoradiation is not routinely used in the UK but may be considered in high-risk patients who have not received neoadjuvant treatment. Patients not suitable for surgery may be considered for chemotherapy with or without radiotherapy.

Squamous cell oesophageal carcinomas are managed differently. Chemoradiotherapy is the treatment of choice for localized squamous cell carcinoma of the proximal oesophagus.[5] Localized tumours of the middle and lower third of the oesophagus may be treated with chemoradiotherapy alone, neoadjuvant chemoradiotherapy or perioperative chemotherapy with surgery.[6]

What other information might influence treatment decisions?

Surgical resection of gastro-oesophageal tumours represents a major physiological challenge to all patients. Concerns about adverse outcome have often resulted in the undertreatment of those with significant comorbidity or advanced age. It is increasingly clear that, although important, cardiorespiratory function is not the only predictor of outcome. Frailty and cognitive impairment also predict surgical complications and these factors may be more important than chronological age. Historically, time pressures have resulted in decision making by cancer multidisciplinary teams (MDTs) without important information that could influence outcomes. Comprehensive Geriatric Assessment (CGA) systematically addresses the medical, cognitive, nutritional, functional, psychological and social issues of the patient. Embedded postoperative medical liaison and addressing reversible problems early in the perioperative setting improve perioperative complication rates and surgical outcomes and reduce inpatient length of stay. CGA has also been shown to be advantageous in the context of systemic chemotherapy, and is becoming more widely used in the field of oncogeriatrics.[7]

What is the relevance of morbid obesity to perioperative management?

Older patients with upper gastrointestinal malignancy are commonly nutritionally impaired at diagnosis. Low BMI is associated with postoperative complications including infection and poor wound healing. High-risk patients (weight loss >10% over 6 months, BMI <18.5 kg/m^2, serum albumin <30 g/l) are likely to require nutritional support prior to surgery.[8] Enteral feeding tubes and oesophageal stents may play a role, since neoadjuvant chemotherapy may worsen nutritional status.

Obese patients face different problems. These commonly include undiagnosed obesity-associated hypoventilation or obstructive sleep apnoea (OSA), both of which can lead to perioperative respiratory failure. Obese patients with OSA may report excess fatigue and daytime somnolence, although these are common in patients recently diagnosed with upper gastrointestinal cancer, who have high rates of coexisting anaemia. Specific screening for OSA is recommended using the Epworth Sleepiness Scale. If the results suggest a sleep disorder, urgent referral for sleep studies before surgery may be indicated. Treatment of obesity in the context of urgent cancer surgery is difficult. There is little opportunity for structured weight loss, so slow ventilator weaning and vigilance for respiratory failure may be necessary.[9]

Musculoskeletal disorders such as osteoarthritis are also more prevalent in obesity. These may result in slow rehabilitation and the need for additional social services support at discharge. In this case, the patient was the primary caregiver for his wife, so the wider social implications of this patient's illness need to be taken into account. A referral to social services was made to ensure the patient's wife was adequately cared for during her husband's hospitalization.

How will stage 3 chronic kidney disease affect his management?

Before chemotherapy, patients with an eGFR <60 ml/min should undergo measurement of EDTA clearance. Platinum-based drugs and fluoropyrimidines may be omitted if the patient demonstrates significant renal impairment. Meticulous attention to fluid balance is needed perioperatively to maintain euvolaemia. Avoidance of nephrotoxins, renal dose adjustment of medication and avoidance of intravenous contrast (wherever possible) are also essential.

What is important specifically about diabetes in this context?

Patients with suboptimal glycaemic control (HbA_{1c} >75 mmol/mol) are at an elevated risk of surgical complications. Perioperative management has recently been standardized by national guidance.[10] This guidance recommends preoperative optimization of HbA_{1c}, which is often made worse by steroids given as an adjunct to chemotherapy. Perioperative target glucose should aim for 6–10 mmol/l, and both oral hypoglycaemic agents and insulin should be modified according to the timeline of surgery.[10]

Diabetes is often complicated by undiagnosed macrovascular complications. Older people (and those with diabetes) are less likely to have typical anginal symptoms in the presence of ischaemic heart disease. Patients should have a 12-lead ECG as part of their preoperative assessment, and exercise tolerance should be assessed using the metabolic equivalent of task (MET) scale (Table 7.3). Our patient has difficulty climbing two flights of stairs in a single attempt, and therefore has MET 3. MET <4 may indicate cardiorespiratory disease.[9] In an obese and diabetic patient, there must be a high suspicion of cardiac failure or reversible ischaemia. Further investigation should be conducted with stress echocardiography, cardiac MRI or coronary CT. Revascularization or optimization before surgery may be indicated. Anthracycline and fluoropyrimidine chemotherapy may need to be avoided due to the risk of cardiac dysfunction with these drugs.[11]

Microvascular complications of diabetes often include subclinical peripheral neuropathy and visual impairment. Neuropathy can be exacerbated by platinum chemotherapy, which may require substitution. Where deficits are present, they may be associated with falls, reduced mobility and slow rehabilitation.

Table 7.3 MET scale.

MET value	Activity
2	Light gardening/walking slowly
3	Vacuuming/walking at average pace
4	Weeding garden/climbing two flights of stairs
5	Mowing lawn/brisk walking
6	Moving heavy objects
7	Swimming
8–10	Running

1 MET = 3.5 ml O_2 uptake per kg per min.

Patient outcome

Both metformin and ibuprofen were stopped due to their association with renal impairment and peptic ulceration, which can potentially be exacerbated by the use of steroid therapy, a common adjunct to chemotherapy. The risk of surgical complications was higher given the previously discussed stage 3 chronic kidney disease, obesity and diabetes, yet cardiorespiratory status was determined to be acceptable after stress echocardiography.

The patient underwent an oesophagogastrectomy supported by perioperative chemotherapy. Neoadjuvant epirubicin, cisplatin and capecitabine chemotherapy was delivered, with a dose reduction in both cisplatin and capecitabine in view of the renal impairment. His inpatient postoperative recovery time was significantly protracted to 7 weeks. His nutritional status was compromised, so he required parenteral nutrition during his stay. On discharge he had re-established satisfactory oral intake and his Eastern Cooperative Oncology Group performance status improved from 4 to 2 with help from the physiotherapy team. Given the time lapse and reduced performance status postoperatively, it was decided not to proceed to adjuvant chemotherapy. He is currently on a clinical surveillance programme. He continues to have regular follow-up, with no evidence of relapse of disease 18 months after surgery.

Conclusion and learning points

Overall life expectancy for an 81-year-old man living in the UK is approximately 7 years. It is increasingly clear that chronological age is not always a true reflection of biological age.

- Comorbidities and frailty may be more important in predicting outcomes; however, disentangling these factors in individual patients can be challenging.

- Deciding where absolute contraindications to surgery exist represents a major challenge for meetings of the cancer MDT.

- CGA and preoperative optimization, combined with embedded perioperative medical support, is proven to improve surgical outcomes.

- Review of medication and dose adjustment of cytotoxic chemotherapy are important to reduce toxicity.

- An individualized approach is necessary.

References

1 Silvera SAN, Mayne ST, Gammon MD, *et al.* Diet and lifestyle factors and risk of subtypes of esophageal and gastric cancer: classification tree analysis. *Ann Epidemiol* 2014; 24: 50–7.

2 Crumley AB, Going JJ, McEwan K, *et al.* Endoscopic mucosal resection for gastroesophageal cancer in a U.K. population. Long term follow-up of a consecutive series. *Surg Endosc* 2011; 25: 543–8.

3 Cunningham D, Allum WH, Stenning SP, *et al.* Perioperative chemotherapy versus surgery alone for resectable gastroesophageal cancer. *N Engl J Med* 2006; 355: 11–20.

4 Stahl M, Walz MK, Stuschke M, *et al.* Phase III comparison of perioperative chemotherapy compared with chemoradiotherapy in patients with locally advanced adenocarcinoma of the esophagogastric junction. *J Clin Oncol* 2009; 27: 851–6.

5 Stahl M, Stuschke M, Lehmann N, *et al.* Chemoradiation with and without surgery in patients with locally advanced squamous cell carcinoma of the esophagus. *J Clin Oncol* 2005; 23: 2310–17.

6 Minsky BD, Pajak TF, Ginsberg RJ, *et al.* INT 0123 (Radiation Therapy Oncology Group 94-05) phase III trial of combined-modality therapy for esophageal cancer: high-dose versus standard-dose radiation therapy. *J Clin Oncol* 2002; 20: 1167–74.

7 Partridge JS, Harari D, Martin FC, *et al.* The impact of pre-operative comprehensive geriatric assessment on postoperative outcomes in older patients undergoing scheduled surgery: a systematic review. *Anaesthesia* 2014: 69 (suppl 1): 8–16.

8 Weimann A, Braga M, Harsanyi L, *et al.* ESPEN guidelines on enteral nutrition: surgery including organ transplantation. *Clin Nutr* 2006; 25: 224–44.

9 Shipway DJH, Harari D, Dhesi JK. Peri-operative management of older people undergoing surgery. *Rev Clin Gerontol* 2014; 24: 78–92.

10 Dhatariya K, Flanagan D, Hilton L, *et al. Management of adults with diabetes undergoing surgery and elective procedures: improving standards.* London: NHS Diabetes, 2011.

11 Poldermans D, Bax JJ, Boersma E, *et al.* Guidelines for pre-operative cardiac risk assessment and perioperative cardiac management in non-cardiac surgery: the Task Force for Preoperative Cardiac Risk Assessment and Perioperative Cardiac Management in Non-cardiac Surgery of the European Society of Cardiology (ESC) and endorsed by the European Society of Anaesthesiology (ESA). *Eur J Anaesthesiol* 2010; 27: 92–137.

Further reading

- European Society for Medical Oncology (2013). *Oesophageal cancer: ESMO clinical practice guidelines.* Available from: www.esmo.org/Guidelines/Gastrointestinal-Cancers/Oesophageal-Cancer (accessed 30 June 2015).

08 Carcinoma of Unknown Primary in a Patient with Multiple Comorbidities

Kiruthikah Thillai, Jacqueline Simms, Sarah Rudman, Jonathan Birns

Case history

An 85-year-old woman with hypertension, ischaemic heart disease and chronic kidney disease presented with a 6 month history of anorexia, malaise and weight loss. She was compliant with antiplatelet and antihypertensive medications. She lived alone, spending most of the day resting, and required a twice-daily carer to help her wash and dress. Physical examination revealed hepatomegaly. Serum haematology and biochemistry showed normocytic anaemia (Hb 8.2 g/dl [normal range 11.5–16.5]); raised aspartate transaminase (262 IU/l [normal range 0–37]); raised creatinine (200 mol/l [normal range 45–84]); and an estimated glomerular filtration rate 21 ml/min (normal range 70–130) (similar to that measured 1 year previously). Abdominal ultrasound revealed a solitary liver lesion in segment VII measuring 4.2×3.7 cm, indicating a possible metastasis. Subsequent CT scanning confirmed three further bilobar metastatic lesions and multiple enlarged abdominal lymph nodes. Histology from an ultrasound-guided liver biopsy confirmed a poorly differentiated adenocarcinoma that stained positive for cytokeratin (CK) 7 and negative for CK20 and oestrogen receptor (ER). No primary tumour was identified on imaging. Comprehensive Geriatric Assessment (CGA) helped to determine optimal management strategies for her new oncological diagnosis, comorbidities and frailty. Supportive care was recommended in view of the unfavourable risk–benefit profile of systemic anticancer treatment. Her fatigue, social isolation and declining functional independence was managed with four-times-daily carer input, a 'meals-on-wheels' service and community-based palliative care.

What are the guidelines and evidence for investigating patients with metastatic disease of unknown primary?

What are the considerations when investigating a frail older patient with suspected cancer of unknown primary (CUP)?

How can prognosis be assessed in this patient?

What evidence-based treatment options are available for this patient?

What are the realistic goals for this patient?

How may CGA help identify and implement best supportive care for this patient?

What are the guidelines and evidence for investigating patients with metastatic disease of unknown primary?

NICE guidelines advise hospitals with a cancer centre to have a dedicated acute oncology service that ensures all patients with a malignancy of unidentified primary origin (MUO) are investigated appropriately (Table 8.1). Routine imaging by CT is supplemented by more dedicated investigations depending on the individual features of each case;[1,2] for example, in a female with isolated axillary lymphadenopathy, breast imaging may be indicated.

If, after a full diagnostic work-up, a primary site is not found, MUO is amended to CUP. CUP accounts for 3–5% of invasive cancers and comprises moderately differentiated adenocarcinomas (60%), poorly differentiated carcinomas or adenocarcinomas (30%), poorly differentiated or undifferentiated malignant neoplasms (5%), squamous cell cancers (5%), and, rarely, neuroendocrine or mixed tumours.[3] Histological diagnosis is advisable with immunohistochemistry, aiding the identification of the site of origin based on the theory that homogeneity remains between occult primary and metastatic sites. By interpreting immunohistochemistry results, it is possible to assign up to 25% of cases with CUP to a primary site of origin. Guidelines suggest initial staining should include CK7, CK20, thyroid transcription factor (TTF-1) and placental alkaline phosphatase. Further staining includes ER for women and prostate-specific antigen (PSA) for men (Table 8.2). Genomic studies are not currently recommended due to the lack of prospective evidence.

Table 8.1   Initial diagnostics for MUO (adapted from NICE guidelines[2]).

Diagnostics test for MUO

- Comprehensive history and physical examination
- Routine bloods
- Chest radiograph
- Myeloma screen (if isolated or multiple lytic bone lesions are present)
- Symptom-directed endoscopy
- CT scan of chest, abdomen and pelvis
- PSA (in men)
- CA-125 in women with peritoneal malignancy or ascites
- AFP and beta-hCG, particularly in presence of midline nodal disease
- Testicular ultrasound if clinically compatible with germ cell tumours
- Biopsy and standard histological examination with immunohistochemistry where necessary

AFP, alpha-fetoprotein; beta-hCG, beta subunit of human chorionic gonadotropin.

Table 8.2   Commonly used immunohistochemistry staining to identify site of origin of malignancy.

Immunohistochemistry stain	Site of origin
beta-hCG, AFP	Germ cell tumour
CK7, CK20, CDX-2, CEA	Colorectal cancer
Hep Par 1	Hepatocellular carcinoma
TTF-1, CK7, napsin-A	Lung
ER, HER2	Breast
Chromogranin, synaptophysin	Neuroendocrine
CK7, CK20, uroplakin III	Urothelial

AFP, alpha-fetoprotein; beta-hCG, beta subunit of human chorionic gonadotropin; CDX, caudal-related homeobox; CEA, carcinoembryonic antigen; Hep Par 1, hepatocyte paraffin 1; HER2, human epidermal growth factor receptor 2; TTF, thyroid transcription factor.

What are the considerations when investigating a frail older patient with suspected CUP?

Managing CUP in the older person poses unique challenges. Compared with the younger population, older patients may present with more widespread metastatic disease and may be relatively asymptomatic until an acute clinical event causes rapid decline. Furthermore, non-specific cancer symptoms such as fatigue may overlap with symptomatic comorbidities such as undiagnosed heart failure.

If a patient is not to receive systemic treatment, certain aspects of the diagnostic work-up may be withheld if they will not alter overall management. For example, tissue confirmation of malignancy may not be warranted if imaging is sufficient to confirm metastatic cancer.[4] However, confirmation of histological subtype may lead to a more accurate prognosis and enable more detailed patient discussions and focused symptomatic care. More invasive investigations such as liver biopsies are often well tolerated in older adults.

How can prognosis be assessed in this patient?

Several prognostic models have been proposed based on retrospective analyses.[5] Factors include site of tumour and metastases, number of metastases, poor differentiation of tumour, performance status (PS) and serum lactate dehydrogenase (LDH). PS is an observation of cancer patients' mobility and overall functional level that is used to facilitate treatment decisions. A number of scoring systems have been used, one being the WHO score, which ranges from 0 to 5, with 0 denoting perfect health and 5 death. Culine et al.[5] suggested that in combination with LDH level, PS may be used to separate patients with CUP into good and poor risk categories; indeed, patients with PS 0–1 and normal LDH were found to have a median overall survival (OS) of 11.7 months compared with patients with PS 2–3 and/or raised LDH, who had a median OS of 3.9 months ($p<0.001$). However, in older people, PS alone is too generic for a meaningful assessment of comorbidities. It is valid in identifying fit patients who have PS 0–1, but those with PS 2 require more extensive CGA.[6]

What evidence–based treatment options are available for this patient?

There is evidence to suggest that survival is improved if a potential primary site is identified and managed accordingly. However, when no clear tumour type is suspected, treatment comprises various surgical, radiotherapy and/or chemotherapy regimens, although the optimum treatment strategy remains unknown due to the lack of prospective randomized trials (Table 8.3). No targeted chemotherapeutic agent has been approved for the management of CUP, with meta-analyses suggesting no superiority among regimens that contained platinum, a taxane or 'new-generation' drugs such as gemcitabine, vinca alkaloids or irinotecan. There is some evidence that lower toxicity profile chemotherapy regimens can be tolerated in older patients with CUP. Whilst genetic analysis is not currently recommended, a prospective study assessing the molecular profiling of 192 patients using a 92 gene assay to predict the site of origin demonstrated a median survival of 12.5 months for patients who received tailored therapy based on the genetic results, suggesting the potential benefit of such testing in the future.[7]

What are the realistic goals for this patient?

Prognosis remains poor for most patients with CUP. Management should be tailored to the individual patient, and honest and frank discussions should take place between clinician(s) and patient. Symptom palliation and maintenance of quality of life are paramount, due to the poor prognosis of these tumours. In this case study, the patient is frail and her renal impairment and

Table 8.3 Examples of managing subgroups of CUP.

CUP subgroup	Management
SCC confined to the inguinal nodes	Refer to specialist surgeon within an appropriate MDT Consider surgery +/– RT for radical treatment
Solitary visceral (e.g. liver/lung) metastases	Refer to appropriate MDT for consideration of surgery/loco-regional therapy
Adenocarcinoma in isolated axillary lymphadenopathy in females	Consider treatment as per breast cancer management
SCC in isolated cervical lymphadenopathy	Consider treatment as per head and neck SCC
Isolated cerebral metastases	Refer to neuro-oncology MDT

MDT, multidisciplinary team; RT, radiotherapy; SCC, squamous cell carcinoma.

poor functional status are likely to preclude the safe administration of chemotherapy. When cure or prolongation of survival is not a realistic treatment goal, good symptom control is imperative. In the case described, supporting 'active' life expectancy may take precedence, as loss of independence is a major threat to quality of life.

How may CGA help identify and implement best supportive care for this patient?

Early CGA is crucial to assess and plan interventions for issues regarding physical and mental health, functional capacity and social circumstances (Figure 8.1). Importantly, frailty may not be permanent and some aspects may be ameliorated, potentially permitting chemotherapy. Comorbidity type and severity should be considered and functional assessments by a physiotherapist, occupational therapist, psychologist and/or social worker may, in addition to those undertaken by geriatric doctors and nurses, help to identify ways to support patient independence. Involvement of palliative care services may also facilitate cancer-related symptom management and end-of-life care. Some issues identified in this case include fatigue, social isolation and declining functional independence. Fatigue, for example, is a common symptom of malignancy, yet it may also be a consequence of anaemia, poor sleep or malnutrition, and such causes should be actively sought and treated if possible.

Home-based multidisciplinary intervention teams (MDTs) can improve functional status in frail older patients following hospital discharge,[8] although evidence for such interventions specifically for older patients with cancer is limited. Best practice guidelines from the British Geriatrics Society for managing frail older adults in the community[9] propose that key elements include: (1) creating an individualized support and care plan, including the patient's wishes and expectations; (2) holistic medical review to diagnose and optimize medical problems (e.g. iron deficiency anaemia); (3) application of evidence-based medication review checklists to rationalize inappropriate or 'no longer beneficial' medications (e.g. statin therapy).[10]

Conclusion and learning points

Metastatic CUP is a unique group of malignancies whose prominence in cancer care is growing. With recent national guidelines offering clearer definitions and management algorithms, a more uniform approach may be taken when treating these patients. Those with a poor PS have a worse prognosis and risk greater toxicities of treatment. The management of CUP in older patients is often compounded by significant underlying

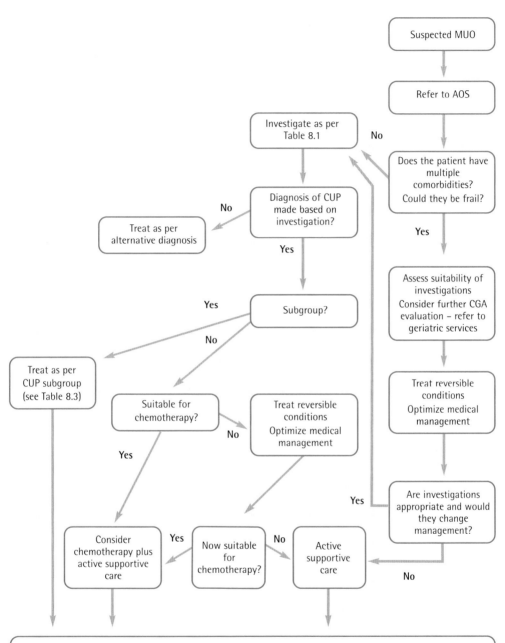

Figure 8.1 Diagnostic and management algorithm for older patients with CUP. AOS, acute oncology service.

morbidity. In patients in whom anticancer treatment is not possible, investigations must be carefully planned to avoid undue discomfort or risk to the patient. However, patients can still receive treatment in the form of palliative care and support from CGA services for symptom control.

- CUP has a poor prognosis for most patients; realistic goals of care must therefore be shared between the patient and the MDT.
- Older patients with MUO/CUP should be carefully assessed to avoid unnecessary investigations.
- Systemic chemotherapy may offer modest survival benefit but diminish quality of life in older frail patients. It should therefore be reserved for those with a favourable PS.
- For patients with a poorer PS, CGA is a useful paradigm to help optimize patients' physical, mental and functional morbidities and guide management decisions.

References

1 Gauri R, Varadhachary MD, Raber MN. Cancer of unknown primary site. *N Engl J Med* 2014; 371: 757–65.

2 National Institute for Health and Care Excellence (2010). *Metastatic malignant disease of unknown primary origin. Diagnosis and management of metastatic malignant disease of unknown primary origin. NICE clinical guideline 104.* Available from: www.nice.org.uk/guidance/cg104/chapter/guidance (accessed 25 February 2015).

3 Bishnoi S, Pittman K, Yeend S, *et al.* Gemcitabine and carboplatin in carcinoma of unknown primary site (CUP) in elderly patients: analysis of a phase 2 Adelaide Cancer Trials and Education Collaborative (ACTEC) study. *J Geriatr Oncol* 2011; 2: 233–8.

4 Taylor MB, Bromham NR, Arnold SE. Carcinoma of unknown primary: key radiological issues from the recent National Institute for Health and Clinical Excellence guidelines. *Br J Radiol* 2012; 85: 661–71.

5 Culine S, Kramar A, Saghatchian M, *et al.* Development and validation of a prognostic model to predict the length of survival in patients with carcinomas of an unknown primary site. *J Clin Oncol* 2002; 20: 4679–83.

6 Extermann M, Aapro M, Bernabei R, *et al.* Use of comprehensive geriatric assessment in older cancer patients: recommendations from the task force on CGA of the International Society of Geriatric Oncology (SIOG). *Crit Rev Oncol Hematol* 2005; 55: 241–52.

7 Hainsworth JD, Rubin MS, Spigel DR, *et al.* Molecular gene expression profiling to predict the tissue of origin and direct site-specific therapy in patients with carcinoma of unknown primary site: a prospective trial of the Sarah Cannon Research Institute. *J Clin Oncol* 2013; 31: 217–23.

8 Nikolaus T, Specht-Leible N, Bach M, *et al.* A randomized trial of comprehensive geriatric assessment and home intervention in the care of hospitalized patients. *Age Ageing* 1999; 28: 543–50.

9 Turner G, Clegg A. Best practice guidelines for the management of frailty: a British Geriatrics Society, Age UK and Royal College of General Practitioners report. *Age Ageing* 2014; 43: 744–7.

10 Gallagher P, Ryan C, Byrne S, Kennedy S, O'Mahony D. STOPP (screening tool of older person's prescriptions) and START (screening tool to alert doctors to right treatment). Consensus validation. *Int J Clin Pharmacol Ther* 2008; 46: 72–83.

09 Incontinence Developing During Chemotherapy in a Patient with Advanced Ovarian Cancer and Diabetes

Jane Hook, Eileen Burns, David Jackson

Case history

An 85-year-old woman presented to her GP with a 3 month history of abdominal pain, bloating and urinary frequency. Past medical history included type 2 diabetes mellitus and vaginal prolapse, managed with a ring pessary. At her recent diabetic review, her HbA_{1c} level was 70 mmol/mol and she had chronic kidney disease (stage 3 with estimated glomerular filtration rate [GFR] 55 ml/min) and mild sensory neuropathy. Regular medications were metformin, gliclazide, ramipril, simvastatin and paracetamol. She lived alone in a bungalow, walked with a stick, and was independent in her activities of daily living (ADL) but required her daughter's help with shopping. GP-measured serum CA-125 was >1000 U/ml; pelvic ultrasound revealed a large adnexal mass. She was referred for urgent investigation for suspected ovarian cancer.

Staging investigations showed a large pelvic mass causing bilateral hydronephrosis, small-volume ascites and omental deposits (International Federation of Gynecology and Obstetrics [FIGO] stage IIIC). Omental biopsy confirmed a high-grade serous adenocarcinoma of ovarian origin. The gynae-oncology multidisciplinary team (MDT) recommended neoadjuvant chemotherapy with interval debulking surgery. Bilateral ureteric stents were inserted to prevent development of renal failure.

At her initial oncology appointment, she had poorly controlled pelvic pain, was opening her bowels on alternate days and getting up twice a night to pass urine with increased urgency and dysuria following the stent insertion. Her Eastern Cooperative Oncology Group (ECOG) performance status (PS) was 2. The patient agreed to treatment with carboplatin. A regular low-dose opiate and laxative were started. She was asked to monitor her blood glucose daily.

Cycles 1 and 2 were well tolerated with mild fatigue and constipation. When she attended for cycle 3, the chemotherapy nurses noticed that she was unkempt and confused. Assessment on the acute oncology unit found that she was incontinent of urine and faeces, had gradually worsening constipation, followed by diarrhoea, and had increasing urinary frequency with a feeling of incomplete voiding and dysuria. Her Abbreviated Mental Test Score (AMTS) was 7/10 and she was unsteady on her feet with postural drop >30 mmHg. Her rectum was loaded with hard stool and her pessary was poorly fitting. Urea, creatinine and blood glucose were elevated. Urinalysis suggested infection, which was confirmed by microscopy and culture. She was diagnosed with delirium due to urinary tract infection (UTI), faecal incontinence due to constipation, poor glycaemic control, and postural hypotension due to dehydration and medication. She was admitted to hospital.

What was the goal of cancer treatment for this patient?

How was her incontinence managed?

What is the evidence base for her cancer treatment?

What patient-related factors influenced her cancer treatment plan?

How can incontinence be identified and managed in cancer services?

What was the goal of cancer treatment for this patient?

In common with 75% of women with ovarian cancer, this patient presented with advanced disease (FIGO stage III or IV). Standard treatment is platinum-based chemotherapy and debulking surgery, performed by a specialist surgeon, given with the aim of prolonging survival and improving symptom control and quality of life. Ovarian cancer is a chemo-sensitive malignancy (the radiological response rate to platinum is >50%); patients >70 years with ovarian cancer are more likely to receive chemotherapy than for other solid tumours.[1] Most patients relapse but respond to further lines of chemotherapy, and a small number are long-term survivors. Five year survival in patients aged over 85 years is 14%.[2] The average life expectancy of an 85-year-old woman is 6.8 years.[3] Studies have shown that older women are less likely to receive standard treatment, but those who do derive the same magnitude of benefit as younger women, although they are at higher risk of complications.[4,5]

The patient and her oncologist had a careful discussion about treatment and prognosis. Her goal was to regain her usual level of well-being. She wanted to reduce the risk of toxicity (including hair loss) and to have time off treatment when she was feeling well. Therefore, her treatment plan was single-agent carboplatin with the potential for surgery, depending on her response to chemotherapy, without addition of paclitaxel or bevacizumab.

How was her incontinence managed?

Our patient had multiple interacting factors contributing to urinary and faecal incontinence, including changes within the genitourinary and gastrointestinal tracts, as well as external factors (Figure 9.1). Her ovarian cancer, comorbidities and treatment all contributed. The key to management was to identify reversible causes. The aim of treatment was to regain continence and usual functional status, and prevent future episodes.

The history focused on: (1) symptoms to identify type of incontinence and causes (Table 9.1); (2) associated symptoms and acute changes in cognition, mobility and ADL; (3) comorbidities; (4) medication; and (5) usual functional status, mobility and access to toilets. Examination assessed hydration, mobility and cognitive impairment, and included abdominal, rectal, vaginal and neurological examinations. Initial investigations were baseline bloods plus urinalysis and midstream specimen of urine. A post-void residual bladder scan was inaccurate due to her pelvic mass. In such a scenario, where urinary retention is a significant possibility, it is reasonable to perform an in–out catheter to clarify post-void residual volumes.

The patient was acutely delirious, resulting in temporary loss of capacity. Initial management was done in her best interests by the medical team in consultation with her daughter. This comprised intravenous fluids for rehydration, antibiotics to treat complex UTI, and optimization of diabetic control to reduce polyuria. The faecal impaction was treated with enemas, an increased

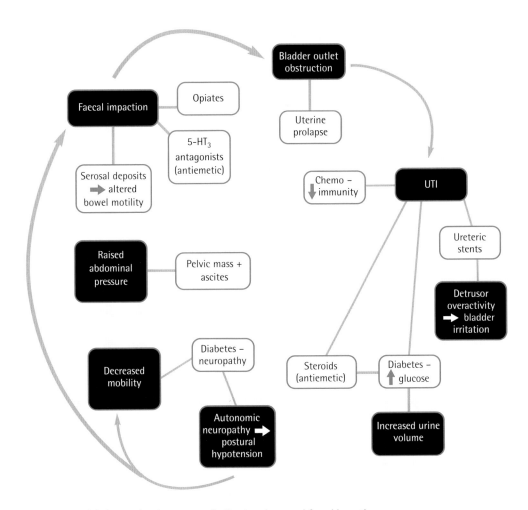

Figure 9.1 Multiple interacting factors contributing to urinary and faecal incontinence.

dose of laxative and the addition of a stool softener. Her ACE inhibitor was stopped because of postural hypotension. While confused, she was unable to find the toilet, so she was prompted and supported to maximize continence.

Her confusion resolved with treatment of the UTI. The vaginal pessary was reinserted by the urogynaecologists. Her urinary incontinence improved but she was still not always able to get to the toilet in time. She did then admit to long-standing problems with urge incontinence, which had worsened when the ureteric stents were inserted. A trial of an antimuscarinic agent was considered but not started at that time. Lifestyle advice and bladder retraining were advised. She was assessed by physio- and occupational therapists and was given a commode to reduce both the distance she had to walk to the toilet at night and the risk of falls, and issued with containment devices to preserve dignity. She was discharged home with increased support and asked to keep a 3 day bladder diary.

Following a 2 week delay, she was reassessed in the clinic. Carboplatin was restarted with a reduced course of dexamethasone to improve glycaemic control. A reassessment CT scan showed

Table 9.1 Classification of urinary and faecal incontinence.

Urinary incontinence	Any involuntary leakage of urine
Stress incontinence	Involuntary leakage of small amounts of urine on effort, exertion, sneezing or coughing
Urgency incontinence	Involuntary urine leakage accompanied or immediately preceded by a compelling desire to urinate that is difficult to delay (urgency)
	Overactive bladder (OAB) is urgency with or without urinary incontinence (wet or dry OAB) and presents as frequency and nocturia
Mixed incontinence	A combination of stress and urgency symptoms
Overflow incontinence	Urinary incontinence due to incomplete bladder emptying, secondary to bladder outflow obstruction or underactive bladder
Functional incontinence	Urinary incontinence due to factors outside the urinary tract, including comorbidities, medications, mobility and other environmental factors
Faecal incontinence	Involuntary leakage of faeces
	Usually due to complex interplay of coexisting factors Causes include damage or weakness of the anal sphincters, faecal loading, neurological motor and/or sensory impairment, cognitive impairment, problems with toilet access, rectal capacity, gut motility or stool consistency

a good response to treatment. Surgery was performed with <1 cm residual disease. She was able to stop her opiates, the ureteric stents were removed and she completed postoperative chemotherapy. At 6 months' follow-up, she was back to her premorbid level of functioning. Ongoing support from an incontinence nurse specialist was improving her chronic urinary incontinence through a bladder-training programme and the use of selective anticholinergic medication.

What is the evidence base for her cancer treatment?

Over 50% of cases of ovarian cancer occur in women aged over 65 years, and 20% in those aged over 80 years. Older women, especially the over-80s, are underrepresented in clinical trials. The evidence base for treating this patient is based on extrapolation from randomized controlled trial (RCT) data in younger women, single-arm studies, and retrospective analyses of institutional and population-based data.

The key decisions in her treatment plan (Figure 9.2) were whether she should have surgery and which chemotherapy regimen should be chosen.

Should she have debulking surgery, and when?

Debulking surgery followed by six cycles of chemotherapy is standard treatment for advanced ovarian cancer. Surgery versus no surgery has not been investigated in an RCT, but meta-analyses of non-randomized studies and analyses of RCT data consistently show that debulking to <1 cm or no macroscopic residual disease (optimal debulking) is a major prognostic factor for survival. The required surgery, however, is extensive: laparotomy with bilateral salpingo-oophorectomy, hysterectomy, omentectomy and resection of peritoneal deposits as a minimum; age >75 years and poor PS or poor nutritional status have been associated with increased morbidity.

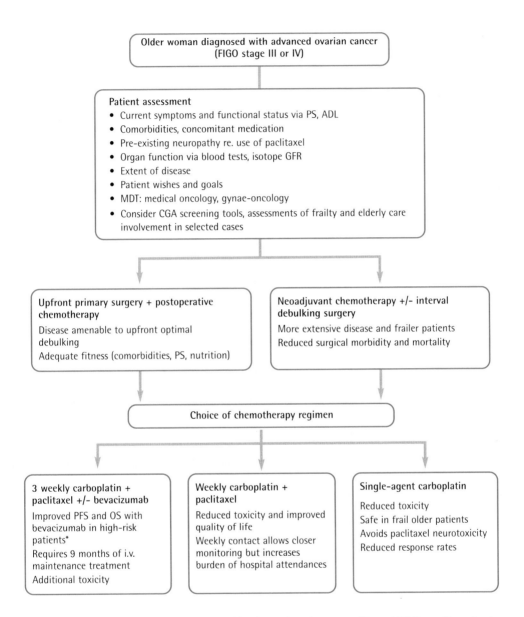

Figure 9.2 Treatment algorithm for older women with advanced ovarian cancer. *Current UK Cancer Drugs Fund approved indications for use of bevacizumab are FIGO stage IV disease, inoperable stage III disease or stage III disease debulked to >1 cm residual disease (i.e. high-risk patients).[13]

An alternative strategy is to give neoadjuvant chemotherapy with interval debulking surgery performed after three cycles. This has been compared with upfront surgery in two RCTs which found similar survival with neoadjuvant chemotherapy but lower postoperative mortality and morbidity.[6,7] On this basis, neoadjuvant chemotherapy is increasingly used, particularly in frailer patients.

Currently, the decision to operate is based on prediction by a specialist gynae-oncology surgeon of the likelihood of achieving optimal debulking using CT imaging +/− laparoscopy, and standard assessments of patient fitness. CT scans underestimate the volume of peritoneal disease. The role of surgery in women who cannot be optimally debulked is questionable. Methods to improve patient selection, including use of preoperative geriatric assessments, such as Comprehensive Geriatric Assessment (CGA), are a focus of current research.

Choice of chemotherapy regimen

Carboplatin plus paclitaxel given every 3 weeks is standard treatment based on a series of RCTs conducted in the early 2000s (median survival range 30–38 months).[8] The febrile neutropenia rate is 5–10%, and 20% of women develop at least moderate peripheral sensory neuropathy. The proportion of older patients in these trials was low. A secondary analysis of one trial suggested that age >70 years is a risk factor for increased toxicity and decreased treatment completion.[9] In one RCT of 2073 women, survival was similar with single-agent carboplatin versus carboplatin plus paclitaxel, but with less toxicity (sensory neuropathy rate 1%).[10] Single-agent carboplatin can be delivered to frail older patients: in a study of 111 frail >70-year-olds (40% >80 years), 74% completed six cycles, with a median survival of 17.4 months and manageable toxicity.[11] A dose-fractionated weekly schedule of carboplatin plus paclitaxel has also been shown to decrease toxicity.[12]

Addition of the anti-vascular endothelial growth factor monoclonal antibody bevacizumab to carboplatin plus paclitaxel, followed by 9 months of maintenance treatment, is associated with a modest improvement in progression-free survival (PFS) and overall survival (OS), with greater benefit in stage IV or suboptimally debulked stage III disease.[13] This should be considered in selected older women, but toxicity includes hypertension, proteinuria, bleeding, arterial and venous thromboembolic events, and gastrointestinal perforation.

What patient–related factors influenced her cancer treatment plan?

Our patient had a good level of premorbid independence and quality of life but with some indicators of frailty and an ECOG PS of 2. Pre-existing sensory neuropathy increased her risk of paclitaxel-related neurotoxicity. These factors and her wish to minimize toxicity led to the selection of carboplatin rather than combination chemotherapy. Neoadjuvant chemotherapy was used to decrease the risk of surgical morbidity.

How can incontinence be identified and managed in cancer services?

Incontinence is a common and underreported problem that causes poor quality of life for patients and carers, a decline in functional status and increased risk of admission to 24 h care. It is therefore important to identify it at baseline and during anticancer treatment. The prevalence of urinary incontinence increases with age and affects up to 30% of independent older women. Diabetes increases the risk of both urinary and faecal incontinence. Patients may not self-report incontinence due to embarrassment or a belief that it is a normal part of ageing. High levels of awareness and actively and sympathetically asking about urinary and faecal incontinence symptoms are key to identifying cases.

Initial assessment should identify the type of incontinence (Table 9.1) and potentially reversible causes. A 3 day bladder diary is a useful assessment tool. Management should concentrate on modification of factors contributing to functional incontinence (medication, comorbidities and environment), as these factors can respond to simple interventions. First-line management of stress and urge urinary incontinence is usually behavioural: pelvic floor-strengthening exercises and bladder-training programmes. These require significant patient involvement over months and may not be feasible during anticancer therapy. Antimuscarinic agents can improve urge urinary incontinence, but their use needs to be carefully considered. Oxybutynin is contraindicated in frail older patients as it is very poorly tolerated and has been reported to be associated with acute confusion in this group. Selective antimuscarinic agents are, however, generally well tolerated and effective in treating overactive bladder (OAB).[14]

Ureteric stents are frequently used in ovarian cancer. Most patients experience dysuria and urgency following insertion, and they are a risk factor for recurrent UTIs. There is no good evidence to guide the management of stent-related symptoms. Alpha$_1$-blockers and antimuscarinic agents are used for irritative symptoms but have only been investigated in small non-cancer-specific studies. Continuous rotating antibiotics can be considered in patients with recurrent UTIs.[15] In patients who require long-term stents, optimum management includes ensuring that they are changed on schedule.

NICE guidance requires that all NHS hospitals have an incontinence MDT to provide specialist input for complex cases and those who do not respond to initial management. The MDT should comprise a urogynaecologist or urologist with a special interest in female urology, a specialist nurse, a physiotherapist, a colorectal surgeon and an elderly care specialist. Indications for referral include combined urinary and faecal incontinence, symptoms of voiding difficulty, and previous pelvic cancer surgery or radiotherapy.

Conclusion and learning points

- Older women with ovarian cancer should be considered for multimodality therapy with a combination of chemotherapy and debulking surgery.

- Urinary and faecal incontinence are common (particularly in those with diabetes) and underreported, and should be actively assessed at baseline and during chemotherapy.

- Causes are multifactorial and management should concentrate on treatment of modifiable factors related to ovarian cancer, comorbidities and treatment.

References

1 Hall P, Handforth C, Spencer K, *et al*. Age as an independent predictor of chemotherapy treatment decisions in 20 common cancers. *J Clin Oncol* 2014; 32 (5 suppl): abstract 9550.

2 National Cancer Intelligence Network (2012). *Overview of ovarian cancer in England: incidence, mortality and survival*. Available from: www.ncin.org.uk/view?rid=1740 (accessed 14 June 2015).

3 Office for National Statistics (2014). *National life tables, United Kingdom, 2010–2012*. Available from: www.ons.gov.uk/ons/rel/lifetables/national-life-tables/2010---2012/stb-uk-2010-2012 (accessed 14 June 2015).

4 Fairfield KM, Murray K, Lucas FL, *et al*. Completion of adjuvant chemotherapy and use of health services for older women with epithelial ovarian cancer. *J Clin Oncol* 2011; 29: 3921–26.

5 Hershman D, Jacobson JS, McBride R, *et al*. Effectiveness of platinum-based chemotherapy among elderly patients with advanced ovarian cancer. *Gynecol Oncol* 2004; 94: 540–9.

6 Vergote I, Tropé CG, Amant F, *et al*. Neoadjuvant chemotherapy or primary surgery in stage IIIC or IV ovarian cancer. *N Engl J Med* 2010; 363: 943–53.

7 Kehoe S, Hook J, Nankivell M, *et al.* Primary chemotherapy versus primary surgery for newly diagnosed advanced ovarian cancer (CHORUS): an open-label, randomised, controlled, non-inferiority trial. *Lancet* 2015; 386: 249–57.

8 National Institute of Health and Clinical Excellence (2003). *Guidance on the use of paclitaxel in the treatment of ovarian cancer. NICE technology appraisal guidance 55.* Available from: www.nice.org.uk/guidance/ta55 (accessed 27 May 2015).

9 Tew WP, Java J, Chi D, *et al.* Treatment outcomes for older women with advanced ovarian cancer: results from a phase III clinical trial (GOG182). *J Clin Oncol* 2010; 28 (suppl): abstract 5030.

10 International Collaborative Ovarian Neoplasm Group. Paclitaxel plus carboplatin versus standard chemotherapy with either single-agent carboplatin or cyclophosphamide, doxorubicin, and cisplatin in women with ovarian cancer: the ICON3 randomised trial. *Lancet* 2002; 360: 505–15.

11 Falandry C, Weber B, Savoye AM, *et al.* Development of a geriatric vulnerability score in elderly patients with advanced ovarian cancer treated with first-line carboplatin: a GINECO prospective trial. *Ann Oncol* 2013; 24: 2808–13.

12 Pignata S, Scambia G, Katsaros D, *et al.* Carboplatin plus paclitaxel once a week versus every 3 weeks in patients with advanced ovarian cancer (MITO-7): a randomised, multicentre, open-label, phase 3 trial. *Lancet Oncol* 2014; 15: 396–405.

13 Perren TJ, Swart AM, Pfisterer J, *et al.* A phase 3 trial of bevacizumab in ovarian cancer. *N Engl J Med* 2011; 365: 2484–96.

14 Wagg A, Khullar V, Marschall-Kehrel D, *et al.* Flexible-dose fesoterodine in elderly adults with overactive bladder: results of the randomized, double-blind, placebo-controlled study of fesoterodine in an aging population trial. *J Am Geriatr Soc* 2013; 61: 185–93.

15 Alber X, Huertas I, Pereiro II, *et al.* Antibiotics for preventing recurrent urinary tract infection in non-pregnant women. *Cochrane Database Syst Rev* 2004; 3: CD001209.

Further reading

• Tew WP, Hyman BM, Kimmick G, *et al.* Breast and ovarian cancer in the older woman. *J Clin Oncol* 2014; 32: 2553–61.

• Alexander L, Shakespeare K, Barradell V, Orme S. Management of urinary incontinence in frail elderly women. *Obstet Gynaecol Reprod Med* 2015; 25: 75–82.

• National Institute of Health and Clinical Excellence (2013). *Urinary incontinence. The management of urinary incontinence in women. NICE clinical guideline 171.* Available from: www.nice.org.uk/guidance/cg171 (accessed 14 July 2015).

• National Institute of Health and Clinical Excellence (2007). *Faecal incontinence. The management of faecal incontinence in adults. NICE clinical guideline 49.* Available from: www.nice.org.uk/guidance/cg49 (accessed 14 July 2015).

10 A Patient with Breast Cancer and Dementia

Debra Josephs, Kimberley Kok, Finbarr Martin, Eleni Karapanagiotou

Case history

A 75-year-old woman with oestrogen receptor-negative, HER2-negative metastatic breast cancer was referred for consideration of palliative treatment. Her metastatic disease (multiple pulmonary nodules only) had recently been diagnosed on routine surgical follow-up, 6 months after radical mastectomy and axillary node clearance. She attended the clinic appointment with her daughter and son-in-law, who said she had moderate Alzheimer's dementia (Mini-Mental State Examination 14/30), but maintained a good level of function. She was independent in basic activities of daily living (ADL), but not in instrumental ADL.

Three months later, a re-staging CT scan revealed evidence of progressive disease. A decision was made to offer the patient systemic therapy with oral capecitabine.

Background

How would you assess this patient's capacity to consent to treatment? What is the definition of 'capacity', and is there a test to determine mental capacity?

What would your management be if this patient were assessed to have no capacity with regards to consenting to the specific decision about her options for treatment?

What is the evidence base for her treatment options?

What other considerations should be made when offering this patient systemic anticancer therapy?

Background

Cancer is an age-related disease, and the prevalence of dementia also increases with age. With a global ageing population, by 2030, 70% of all cancers will occur in older people, and 63 million people worldwide will have dementia.[1] Dementia is a progressive neurodegenerative condition characterized by impairment in memory and at least one other cognitive domain (aphasia, apraxia, agnosia or disturbances in executive functioning), as well as a compromised ability to perform daily functions.[2] Patients with dementia who are diagnosed with cancer pose a unique challenge, owing to the potential for impaired decision-making capacity, poor communication and difficulties following medication regimens.

How would you assess this patient's capacity to consent to treatment? What is the definition of 'capacity', and is there a test to determine mental capacity?

Decision-making 'capacity' refers to an individual's ability to make decisions or to take actions that influence his or her life. Capacity has to be assumed unless proven it is lacking. It is decision-specific (e.g. the patient may have capacity to decide which flavour ice cream she would prefer, but may lack capacity with regards to consenting for treatment), and a person is allowed to make an 'unwise' decision provided they have the capacity to do so. Progressive dementia may interfere with decision-making abilities involved in any aspect of life. An assessment of cognitive function may alert the clinician to the possibility of impaired decision-making capacity but cannot be used to assume incapacity. As there is no uniformity in the illness progression, specific capacities may be lost at different periods during the course of each person's disease; therefore it is important to assess each patient individually and regularly.

In 2007, the Mental Capacity Act (MCA) 2005 came into force in England and Wales. It provided a legal framework for decision making on behalf of adults who cannot make decisions themselves.[3] In Scotland, decision making in this area is covered by the Adults with Incapacity (Scotland) Act 2000, and in Northern Ireland, it is governed by the common law.

For the purpose of the MCA, a person lacks capacity if, at the time the decision needs to be made, he or she is unable to make or communicate the decision because of an 'impairment of, or a disturbance in the functioning of, the mind or brain'. The test set out by the MCA to assess capacity is a two-stage 'functional' one, with the purpose of examining the process of decision making (Table 10.1). All efforts should be made to enhance decision-making capacity by ensuring sensory impairments are addressed and the process is described in simple language without medical jargon. Where an individual fails one or more parts of this test, then they have failed to demonstrate capacity for that particular decision.

In this case, the patient must be supported in decision making by using appropriate language and by ensuring she is supported by her family, to reduce any associated anxiety. Breaking down the information may also enhance the patient's ability to make a decision. For example, using questions such as:

'Tell me what you believe is wrong with your health now?'

'What do you think will happen if you do not continue with treatment?'

'Help me understand how you have decided on refusing/accepting treatment?'

What would your management be if this patient were assessed to have no capacity with regards to consenting to the specific decision about her options for treatment?

First, it is important to ascertain whether the patient has a valid advance directive declining treatment for breast cancer. If she does, then this must be respected, as long as this decision was

Table 10.1 Mental Capacity Act: two-stage capacity assessment.

Stage 1: Does the person have an impairment of, or a disturbance in the function of, the mind or brain?
Examples of impairment or disturbance in the function of the mind or brain may be temporary or permanent. This includes unconsciousness, stroke, dementia, delirium, brain injury, learning disability and the symptoms of drug or alcohol use (see MCA *Code of practice*, 4.12, in Further reading section)

Stage 2: Does the impairment or disturbance mean that the person is unable to make a specific decision when needed? Is the person unable to:
1. Understand the information relevant to the decision
2. Retain that information
3. Use or weigh that information as part of the process of making the decision, or
4. Communicate his/her decision (whether by talking, using sign language or any other means)
   [MCA, section 3(1)]

made with information still pertinent to the current situation and was not made under duress. In the absence of an advance directive, a decision will need to be made in her 'best interests' with the involvement of her family.

What constitutes an individual's best interests will depend upon the circumstances of each case. A best interest judgement is not an attempt to determine what the person would have wanted, although this must be taken into account. It is as objective a test as possible of what would be in the person's actual best interests, taking into consideration all relevant factors. This test involves consideration of the likely consequences – intended or not – of receiving a treatment under consideration, the consequences of having this treatment, and a judgement about the value to the patient of the difference. A crucial part of any best interest judgement will involve a discussion with those close to the individual, including family, friends or carers, where it is practical or appropriate to do so, bearing in mind the duty of confidentiality.

On some occasions, a patient with dementia may have appointed someone an 'attorney', by making a Lasting Power of Attorney (LPA) for health and welfare. The attorney would make best interest decisions when the person lacks capacity with respect to the proposed treatment. With the increasing use of LPA orders, the treating team should check whether an incapacitated person has made an LPA that includes health and welfare decisions.

In the event that there is no LPA and there are no available family members or friends willing to be consulted about treatment decisions, an independent mental capacity advocate (IMCA) should be appointed. An IMCA supports and represents vulnerable adults who lack capacity to make certain decisions. They are independent of the healthcare professional making the decision and represent the patient in discussions about whether the proposed decision is in the patient's best interests.

What is the evidence base for her treatment options?

According to current guidelines, older patients with metastatic breast cancer should not be excluded from chemotherapy, especially in cases of hormone receptor-negative (as in this case, where oral endocrine therapy is not a therapeutic option) or hormone-refractory tumours, or rapidly progressive disease.[4] The guidelines also support single-agent chemotherapy rather than combination regimens, which are usually more toxic. Preference should be given to chemotherapy agents with better safety profiles that have been studied in older patients.[4] Oral therapy is attractive since it eliminates the constraints and risks of parenteral therapy, but it is important to take into consideration that efficacy and tolerability may be compromised by concomitant medications and errors in compliance.[4] Given the impact of dementia on prognosis and quality of life, however, the level of cognitive function of an older patient must be taken into account when deciding whether to pursue toxic anticancer therapy.

Capecitabine, an oral cytotoxic, has shown efficacy in advanced breast cancer, with a favourable toxicity profile.[5,6] Notwithstanding these important advantages, there are some challenges in the use of capecitabine in this patient, including difficulty ensuring her compliance (see below), and potentially large interindividual variability in tolerance, which could result in her experiencing significant toxicities (such as diarrhoea or palmar-plantar erythema). Since the registered dose of capecitabine is widely acknowledged to be too high, a reduction in the starting dose would be recommended, e.g. 1000 mg/m^2 twice daily.

For this patient, a discussion between the oncologist and the patient's daughter and son-in-law regarding the expected benefits and possible toxicities of capecitabine would be paramount in the decision-making process.

What other considerations should be made when offering this patient systemic anticancer therapy?

Life expectancy in dementia has a bearing on clinical decision making. Studies have found that survival of patients with dementia is shorter than previously reported, with both clinicians and family members overestimating life expectancy in patients with dementia.[7] However, there is a significant minority of patients with dementia (especially Alzheimer's) who do not have significant medical comorbidities and have good functional reserves. A diagnosis of dementia should not preclude a decision not to offer patients anticancer treatment if they may otherwise be suitable for treatment.

When offering a patient with dementia cytotoxic chemotherapy, careful consideration of safety is of critical importance. It is essential that the multidisciplinary team ascertain whether the patient is able to understand when to seek help and that any necessary support is available. Robust plans must be communicated with the family. This is particularly important with respect to monitoring for, and timely reporting of, toxicities. Furthermore, for oral chemotherapy, the likelihood of adherence to the treatment schedule must be addressed, and steps should be taken to promote concordance, such as the use of 'pill organizers' or supervision and administration of medication.

Conclusion and learning points

- Patients with dementia and cancer pose a unique challenge, due to the potential for impaired decision-making capacity, poor communication and difficulties following treatment regimens.

- Decision-making capacity should be assessed frequently using the two-stage 'functional' test set out by the MCA.

- In patients with limited decision-making capacity, and in the absence of an advance directive, a decision must be made in his or her 'best interests' with the involvement of family or, if appointed, an attorney.

- A risk–benefit analysis must be considered individually for each patient, with careful consideration of safety.

- In some cases, the risks of treatment outweigh the benefits; however, in individuals with mild dementia and longer life expectancy, the potential benefits could be significant and the person should not be denied them based on the diagnosis of dementia.

References

1 Solomons L, Solomons J, Gosney M. Dementia and cancer: a review of the literature and current practice. *Aging Health* 2013; 9: 307–19.

2 Budson AE, Solomon PR. *Memory loss: a practical guide for clinicians.* Philadelphia, PA: Elsevier Saunders, 2011.

3 British Medical Association (2012). *Mental Capacity Act tool kit.* Available from: http://bma.org.uk/practical-support-at-work/ethics/mental-capacity-tool-kit (accessed 17 March 2015).

4 Biganzoli L, Wildiers H, Oakman C, *et al.* Management of elderly patients with breast cancer: updated recommendations of the International Society of Geriatric Oncology (SIOG) and European Society of Breast Cancer Specialists (EUSOMA). *Lancet Oncol* 2012; 13: e148–60.

5 Blum JL, Dieras V, Lo Russo PM, *et al.* Multicenter, phase II study of capecitabine in taxane-pretreated metastatic breast carcinoma patients. *Cancer* 2001; 92: 1759–68.

6 O'Shaughnessy JA, Blum J, Moiseyenko V, *et al.* Randomized, open-label, phase II trial of oral capecitabine (Xeloda) vs. a reference arm of intravenous CMF (cyclophosphamide, methotrexate and 5-fluorouracil) as first-line therapy for advanced/metastatic breast cancer. *Ann Oncol* 2001; 12: 1247–54.

7 Wolfson C, Wolfson D, Asgharian M, *et al.* A reevaluation of the duration of survival after the onset of dementia. *N Engl J Med* 2001; 344: 1111–16.

Further reading

· General Medical Council (2008). *Consent: patients and doctors making decisions together.* Available from: www.gmc-uk.org/guidance/ethical_guidance/consent_guidance_index.asp (accessed 17 March 2015).

· Department of Health (2009). *Reference guide to consent for examination or treatment.* 2nd ed. Available from: www.gov.uk/government/uploads/system/uploads/attachment_data/file/138296/dh_103653__1_.pdf (accessed 17 March 2015).

· Department of Health. *Mental Capacity Act.* London: HMSO, 2005.

· Department for Constitutional Affairs. *Mental Capacity Act 2005. Code of practice.* London: TSO, 2007.

11 A Patient with Acute Myeloid Leukaemia, Comorbidities and Fatigue

Emma Drasar, Emily Bart-Smith, Gulnaz Shah, Tania Kalsi, Timothy Chevassut

Case history

A 71-year-old man presented to his GP with gum bleeding and easy bruising. On further questioning he admitted to feeling fatigued for several months, had lost weight and had a poor appetite. His past medical history included a myocardial infarction 8 years ago (no ongoing angina), type 2 diabetes, hypothyroidism and benign prostatic hypertrophy (BPH). Medications were levothyroxine, metformin, tamsulosin and aspirin. His new GP had also recently started bisoprolol and ramipril at his annual ischaemic heart disease review.

He was married but lived alone, as his wife had severe dementia and resided in a nearby nursing home. He was independent and could walk 100 yards with a stick. Eastern Cooperative Oncology Group performance status (PS) was 0. On examination, he was pale, BP 110/75 mmHg, pulse 70 bpm. His abdominal examination revealed some suprapubic fullness.

Full blood count revealed pancytopenia (white cell count $3\times10^9/l$, Hb 83 g/l, platelets $35\times10^9/l$), and a blood film demonstrated macrocytic anaemia, hypogranular neutrophils and occasional blasts. Bone marrow examination confirmed a diagnosis of acute myeloid leukaemia (AML) with background myelodysplastic changes; a cytogenetic abnormality of monosomy 7 was detected. Fms-related tyrosine kinase 3 status was wild type. HbA_{1c} was 45 mmol/mol.

What was his likely prognosis and how can it be determined?

What are the treatment options?

Which patient factors and comorbidities should be assessed and modified?

Can anything be done for his fatigue?

What was his likely prognosis and how can it be determined?

AML is a disease of older patients: the median age at presentation is 70 years.[1] The goal of pretreatment assessment is to determine whether a patient will benefit from intensive (and therefore curative) therapy. Prognostic factors in older patients with AML have been identified from cohort studies, prospective trials and international databases. This has resulted in the development of a number of prognostic scores,[2–6] although none is widely accepted as a gold standard tool.[7] These scores are based around a combination of cytogenetics, PS, age, white cell count and other laboratory variables. For example, Kantarjian *et al.*[4] found patients aged >60 years with poor-risk disease had a less than 10% chance of being alive at 1 year compared with 30% and >50% for standard- and good-risk disease, respectively. Age >75 years was an adverse risk factor in this analysis.

Our patient has poor prognostic factors including monosomal karyotype, possible preceding myelodysplastic syndrome (indicated by the dysplastic morphology and longer history of fatigue), medical comorbidities and age ≥60 years. Based on trial data analysis, the poor prognostic factors in this case would result in a predicted 5 year survival of only 2% even with curative intent aggressive treatment.[3]

What are the treatment options?

Therapeutic options in AML should not be determined by a patient's chronological age. Consideration, however, should be given to comorbidities which may limit the delivery of effective chemotherapy and potentially increase the risk of toxicity, such as the risk of cardiac toxicity with anthracyclines. Therapy-related mortality is increased in older patients, and the likelihood of a cure should be balanced against the risk of toxicity. In addition, treatment decisions should clearly take into account the patient's views and goals.

The patient in this case is unlikely to be cured. Even with aggressive treatment, his predicted prognosis is poor. He was not keen on prolonged inpatient treatment options, as he was concerned about the impact on his wife's mental health of the loss of his visits to her nursing home. He was, however, keen to explore life-extending treatment options and he agreed to treatment with low-dose cytarabine. The possible treatment options are given below.

Clinical trials and novel agents

All patients, whatever their treatment pathway, should be considered for enrolment in clinical trials. The UK National Cancer Research Institute's AML LI (less intensive)-1 study is a rolling programme of trials in older patients and those not suitable for more intensive conventional therapy.

Intensive induction chemotherapy with curative intent including consolidation with allogeneic stem cell transplant from a related or unrelated donor

- High-dose inpatient chemotherapy: each cycle of chemotherapy requires an inpatient stay of approximately 4–6 weeks.
- Common complications include neutropenic sepsis, prolonged cytopenias and invasive fungal infections.

Intermediate non-curative but life-extending approaches with hypomethylating agents (azacitidine or decitabine) or low-dose cytarabine

- Hypomethylating agents may improve disease control:[8,9] a good response with improved PS and organ function may enable subsequent curative intent reduced-intensity allogeneic haematopoietic stem cell transplant.
- Low-dose cytarabine is not associated with significant toxicity and produces a higher complete response rate than best supportive care (18% vs 1%).[10]
- Both regimens can be given on an outpatient basis.

Best supportive care

Best supportive care is used in conjunction with all the above approaches but can also be used in isolation for patients who are unsuitable for or unwilling to have chemotherapy.

- Best supportive care may include oral cytoreductive drugs, e.g. hydroxycarbamide for management of leucostasis. Blood and platelet transfusions may be indicated for symptomatic anaemia and bleeding, respectively. Prophylactic antibiotics and antifungals may also be used to reduce infective episodes and avoid inpatient stays. Patients and their families should be encouraged to engage in end-of-life planning with the support of palliative care.

Which patient factors and comorbidities should be assessed and modified?

A thorough assessment of comorbidities and wider needs with resulting intervention plans are important for the patient and for clinical decision making, to prevent complications and to optimize quality of life.

Cardiac disease

As the patient was asymptomatic, his cardiac disease did not preclude chemotherapy or immunomodulatory agents including anthracyclines and antithymocyte globulin. A pretreatment echocardiogram to evaluate left ventricular ejection fraction would be useful if the planned treatment were potentially cardiotoxic. His platelets were 35×10^9/l, so his aspirin was discontinued. His GP had recently started a beta-blocker and an ACE inhibitor for his heart disease in order to improve long-term cardiac outcomes. There is likely little prognostic benefit from these drugs in the context of his AML prognosis; therefore, it would be sensible to discuss discontinuing them with his GP. His beta-blocker should not be stopped if he had ongoing angina, to avoid chest pain which may affect his quality of life.

Diabetes

The impact on his diabetes of chemotherapy-related nausea/vomiting and declining appetite should be pre-empted. Had he opted for curative treatment, the impact of the change in diet and exercise during prolonged inpatient stays should also have been considered. This man already had a poor appetite, was losing weight and his HbA_{1c} was 46 mmol/mol on metformin 500 mg/day (i.e. very tight control). Metformin can reduce appetite and weight and may cause nausea. In this case, because of his poor AML life expectancy, looser pragmatic blood sugar control would be a reasonable approach. For the delivery of his outpatient intermediate treatment, provisions were made for blood glucose monitoring during chemotherapy (blood glucose monitoring machine provided, and district nurse and enhanced GP input arranged). Evidence of diabetic end-organ damage was excluded (diabetic-related renal impairment may affect the choice of chemotherapy agent and/or the monitoring of renal function; diabetic-related peripheral neuropathy and significant retinopathy are relevant to falls risk assessment, especially for planned prolonged inpatient stays).

Nutrition

The impact of chemotherapy toxicities such as mucositis should be anticipated. The patient was referred to a dietitian prior to commencing chemotherapy. The clinical history identified that he was currently not cooking (as it required standing for too long) or shopping, due to fatigue. Arrangements were made with his daughter to order his shopping delivery online with ready-made meals and to purchase a microwave oven. Occupational therapy provided him with a kitchen perching stool.

BPH

The patient described poor stream, symptoms of incomplete emptying and 5× nocturia. Clinical examination indicated suprapubic fullness. A bladder scan demonstrated a post-void residual volume of 200 ml, indicating an increased risk of urinary infections during chemotherapy which may cause renal impairment if he develops frank retention. Finasteride was started and he was taught the double-voiding technique (voiding, then waiting 1 min while pushing down into the bladder with both hands before voiding again) to reduce residual volumes.

Functional assessment

A thorough history of his current (not historical) ability was carried out, which identified difficulties cooking and shopping, and that he strip-washed in the morning as he was unable to get out of the bath due to fatigue. Occupational therapy provided him with a bath seat. If he had chosen curative inpatient treatment, plans should have been made to counter the risk of functional decline associated with prolonged inpatient stays. Maintenance physiotherapy and nursing encouragement to perform functional tasks may reduce this decline.

Can anything be done for his fatigue?

The National Comprehensive Cancer Network recommends all cancer patients are screened for fatigue at their first oncology appointment.[11] Although his fatigue may largely be a result of his AML and pancytopenia, a number of other potentially modifiable factors/comorbidities might have been contributing to his fatigue:

- Hypothyroidism: his medications were adjusted, as thyroid function tests indicated suboptimal control.

- Mood: his mood was low, as his fatigue precluded his daily visits to his wife and he was worried about what would happen to her if he died. The voluntary sector was used to provide transport for him to visit her care home. Counselling was arranged and he was encouraged to discuss his wife's future care with his daughter. Had he opted for curative treatment, the impact of the isolation of prolonged hospital admissions on his mood should be considered. There are often limitations on visitors due to the distance to tertiary centres, and protocols regarding infection may preclude routine visits from grandchildren on the ward.

- Sleep: the optimization of his BPH may improve his nocturia and, thus, his sleep. History identified that he drank tea late at night and he was advised to replace this with decaffeinated alternatives. The strategies to improve his mood may also improve his sleep. He was given advice about good sleep hygiene.

- Medications: beta-blockers can cause fatigue in some patients. Their discontinuation may help to reduce fatigue.

- Nutritional: improving calorific intake may also improve his symptoms.

- Anaemia: a higher threshold of Hb 10 g/l was set for blood transfusion in view of his fatigue and cardiac disease. For solid tumours, it would also be worthwhile to identify and treat other causes of anaemia (vitamin B_{12}, folate, iron).

- Pain: on direct questioning, he described left knee pain that indicated osteoarthritis on examination. He was prescribed regular analgesia.

- Exercise: advice on improving exercise tolerance was given.[12]

Conclusion and learning points

- Despite older patients having a higher frequency of poor prognostic markers in AML, they can nonetheless tolerate intensive and potentially curative chemotherapy if comorbidities are appropriately managed.

- The decision to undertake aggressive curative intent treatment in older patients should be made by evaluating: (1) the chances of prolonged remission, (2) the patient's willingness to undergo intensive treatment, and (3) the risk of potential treatment-associated morbidity.
- Whichever treatment approach is taken, patient optimization and individualized support are key and should occur before, during and after any treatment offered.
- Proactively search out fatigue symptoms in patients presenting to cancer services.
- Identify and manage modifiable contributors to fatigue.

References

1 Juliusson G, Lazarevic V, Horstedt AS, *et al.*; Swedish Acute Leukemia Registry. Acute myeloid leukemia in the real world: why population-based registries are needed. *Blood* 2012; 119: 3890–9.

2 Giles FJ, Borthakur G, Ravandi F, *et al.* The haematopoietic cell transplantation comorbidity index score is predictive of early death and survival in patients over 60 years of age receiving induction therapy for acute myeloid leukaemia. *Br J Haematol* 2007; 136: 624–7.

3 Grimwade D, Walker H, Harrison G, *et al.* The predictive value of hierarchical cytogenetic classification in older adults with acute myeloid leukemia (AML): analysis of 1065 patients entered into the United Kingdom Medical Research Council AML11 trial. *Blood* 2001; 98: 1312–20.

4 Kantarjian H, O'Brien S, Cortes J, *et al.* Results of intensive chemotherapy in 998 patients age 65 years or older with acute myeloid leukemia or high-risk myelodysplastic syndrome: predictive prognostic models for outcome. *Cancer* 2006; 106: 1090–8.

5 Malfuson JV, Etienne A, Turlure P, *et al.* Risk factors and decision criteria for intensive chemotherapy in older patients with acute myeloid leukemia. *Haematologica* 2008; 93: 1806–13.

6 Wheatley K, Brookes CL, Howman AJ, *et al.* Prognostic factor analysis of the survival of elderly patients with AML in the MRC AML11 and LRF AML14 trials. *Br J Haematol* 2009; 145: 598–605.

7 Ossenkoppele G, Lowenberg B. How I treat the older patient with acute myeloid leukemia. *Blood* 2015; 125: 767–74.

8 Cashen AF, Schiller GJ, O'Donnell MR, DiPersio JF. Multicenter, phase II study of decitabine for the first-line treatment of older patients with acute myeloid leukemia. *J Clin Oncol* 2010; 28: 556–61.

9 Fenaux P, Mufti GJ, Hellstrom-Lindberg E, *et al.* Azacitidine prolongs overall survival compared with conventional care regimens in elderly patients with low bone marrow blast count acute myeloid leukemia. *J Clin Oncol* 2010; 28: 562–9.

10 Burnett AK, Milligan D, Prentice AG, *et al.* A comparison of low-dose cytarabine and hydroxyurea with or without all-trans retinoic acid for acute myeloid leukemia and high-risk myelodysplastic syndrome in patients not considered fit for intensive treatment. *Cancer* 2007; 109: 1114–24.

11 Berger AM, Abernethy AP, Atkinson A, *et al.* Cancer-related fatigue. *J Natl Compr Canc Netw* 2010; 8: 904–31.

12 Cramp F, Byron-Daniel J. Exercise for the management of cancer-related fatigue in adults. *Cochrane Database Syst Rev* 2012; 11: CD006145.

12 A Frail Patient with Colorectal Cancer Considered for Chemotherapy Who Struggles to Complete Activities of Daily Living

Sharmistha Ghosh, Joanna Hardwick, Peter Diem, Debashis Sarker

Case history

An 82-year-old man presented to his GP with rectal bleeding and weight loss of 2 st over 6 months. He admitted to having increased fatigue and had become housebound. He lived alone and struggled to complete activities of daily living (ADL) such as cooking and cleaning. He had a past medical history of hypertension for which he took ramipril 5 mg and bendroflumethiazide 2.5 mg daily. On examination, he appeared thin, dishevelled and had palpable hepatomegaly. From the history and examination, it was clear that his performance status (PS) had deteriorated from a baseline of 1 to 2 over a period of just 3 months.

He agreed to a referral for a Comprehensive Geriatric Assessment (CGA) along with initial investigations. Flexible sigmoidoscopy and biopsy revealed a proximal rectal adenocarcinoma. A CT scan of the chest, abdomen and pelvis, and an MRI scan of the pelvis, confirmed this diagnosis and demonstrated liver metastases.

His case was discussed at the colorectal cancer multidisciplinary team (MDT) meeting, and his disease was staged T3N1M1. The patient was provided with a clinical nurse specialist to act as a key worker across the whole care pathway. A clinical nurse specialist is the first point of contact for cancer patients and acts as a coordinator between the patient and different medical specialties.[1] An appointment was given to see an oncologist to discuss palliative systemic treatment options and suitability for palliative radiotherapy to the rectal primary. It was felt that initial surgery and local therapy for the metastases would not be appropriate due to his PS and the distribution of the metastatic disease. In addition, a referral was made to the community palliative care team.

Background

Role of the CGA

What systemic treatments are available for this patient?

What are the potential toxicities of treatment?

Local treatment for liver metastases

Why is it important to identify and manage functional impairment?

Background

Colorectal cancer is one of the commonest cancers in the UK: around 40,000 new cases are diagnosed each year.[2] One of the main risk factors for developing colorectal cancer is age: almost 75% of new cases diagnosed are in those aged over 65 years.[2] This presents clinicians with a unique set of challenges. For example, clinic appointments may take longer if the patient has impaired hearing, vision or cognition. Likewise, physical disabilities or frailties, problems with transport, and a lack of carers, friends or nearby family members can make attendance at clinic a significant challenge.

Role of the CGA

In the CGA clinic it became apparent that since the patient lost his wife 3 years earlier, he had found it difficult to cope with ADL. Cooking and other household chores had been taken care of by his wife and he had struggled to adapt. His hot water supply and washing machine were broken and he had not been able to negotiate the necessary repairs with the housing association. An occupational therapy home visit revealed his flat to be cluttered, messy and in poor condition.

It was obvious from his evaluation that he was depressed, felt very lonely and struggled to see a reason for living. Other issues such as poor hearing and impaired eyesight due to cataracts were also identified. Although his memory appeared intact, he showed evidence of mild executive dysfunction in cognitive testing. He was referred to the audiology and ophthalmology services at the hospital where he was being seen; hearing aids were supplied and cataract surgery was arranged. The geriatrician explained how serotonin levels in the brain can fall, causing low mood in situations such as his, and with his agreement citalopram was started for depression. He was advised to visit his GP regularly for follow-up of all these issues.

A referral was made to social services for his borough (which can be done by letter or telephone call from cancer services) and the social worker made arrangements to clean the house and fix the hot water. With the help of Age Concern (contact details for local services found on website), a local veterans' club was found and he was booked into a daily lunch club. Age UK volunteers also helped him to get his washing machine repaired. In the course of these interventions the patient regained hope and was willing to discuss systemic treatment options. Because of his mild executive dysfunction and hearing impairment, transport to the oncology unit was arranged for him.

What systemic treatments are available for this patient?

Cytotoxic chemotherapy

In fit, healthy people, even those with advanced disease, metastatic disease may be resectable; thus, the aim of treatment is cure. In these patients, chemotherapy is given with the intent of obtaining a good response to allow future surgery.

If the metastatic disease is not resectable, the aim of treatment is palliation. Factors that are taken into consideration when making this decision are the volume and sites of disease, the patient's symptoms, the quality of life currently experienced and the potential toxicity of proposed treatments. The aim of treatment for this group of patients is to achieve control of the disease and maintain this control with minimal toxicity.

In metastatic colorectal cancer, doublet therapy with fluorouracil (5-FU) should be considered, although there is dubiety over treatment sequencing.[2] Folinic acid, 5-FU and irinotecan (FOLFIRI) has been shown to be equivalent to folinic acid, 5-FU and oxaliplatin (FOLFOX),[3] and FOLFOX equivalent to oral capecitabine and oxaliplatin (CAPOX).[4]

The efficacy and toxicity profiles of 5-FU are similar in younger and older populations. Evidence has shown that older patients who have tolerated the full dose of planned chemotherapy gain as much benefit from treatment as do younger patients.[5] In a study which looked specifically at the older population, the addition of oxaliplatin to either infusional 5-FU or capecitabine, or irinotecan to 5-FU, did not result in a significant increase in progression-free survival (PFS) or overall survival (OS). There was, however, a significant improvement in response rate when patients received irinotecan in combination with 5-FU, in comparison with those who received 5-FU alone. Grade 3 or 4 toxicities were experienced by 58% of patients, especially those who were not independent in their ADL and in those who had cognitive impairment.[6,7]

Molecularly targeted therapy

Bevacizumab is an anti-vascular endothelial growth factor (VEGF) antibody. Although the improvement in PFS and OS is modest, its efficacy in combination with FOLFOX,[8,9] CAPOX[9] and single-agent capecitabine in metastatic colorectal cancer has been demonstrated. A trial assessing the addition of bevacizumab to capecitabine alone in older patients demonstrated a significant increase in response rate and PFS, but not in OS. Although toxicities were worse in the combination arm, they were felt to be tolerable.[10]

Cetuximab is an epidermal growth factor receptor (EGFR)-targeted treatment which is effective only in EGFR wild-type KRAS disease. KRAS status is ascertained prior to treatment, and EGFR inhibitor therapy, such as cetuximab, may be considered in combination with FOLFIRI or FOLFOX.[11,12] Patients who received FOLFIRI with cetuximab had an improved OS in comparison with those taking FOLFIRI with bevacizumab.[13]

Aflibercept is a VEGF inhibitor which may be considered in combination with irinotecan as second-line treatment on progression or resistance to oxaliplatin. The VELOUR trial[14] demonstrated an increased OS for patients in the combination arm (FOLFIRI and aflibercept) in comparison with FOLFIRI alone.

What are the potential toxicities of treatment?

Potential toxicities are the major limiting factor when deciding appropriate treatment. Any of the toxicities detailed in Table 12.1 can severely affect ADL.

Local treatment for liver metastases

For patients with liver-predominant metastatic disease, there are a number of potential loco-regional therapeutic options that can be considered as part of a broader treatment strategy

Table 12.1 Systemic treatments and commonly experienced toxicities.

Regimen	Potential toxicity
Irinotecan	Diarrhoea, alopecia, liver dysfunction
Capecitabine	Diarrhoea, palmar-plantar erythema, neuropathy, minimal neutropenia[15]
FOLFOX	Neutropenia (almost 50%), palmar-plantar erythema, diarrhoea[15]
FOLFIRI	Neutropenia, diarrhoea
Bevacizumab	Hypertension, gastrointestinal perforation, wound healing complications, arterial thromboembolism (especially in those aged >65)
Cetuximab	Acne-form rash, diarrhoea[16]
Aflibercept	Hypertension, diarrhoea, increased severity of chemotherapy-related neutropenia, anaemia

Table 12.2 Considerations to be taken into account when deciding on local treatment for liver metastases.

Treatment	Considerations
Standard open surgery	Treatment with curative intent Patients must be fit for surgery Multiple liver metastases
Laparoscopic surgery	Patient must be fit for surgery Single liver metastasis
Microwave ablation	Multiple liver metastases Can be used in isolation or as an adjunct in surgery Proximity to vasculature requires consideration
Cryotherapy	For patients in whom surgery is not appropriate or for use in post-resection recurrence Not recommended for hepatic tumours >4 cm in size
Radiofrequency ablation	For patients who are unfit for surgery or for use in post-resection recurrence Can be used in combination with hepatic resection to small volume metastatic disease in remnant liver
Selective internal radiation therapy	For patients who have limited or no extrahepatic disease For liver metastases not suitable for resection or ablation Can be used alone or in combination with chemotherapy

encompassing systemic therapy (Table 12.2), although clear guidelines are lacking. Thus, it is imperative that such cases are discussed at a hepato-biliary MDT meeting. Characteristics assessed when making recommendations include the number, size and site of metastatic lesions, and the presence of portal lymph node involvement or extrahepatic disease, together with the overall fitness and PS of the patient.

There are an increasing number of options for local treatment, some of which are suitable for those who are less fit.[17,18] These are summarized in Table 12.2

Why is it important to identify and manage functional impairment?

1. It is important to improve quality of life and psychological well-being.

2. Functional impairment may affect how patients tolerate treatment and what treatment can be offered. Patients may decline treatment due to fears and concerns which can often be easily alleviated. Clearly, in this case, chemotherapy-related diarrhoea could have been difficult to manage without appropriate counselling and assessment of wider needs.

3. Impairment of ADL often has important underlying contributors which need to be identified as part of the clinical assessment in the oncology clinic. The causes may inform decision making and may be modifiable or supportable to improve treatment tolerance and/or quality of life. These include:

   • Depression: consider antidepressants, counselling, befriending services and increasing support network.

- Cognitive impairment: consider treatable causes, e.g. drug side effects, hypothyroidism, dementia medication; think how the patient will manage treatment complications; assess whether the patient has capacity to consent; make arrangements for transport.
- Poor eyesight: cataract surgery, optician.
- Poor hearing: hearing aid, removal of wax, help with transport.
- Poor mobility: walking aids, physiotherapy, analgesia, joint replacement.

Conclusion and learning points

- Patients should receive the most intensive and appropriate treatment thought to be safe and effective according to their comorbidities.

- The aim should be to maximize OS while minimizing toxicity to achieve the greatest patient benefit.[19]

- Difficulties coping with daily tasks at 'baseline' may make the complications of chemotherapy difficult for some patients: such functional issues should be identified early and managed throughout treatment.

- Access to social services, therapies and voluntary aid organizations is available to oncologists.

- In patients with multiple needs, joint working with a geriatrician may be helpful.

References

1 National Cancer Action Team (2010). *Quality in nursing. Excellence in cancer care: the contribution of the clinical nurse specialist.* Available from: www.macmillan.org.uk/ Documents/AboutUs/Commissioners/ExcellenceinCancerCaretheContributionoftheClinical NurseSpecialist.pdf (accessed 2 February 2015).

2 National Institute of Health and Care Excellence (2011). *Colorectal cancer. The diagnosis and management of colorectal cancer. NICE clinical guideline 131.* Available from: www.nice.org.uk/ guidance/cg131 (accessed 2 February 2015).

3 Colucci G, Gebbia V, Paoletti G, *et al.* Phase III randomized trial of FOLFIRI versus FOLFOX4 in the treatment of advanced colorectal cancer: a multicenter study of the Gruppo Oncologico Dell'Italia Meridionale. *J Clin Oncol* 2005; 23: 4866–75.

4 Cassidy J, Clarke S, Díaz-Rubio E, *et al.* XELOX vs FOLFOX-4 as first-line therapy for metastatic colorectal cancer: NO16966 updated results. *Br J Cancer* 2011; 105: 58–64.

5 Folprecht G, Seymour MT, Saltz L, *et al.* Irinotecan/fluorouracil combination in first-line therapy of older and younger patients with metastatic colorectal cancer: combined analysis of 2,691 patients in randomized controlled trials. *J Clin Oncol* 2008; 26: 1443–51.

6 Seymour MT, Thompson LC, Wasan HS, *et al.* Chemotherapy options in elderly and frail patients with metastatic colorectal cancer (MRC FOCUS2): an open-label, randomised factorial trial. *Lancet* 2011; 377: 1749–59.

7 Aparicio T, Jouve JL, Teillet L, *et al.* Geriatric factors predict chemotherapy feasibility: ancillary results of FFCD 2001–02 phase III study in first-line chemotherapy for metastatic colorectal cancer in elderly patients. *J Clin Oncol* 2013; 31: 1464–70.

8 Hurwitz H, Fehrenbacher L, Novotny W, *et al.* Bevacizumab plus irinotecan, fluorouracil and leucovorin for metastatic colorectal cancer. *N Engl J Med* 2004; 350: 2335–42.

9 Saltz LB, Clarke S, Díaz-Rubio E, *et al.* Bevacizumab in combination with oxaliplatin-based chemotherapy as first-line therapy in metastatic colorectal cancer: a randomized phase III study. *J Clin Oncol* 2008; 26: 2013–19.

10 Cunningham D, Lang I, Marcuello E, *et al.* Bevacizumab plus capecitabine versus capecitabine alone in elderly patients with previously untreated metastatic colorectal cancer (AVEX): an open-label randomised phase 3 trial. *Lancet Oncol* 2013; 14: 1077–85.

11 Van Cutsem E, Köhne CH, Lang I, *et al.* Cetuximab plus irinotecan, fluorouracil and leucovorin as first-line treatment for metastatic colorectal cancer: updated analysis of overall survival according to tumor KRAS and BRAF mutation status. *J Clin Oncol* 2011; 29: 2011–19.

12 Bokemeyer C, Bondarenko I, Hartmann JT, *et al.* Efficacy according to biomarker status of cetuximab plus FOLFOX-4 as first line treatment for metastatic colorectal cancer: the OPUS study. *Ann Oncol* 2011; 22: 1535–46.

13 Heinemann V, von Weikersthal LF, Decker T, *et al.* FOLFIRI plus cetuximab versus FOLFIRI plus bevacizumab as first-line treatment for patients with metastatic colorectal cancer (FIRE-3): a randomised, open label, phase 3 trial. *Lancet Oncol* 2014; 15: 1065–75.

14 Van Cutsem E, Tabernero J, Lakomy R, *et al.* Addition of aflibercept to fluorouracil, leucovorin, and irinotecan improves survival in a phase III randomized trial in patients with metastatic colorectal cancer previously treated with an oxaliplatin-based regimen. *J Clin Oncol* 2012; 30: 3499–506

15 Grenon NN, Chan J. Managing toxicities associated with colorectal cancer chemotherapy and targeted therapy: a new guide for nurses. *Clin J Oncol Nurs* 2009; 13: 285–96.

16 Lacouture ME, Anadkat MJ, Bensadoun RJ, *et al.* Clinical practice guidelines for the prevention and treatment of EGFR inhibitor-associated dermatologic toxicities. *Support Care Cancer* 2011; 19: 1079–95.

17 Golfieri R, Bilbao JI, Carpanese L, *et al.* Comparison of the survival and tolerability of radioembolisation in elderly vs younger patients with unresectable hepatocellular carcinoma. *J Hepatol* 2013; 59: 753–61.

18 Romero Gutierrez M, Ruano Diaz L, Munoz Lopez D, *et al.* Percutaneous ablation of hepatocellular carcinoma in older patients in clinical practice. *Gastroenterol Hepatol* 2015; 38: 54–61.

19 Papmichael D, Audisio RA, Glimelius B, *et al.* Treatment of colorectal cancer in older patients: International Society of Geriatric Oncology (SIOG) consensus recommendations. *Ann Oncol* 2013; 26: 463–76.

13 Optimal First-Line Management of a Patient with Metastatic Renal Cell Carcinoma

Michael Davidson, Samantha Keeling, Lisa Pickering

Case history

An 84-year-old woman presented with a 6 month history of fatigue and haematuria. She had a background history of hypertension, type 2 diabetes, chronic kidney disease stage 3a (glomerular filtration rate 45–59 ml/min) and heart failure New York Heart Association class II. Her medications were metformin, gliclazide, amlodipine, ramipril, simvastatin, bendroflumethiazide and aspirin. Physical examination revealed a left-sided flank mass but was otherwise unremarkable. Her Karnofsky performance status (PS) was 80%. A staging CT scan showed an 8 cm renal mass with multiple metastases throughout both lung fields. Image-guided biopsy confirmed clear cell metastatic renal cell carcinoma (mRCC).

She was referred to a geriatrician for optimization of medical comorbidities and for oncology assessment. After discussion with the patient and family, the decision was made to commence pazopanib. After 2 weeks of pazopanib she described grade 1 fatigue, grade 1 diarrhoea, grade 1 hand-foot syndrome and grade 3 hypertension. A treatment break was initiated, her ACE inhibitor and calcium channel blocker were escalated to maximum dose and loperamide was recommended. Repeat BP monitoring after 7 days showed adequate control, and pazopanib was reintroduced with a dose reduction.

Is systemic anticancer treatment indicated in this case?

What are the first-line treatment options for mRCC and what is the evidence for their use?

What impact do the patient's age and comorbidities have on treatment decision making?

How could the patient's comorbidities be optimized prior to tyrosine kinase inhibitor (TKI) therapy?

How can toxicities be pre-emptively managed in this patient?

Is systemic anticancer treatment indicated in this case?

The incidence of renal cell cancer has risen by almost a third in the last 10 years and predominantly affects an older population: three-quarters of new cases in the UK are diagnosed in those aged over 60 and a third in those aged over 75.[1] The clinical course of mRCC is known to be variable and at times it can behave in an indolent manner. Several retrospective and one prospective series have demonstrated that selected patients with intermediate- or favourable-risk mRCC and low-volume disease can safely be observed with a surveillance strategy for a period of time with no detriment to their outcome.[2] Therefore, the first consideration in an older patient is whether to commence systemic treatment or whether an observation strategy is appropriate. This decision should be made with understanding of the patient's expected prognosis. The International Metastatic Renal Cell Carcinoma Database Consortium criteria form the most commonly used prognostic model for mRCC and have been validated for the current era of targeted TKI therapies.[3] Patients are stratified according to the presence of six risk factors, as shown in Table 13.1.

Patients with a favourable prognosis displaying none of the risk factors shown in Table 13.1 have a 2 year overall survival (OS) of 75%, compared with patients with more than three risk factors, who have a 2 year survival of only 7%. Our patient had impaired PS and anaemia, putting her into an intermediate-risk category, which carries an estimated median OS of 27 months with treatment. Owing to the presence of multiple, bilateral pulmonary metastases, the disease could not be considered 'low volume'; therefore, systemic first-line anticancer treatment was indicated. It should be remembered when considering PS as a predictive prognostic factor for older patients that it is principally an observation of their current activity level, mobility and ability to care for themselves. In older people, PS may be limited by modifiable factors: for example, poorly controlled pain from osteoarthritis and reversible causes of functional impairment should be considered when evaluating PS in this group.

What are the first-line treatment options for mRCC and what is the evidence for their use?

In phase III trials, three regimens have been shown to be effective for first-line treatment of favourable- or intermediate-risk mRCC, two of which, sunitinib and pazopanib, are approved by NICE and the Scottish Medicines Consortium for use in the UK.[4,5] Sunitinib is an oral multi-targeted kinase inhibitor which primarily exerts its anticancer effect through inhibition of the vascular endothelial growth factor (VEGF) receptor. A pivotal randomized phase III trial compared sunitinib with the then standard-of-care interferon-alpha in treatment-naive mRCC. Significant improvement in median progression-free survival (PFS) from 5.0 to 11.0 months (HR 0.42, 95% CI 0.32–0.454; $p<0.001$) was seen. OS also favoured sunitinib, although interpretation was challenging due to subsequent treatment crossover in many patients.[4] Sunitinib was approved for use in 2007 and has since become an international reference for first-line treatment of mRCC. In the phase III trial,[4] the most common treatment-related adverse events were diarrhoea (61%; grade 3–4: 9%), fatigue (54%; grade 3–4: 11%), hypertension (30%; grade 3–4: 12%) and hand-foot syndrome (29%; grade 3–4: 9%). Currently there is interest in a modified

Table 13.1 Prognostic factors for OS in patients with mRCC treated with VEGF-targeted agents (adapted from Heng et al.[3]).

- Karnofsky PS <80%
- Hb below the lower limit of normal
- Time from diagnosis to treatment <1 year
- Corrected calcium above the upper limit of normal
- Platelets greater than the upper limit of normal
- Neutrophils greater than the upper limit of normal

sunitinib schedule of 2 weeks' treatment followed by a 1 week break. A number of case series and a randomized phase II trial have reported that this schedule seems to have similar efficacy to that of conventionally scheduled sunitinib but with improved tolerability.[6] Pazopanib, another oral multi-targeted TKI, was licensed in 2010. Data from its registration trial reported a median PFS of 11.1 months in the treatment-naive population.[5] A further trial directly comparing the two agents confirmed comparable efficacy; therefore, the choice of TKI is informed by differing scheduling, toxicity and tolerability profiles.[7] Pazopanib is given by continuous once-daily oral dosing and has a slightly different toxicity profile. For example, it has been found to have lower rates of fatigue and skin toxicity but a higher incidence of liver function derangement and alopecia. There was no difference in the rates of cardiovascular adverse events.[7] In a phase II crossover trial,[8] patients received the two drugs sequentially for a 10 week period each: 70% of patients preferred pazopanib versus 22% who preferred sunitinib.

What impact do the patient's age and comorbidities have on treatment decision making?

The efficacy of sunitinib in an older population was examined in a subgroup analysis of 1414 patients aged over 65 years from a large expanded-access trial which reported PFS and OS of 11.3 and 18.2 months, respectively. This compared favourably with outcomes seen in the trial as a whole.[9] Furthermore, a pooled analysis from seven large trials compared sunitinib efficacy and safety in patients below and above 70 years of age.[10] It reported equivalent efficacy and largely equivalent safety, although fatigue, decreased weight and appetite, cough, peripheral oedema and thrombocytopenia were significantly more common in the older cohort.

There are fewer data addressing pazopanib use in an older population. The registration trial, however, included 196 patients aged over 65 and 34 patients aged over 75: no difference in safety or efficacy was seen in a preplanned subgroup analysis.[5] There is a specific safety consideration regarding higher rates of liver toxicity in older people.

Based on these collective data, pazopanib is often the preferred choice in older patients if their comorbidities allow. Nevertheless, some older patients tolerate sunitinib well, and implementation of a modified sunitinib schedule may further improve tolerability.

How could the patient's comorbidities be optimized prior to TKI therapy?

An optimal management plan for older adults with malignancy involves holistic assessment of existing medical problems with consideration and anticipatory management of potential complications of both the disease and the treatment. The patient's mental health, functional capacity, social circumstances and support networks should be taken into consideration. These issues are best addressed by Comprehensive Geriatric Assessment (CGA), which assesses capacity and cognition in a patient-centred, multidisciplinary approach and includes the involvement of a geriatrician.[11] CGA was conducted for this patient. Initiating discussions about advance care planning in a supportive environment is also a key part of the first assessment. This was introduced in the presence of the patient's daughter and a Macmillan nurse who planned to have ongoing discussions and provide community support.

Due to the cardiac risks associated with TKI treatment, an ECG, echocardiogram and functional assessment were performed at baseline. This patient had heart failure with a reduced ejection fraction of 40%, so a selective beta-blocker, bisoprolol, was introduced at a low dose and gradually increased. Repeat cardiac assessment was performed at 3 monthly intervals during treatment.

There is a risk of increasing hypertension during TKI therapy. This patient had a baseline clinic BP of 160/90 mmHg. Her antihypertensive therapy was optimized by first increasing the dose of ramipril, rather than that of amlodipine, in view of her history of chronic kidney disease, heart failure and diabetes. Bendroflumethiazide was stopped because of the risk that it may exacerbate any diarrhoea-induced electrolyte abnormalities that resulted from TKI therapy. Loop diuretics could be used if required for symptomatic management of her heart failure. Despite these measures the patient still experienced grade 3 hypertension during therapy, which required a dose delay and subsequent dose reduction. With appropriate management of cardiac risk factors and close monitoring at baseline and during follow-up, however, treatment can often be maintained and continued safely, as was subsequently achieved in this patient.

Anaemia is common in renal cell carcinoma and can be multifactorial. Our patient had iron deficiency anaemia secondary to haematuria and reduced erythropoietin synthesis, which may be seen in mRCC. She had previously experienced severe constipation and nausea with oral iron supplementation, so a day-case intravenous iron infusion was arranged.

How can toxicities be pre-emptively managed in this patient?

Older patients have reduced physiological reserve and can suffer debilitating morbidity and loss of independence from relatively mild side effects. Pre-empting potential treatment-related toxicity was therefore a crucial part of the management plan. TKI therapies can cause diarrhoea, so it is important to consider pre-existing problems such as constipation, diarrhoea, incontinence or impaired nutritional status. The Malnutrition Universal Screening Tool (MUST) can be used to screen for risk of malnutrition.[12] Because this patient's BMI was 20 kg/m^2 and she had a high-risk MUST score, she was referred to the community dietitian. An occupational therapist assessed her home environment and arranged a downstairs commode in case she experienced problematic diarrhoea. Advice was given about the risks of diarrhoea, such as dehydration and skin damage, and anticipatory loperamide was prescribed. She was advised to stop ramipril and contact her doctor if she developed profuse diarrhoea, to minimize the risk of acute kidney injury. On examination she had dry skin, which is very common in older adults, so an emollient was prescribed. TKI-induced hand-foot syndrome could exacerbate this and be potentially very disabling for older adults.

Conclusion and learning points

- Prior to consideration of treatment for mRCC, risk should be stratified and treatment commenced only if indicated. For lower risk patients an imaging surveillance strategy may be appropriate.

- Sunitinib and pazopanib are both effective evidence-based first-line treatments; however, their toxicity profiles differ, and pazopanib may prove more tolerable than conventionally scheduled sunitinib for many older patients.

- TKIs have characteristic toxicities. Treatment of older patients should be commenced only after consideration and optimization of comorbidities and anticipatory management of potential treatment toxicities. Multidisciplinary input from specialist geriatric services, including CGA, may be required for this.

References

1 Cancer Research UK. *Kidney cancer statistics.* Available from: www.cancerresearchuk.org/cancer-info/cancerstats/keyfacts/kidney-cancer/ (accessed 6 July 2015).

2 Rini B, Dorff T, Elson P, *et al.* A prospective observational study of metastatic renal cell carcinoma (mRCC) prior to initiation of systemic therapy (abstract). *J Clin Oncol* 2014; 32 (suppl 5): 4520.

3 Heng DY, Xie W, Regan MM, *et al.* Prognostic factors for overall survival in patients with metastatic renal cell carcinoma treated with vascular endothelial growth factor-targeted agents: results from a large, multicenter study. *J Clin Oncol* 2009; 27: 5794–9.

4 Motzer RJ, Hutson TE, Tomczak P, *et al.* Sunitinib versus interferon alfa in metastatic renal-cell carcinoma. *N Engl J Med* 2007; 356: 115–24.

5 Sternberg CN, Davis ID, Mardiak J, *et al.* Pazopanib in locally advanced or metastatic renal cell carcinoma: results of a randomized phase III trial. *J Clin Oncol* 2010; 28: 1061–8.

6 Lee, J, Kim M, Park I, *et al.* Randomized phase II trial of sunitinib four-week on and two-week off versus two-week on and one-week off in metastatic clear cell type renal cell carcinoma: RESTORE trial (abstract). *J Clin Oncol* 2015; 33 (suppl 7): 427.

7 Motzer RJ, Hutson TE, Cella D, *et al.* Pazopanib versus sunitinib in metastatic renal-cell carcinoma. *N Engl J Med* 2013; 369: 722–31.

8 Escudier B, Porta C, Bono P, *et al.* Randomized, controlled, double-blind, cross-over trial assessing treatment preference for pazopanib versus sunitinib in patients with metastatic renal cell carcinoma: PISCES Study. *J Clin Oncol* 2014; 32: 1412–18.

9 Gore ME, Szczylik C, Porta C, *et al.* Safety and efficacy of sunitinib for metastatic renal-cell carcinoma: an expanded-access trial. *Lancet Oncol* 2009; 10: 757–63.

10 Hutson TE, Bukowski RM, Rini B, *et al.* Efficacy and safety of sunitinib in elderly patients with metastatic renal cell carcinoma. *Br J Cancer* 2014; 110: 1125–32.

11 International Society of Geriatric Oncology (2011). *Practice guideline. Comprehensive Geriatric Assessment (CGA) in oncological patients.* Available from: www.siog.org/images/SIOG_documents/cga_practice_guideline_wildiers_jul2011.pdf (accessed 6 July 2015).

12 Elia M, ed.; Malnutrition Advisory Group (MAG), a Standing Committee of the British Association for Parenteral and Enteral Nutrition (2003). *The 'MUST' report. Nutritional screening of adults: a multidisciplinary responsibility.* Available from: www.bapen.org.uk/pdfs/must/must_exec_sum.pdf (accessed 6 July 2015).

14 Lymphoma in a Patient with Pre-existing Depression and Parkinson's Disease Who Struggles to Complete Activities of Daily Living

Hazel Lote, Andrew Webb, Edward Spilg

Case history

A 76-year-old white woman presented with a 2 month history of fever, weight loss, fatigue, drenching night sweats and new lumps in the neck, axillary region and groin. Her past medical history included depression, for which she took citalopram, and Parkinson's disease, for which she took co-beneldopa (levodopa and benserazide hydrochloride). She lived alone and had no family nearby. She had struggled with her activities of daily living (ADL) and her instrumental ADL (IADL) for the past few years, even prior to the onset of her new symptoms. She also had mild cognitive impairment (Montreal Cognitive Assessment, 22/30). Prior to her diagnosis, her Eastern Cooperative Oncology Group (ECOG) performance status (PS) was 2, but over the last month it had dropped to 3.

On examination, there was peripheral lymphadenopathy in the cervical, supra-clavicular, axillary and inguinal regions. There was also palpable hepatosplenomegaly.

Blood tests revealed Hb 96 g/l and platelets 84×10^9/l. Her lactate dehydrogenase (LDH) was above the normal range, but electrolytes, renal and liver function were all normal. CT and PET-CT imaging confirmed FDG-avid lymphadenopathy above and below the diaphragm, along with splenic and liver involvement. Excision biopsy of an axillary lymph node confirmed a diagnosis of diffuse large B cell lymphoma (DLBCL). The cells were positive for CD20 on immunohistochemistry. Bone marrow biopsy and trephine did not show any evidence of lymphoma. An echocardiogram revealed a normal ejection fraction. The overall staging was recorded as stage IVB DLBCL.

Following discussion among the multidisciplinary team (MDT), she was treated with six cycles of R-mini-CHOP (full-dose rituximab in combination with low-dose cyclophosphamide, doxorubicin, vincristine and prednisolone [CHOP]) to a complete metabolic response. She is currently in remission.

What is the goal of cancer treatment for this patient?

What prognostic tools are available, and what staging investigations are required?

Which key questions would you address in this patient prior to making a decision on her treatment?

> What is the evidence base for the patient's treatment options, taking into account her age, PS and comorbidities?

What is the goal of cancer treatment for this patient?

Non-Hodgkin's lymphoma is the sixth most common cancer in the UK,[1] with an incidence of 22 new cases per 100,000 males and 18 per 100,000 females per year in the UK.[1] DLBCL is the most common subtype, accounting for nearly half of all non-Hodgkin's lymphoma diagnoses.[1] It predominantly affects older age groups, with 63% of cases occurring in patients aged 65 or over.[1]

DLBCL is an aggressive disease and, if left untreated, is rapidly fatal.[2] Surgery or radiotherapy alone are not suitable curative options for first-line treatment of this stage of disease.[2,3] It is, however, extremely chemo-responsive and the majority of patients (60% of all patients diagnosed with DLBCL) are cured.[2] Therefore, the aim of treatment in this patient is curative.

What prognostic tools are available, and what staging investigations are required?

Prior to making a treatment recommendation, key information is required regarding the lymphoma and its stage.

International Prognostic Index (IPI) and Revised IPI[2,4]

The International Prognostic Index (IPI) helps calculate prognosis when non-Hodgkin's lymphoma is treated with chemotherapy[2] (Figure 14.1). In the rituximab era, the Revised IPI (R-IPI) characterizes prognosis when chemotherapy is given with rituximab (Figure 14.1).[4]

1 point for each of the following factors:

- Age >60 years
- LDH raised above the upper limit of normal
- ECOG PS ≥2
- Stage 3 or 4 disease
- More than one extranodal disease site involved

Risk	Low	Low to intermediate	High to intermediate	High
IPI score	0, 1	2	3	4, 5
3 year survival	91%	81%	65%	59%

Risk	Very good	Good	Poor
R-IPI score	0	1, 2	3, 4, 5
4 year survival	94%	79%	55%

Figure 14.1 IPI[2] (upper panel) and R-IPI[4] (lower panel). Patients score 1 point for each of the prognostic factors and can then be risk-stratified to provide chances of survival at 3 years (IPI)[2] and 4 years (R-IPI).[4] When assessing the ECOG PS score for lymphoma patients, many patients have a poor PS at presentation due to the extent of their disease, which can cause significant symptoms such as weight loss and night sweats in addition to enlarged lymph nodes.[2] Usually, following treatment, symptoms improve and the PS returns to baseline.

Alternative adaptations include age-adjusted IPI.[3] Even with full treatment, the patient in our case has high-risk disease, with a 60% 3 year survival using IPI criteria, and a 55% 4 year survival using R-IPI criteria.[2]

The Lugano classification[5]

Updated recommendations on initial evaluation, staging and response assessment for Hodgkin's and non-Hodgkin's lymphoma were published in September 2014.[5] Key changes were:
- PET-CT scans are now included.
- Ann-Arbor staging system no longer includes subtypes A or B depending on the presence (B) or absence (A) of B symptoms for non-Hodgkin's lymphoma.
- Bone marrow biopsy is no longer mandatory.[5]
- Despite this, in clinical practice lymphoma staging continues to include A or B subtypes.[2]

Which key questions would you address in this patient prior to making a decision on her treatment?

The first question to address is whether this patient should be treated with chemotherapy. Evidence is emerging that Comprehensive Geriatric Assessment (CGA) may allow identification of older patients who would benefit from further optimization prior to receiving chemotherapy.[6-8]

Issues to address when deciding oncological treatment include:
- Why does this patient struggle to complete ADL (e.g. dressing, eating, ambulation, transfers and hygiene) and IADL (e.g. shopping, housework, medicines management, managing finances, food preparation and telephone use)? Is it predominantly due to Parkinson's disease or depression, or is it related to current lymphoma symptoms? Would occupational therapy or physiotherapy to assess and optimize physical function, cognition and mobility be of benefit in her case? There is increasing evidence from multiple studies in older patients with cancer demonstrating that evaluation of IADL adds substantially to the functional information provided by ECOG.[6]
- Is the Parkinson's disease being optimally treated with co-beneldopa, or are medication adjustments required?[6]
- Is the depression caused by undertreatment of the Parkinson's disease? Are there any reversible causes for the depression? Is the depression being adequately treated? Should any medications be started/adjusted?[6]
- What are the likeliest causes contributing to the mild cognitive impairment?[6] Is it related to the Parkinson's disease, the depression, their treatments, or is there another underlying cause which should be investigated and treated?[6]
- Consider possible drug interactions and modify medications if necessary.[6] For example, metoclopramide antiemetic interacts with Parkinson's disease medications.
- Is nutritional intake adequate?[6] Should a dietitian provide nutritional support to optimize oral intake and correct any nutritional deficiencies that may affect physical or cognitive function?[6]
- Assessment of the level of social support:[6] the patient currently lives alone, but are there family members who could stay for the duration of her chemotherapy regimen? Are carers required? Is community support available? What modes of transport are available and accessible?

- What are the patient's views about embarking on intensive chemotherapy on a background of comorbid disease? What is the patient's mental capacity to inform decision making? Is a Power of Attorney in place?

What is the evidence base for the patient's treatment options, taking into account her age, PS and comorbidities?

The current gold standard therapy for DLBCL is combination chemotherapy combined with rituximab.[3] Major complications of chemotherapy for DLBCL include neutropenic sepsis, rituximab drug reaction, cardiotoxicity, venous thromboembolism, neurotoxicity and, rarely, tumour lysis syndrome. Chemotherapy may also be associated with other side effects that may have a significant impact on quality of life, including: fatigue, nausea and hair loss.[2]

European Society for Medical Oncology clinical practice guidelines[3]

Choice of chemotherapy regimen depends upon the patient's age, comorbidities, frailty, cardiac function and IPI.[3] In healthy patients aged 60–80 years with a high IPI score, the standard chemotherapy is R-CHOP (rituximab, cyclophosphamide, doxorubicin, vincristine and prednisolone). The standard approach would be to offer six to eight cycles (or six cycles of R-CHOP and two additional cycles of rituximab), delivered every 21 days.[3] Clinical practice in the UK is to deliver six cycles of R-CHOP, based on the results of the RICOVER-60 trial.[3,9,10]

European Society for Medical Oncology guidelines recommend CNS prophylaxis in patients with high IPI, potentially delivered via high-dose intravenous rather than intrathecal methotrexate.[3] However, in practice, the delivery of intravenous methotrexate in a patient >70 years old with a poor PS is generally regarded as too toxic. Additionally, there is not a high level of evidence for either intravenous or intrathecal methotrexate.

International Society of Geriatric Oncology expert position commentary[10]

DLBCL prevalence in older patients is increasing, yet these patients are under-represented in clinical trials.[10] R-CHOP is superior to CHOP alone in older people.[10,11] Large phase III clinical trials have shown that the majority of older patients may be treated with full-dose R-CHOP chemotherapy, although there is potential selection bias amongst a trial population versus the standard population.[10] Phase III trials (Groupe d'Etude des Lymphomes de l'Adulte [GELA] and R-CHOP 14 Versus 21[10]), exploring a 21 day versus a 14 day regimen of R-CHOP, did not show any benefit from the 14 day regimen.[3,10] R-CHOP in a 21 day regimen therefore remains the gold standard first-line treatment for all patients in whom there is no contraindication.[3]

In the older population, anthracycline-based chemotherapy may worsen comorbidity and have a detrimental effect on functional status.[7,10] Levels of evidence for attenuated R-CHOP regimens or alternative chemotherapy regimens in first-line treatment of DLBCL are limited to phase II clinical trials.[10] Several of these demonstrate complete remission rates >50%.[10] In the over-80 age group, attenuated regimens such as R-mini-CHOP 21×6 may be appropriate.[3] For patients unable to tolerate anthracyclines, a regimen such as rituximab, cyclophosphamide, vincristine + prednisolone could be considered.[10]

Conclusion and learning points

- Untreated DLBCL is rapidly fatal.
- Even in high-risk, extensive stage DLBCL, the majority of patients can be cured with chemotherapy.
- A proposed algorithm for the assessment and treatment of DLBCL in the older patient is shown in Figure 14.2.

- Chemotherapy is given in an intensive regimen and there is a significant risk of side effects with treatment.
- Effective assessment and optimal management of comorbidities, physical and cognitive function, medication, nutrition, psychological status and social support, potentially inviting the input of a geriatrician, may increase the chances of being able to successfully deliver chemotherapy or guide alternative management when assessment indicates chemotherapy may not be appropriate.
- Ultimately the decision regarding oncological treatment will involve weighing up the risks of treating with the risks of not treating, and discussing these risks openly and honestly with the patient.
- Age alone should not be a contraindication to R-CHOP chemotherapy. Functional assessment, as part of CGA, is a better marker of biological ageing and should be used to assist the selection of patients requiring optimization for appropriate treatments.
- Be aware of possible drug interactions and work closely with geriatricians and other health professionals such as pharmacists to ensure that adverse drug interactions are avoided.
- If the patient has full capacity, he or she will have the final decision regarding the choice of treatment and care.

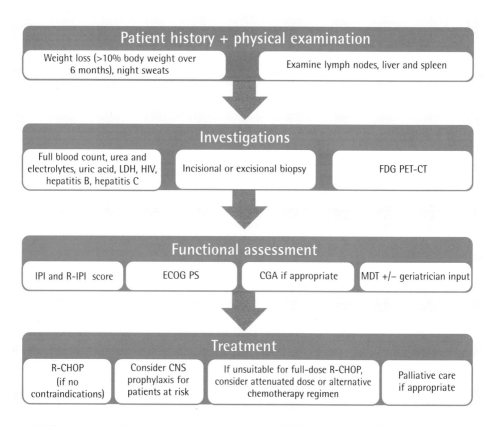

Figure 14.2 Suggested algorithm for assessment and treatment of DLBCL in the older patient.

References

1 Cancer Research UK. *Non-Hodgkin lymphoma incidence statistics.* Available from: www.cancerresearchuk.org/cancer-info/cancerstats/types/nhl/incidence/uk-nonhodgkin-lymphoma-incidence-statistics (accessed February 2015).

2 Freedman AS, Friedberg JW (2015). *Patient information: diffuse large B cell lymphoma in adults (beyond the basics).* Available from: www.uptodate.com/contents/diffuse-large-b-cell-lymphoma-in-adults-beyond-the-basics (accessed 17 March 2015).

3 Tilly H, Vitolo U, Walewski J, *et al.* Diffuse large B-cell lymphoma (DLBCL): ESMO clinical practice guidelines for diagnosis, treatment and follow-up. *Ann Oncol* 2012; 23 (suppl 7): vii78–82.

4 Sehn LH, Berry B, Chhanabhai M, *et al.* The revised international prognostic index (R-IPI) is a better predictor of outcome than the standard IPI for patients with diffuse large B-cell lymphoma treated with R-CHOP. *Blood* 2007; 109: 1857–61.

5 Cheson BD, Fisher RI, Barrington SF, *et al.* Recommendations for initial evaluation, staging, and response assessment of Hodgkin and non-Hodgkin lymphoma: the Lugano classification. *J Clin Oncol* 2014; 32: 3059–68.

6 Extermann M, Hurria A. Comprehensive geriatric assessment for older patients with cancer. *J Clin Oncol* 2007; 25: 1824–31.

7 Morrison VA, Hamlin P, Soubeyran P, *et al.* Diffuse large B-cell lymphoma in the elderly: impact of prognosis, comorbidities, geriatric assessment, and supportive care on clinical practice. An International Society of Geriatric Oncology (SIOG) expert position paper. *J Geriatr Oncol* 2015; 6: 141–52.

8 Owusu C, Berger NA. Comprehensive geriatric assessment in the older cancer patient: coming of age in clinical cancer care. *Clin Pract (Lond)* 2014; 11: 749–62.

9 Pfreundschuh M, Schubert J, Ziepert M, *et al.* Six versus eight cycles of bi-weekly CHOP-14 with or without rituximab in elderly patients with aggressive CD20+ B-cell lymphomas: a randomised controlled trial (RICOVER-60). *Lancet Oncol* 2008; 9: 105–16.

10 Morrison VA, Hamlin P, Soubeyran P, *et al.* Approach to therapy of diffuse large B-cell lymphoma in the elderly: the International Society of Geriatric Oncology (SIOG) expert position commentary. *Ann Oncol* 2015; 26: 1058–68.

11 Coiffier B, Lepage E, Briere J, *et al.* CHOP chemotherapy plus rituximab compared with CHOP alone in elderly patients with diffuse large-B-cell lymphoma. *N Engl J Med* 2002; 346: 235–42.

Further reading

• Nasreddine ZS, Phillips NA, Bédirian V, *et al.* The Montreal cognitive assessment, MoCA: a brief screening tool for mild cognitive impairment. *J Am Geriatr Soc* 2005; 53: 695–9.

15 A Patient with Carcinoma of the Thyroid and Delirium

Cressida Lorimer, James Fleet, Kate Newbold

Case history

A 76-year-old woman with known papillary thyroid cancer was admitted to the oncology ward following thyroidectomy. She had no significant past medical history. She became acutely confused and her family were concerned about her management on the ward. A urinary tract infection was subsequently diagnosed and she recovered with antibiotics. The nursing staff raised concerns about the future planned treatment with radioactive iodine should she have further episodes of confusion.

What is delirium and who is most at risk?

How is delirium diagnosed?

What are the common causes of delirium and how do these particularly relate to older patients with cancer?

How can delirium be prevented?

What measures should be implemented on wards when treating a patient with delirium?

What are the factors to consider in treating older patients with radioactive iodine who are at risk of delirium?

What is delirium and who is most at risk?

Delirium is the most common neuropsychiatric condition seen in oncology patients and is characterized by a rapid onset of fluctuating inattention and global cognition deficits. Often precipitated by multiple triggering factors, it can affect people at any stage of their life; however, it is more common in older people, those with pre-existing cognitive or functional impairment and those with multiple comorbidities. As the population ages, the number of older people with cancer who are at risk of delirium is rising. Delirium is associated with increased risk of death, institutionalization and cognitive decline, even in those without prior cognitive impairment, and its onset is associated with increasing healthcare costs.[1] The incidence in patients with cancer has been reported to be between 8% and 85% depending on the setting.[2] This is explained by the interaction of patient factors and precipitants of varying severity, whereby those with intrinsic risk factors for delirium (representing a vulnerable brain) may develop delirium with mild precipitants, whereas severe illness is often required in those whose brains are less vulnerable.

How is delirium diagnosed?

The diagnosis of delirium rests on clinical assessment and it should be distinguished from other neuropsychiatric disorders such as dementia, depression and psychosis. The gold standard is the

Table 15.1 The Confusion Assessment Method.[3] The diagnosis of delirium requires a present or abnormal rating for features 1 and 2 and for either 3 or 4.

Feature	Assessment
1. Acute onset and fluctuating course	Usually derived from collateral history. Is there evidence of an acute change in mental status with abnormal behaviour that varies in severity through the day?
2. Inattention	Is the patient unable to maintain attention or easily distracted, with difficulty keeping track of conversation?
3. Disorganized thinking	Is the patient's speech incoherent or disorganized, with illogical and unpredictable switching of thoughts and/or irrelevant conversation?
4. Altered level of consciousness	Is the patient 'alert' (normal) or displays an abnormal level of consciousness: vigilant or hyper-alert (hyperactive delirium), lethargic or drowsy, stuporous or comatose (hypoactive delirium); may fluctuate between states (mixed type delirium)

application of DSM-5 criteria, but its use requires experience and time. Therefore, a number of different diagnostic tools have been developed, of which the Confusion Assessment Method[3] (Table 15.1) is the most widely used and has been found to have the best diagnostic utility.

What are the common causes of delirium and how do these particularly relate to older patients with cancer?

Almost any medical illness or inflammatory process may precipitate a delirious episode. Many of these are particularly relevant to patients with cancer (Table 15.2). Many drugs used in oncology have been associated with delirium, including benzodiazepines, steroids, opiates and drugs with a high anticholinergic load (e.g. first-generation antihistamines and tricyclic antidepressants). The relationship is, however, complex: for example, uncontrolled pain is a more significant risk factor for delirium compared with opiates. Therefore, judicious prescribing with consideration of the risks and benefits and use at the lowest therapeutic dose are recommended. With the multitude of potential precipitants, investigation requires a broad approach, including history and clinical examination, infective screen and blood tests. Neuroimaging is mandatory in patients with localizing neurology and is often required in those with an elusive aetiology.

Table 15.2 Common precipitants to delirium and their particular significance in oncology patients.

Precipitant	Oncological relevance
Cardiac disease	Induced by chemotherapy
CNS irritation	Cerebrovascular accident, cerebral metastases, leptomeningeal disease
Constipation/urinary retention	Induced by opiates, antiemetics or tricyclic antidepressants
Dehydration	Chemotherapy-induced diarrhoea and vomiting
Electrolyte disturbance	Hypercalcaemia, malnutrition
Endocrinopathies	Thyroid, adrenal
Hypo/hyperglycaemia	Steroid use
Hypoxaemia	Pneumonia, pulmonary embolism, lung cancer/metastases
Infection	Urinary tract infection, chest infection, neutropenic sepsis

Further tests may include lumbar puncture or electroencephalogram to identify rarer causes such as infective encephalitis or non-convulsive status epilepticus.

How can delirium be prevented?

Prevention of delirium is the most important intervention in minimizing its impact. Randomized controlled trial data have shown that delirium is approximately 30% preventable in surgical and medical groups. As delirium is mostly multifactorial, prevention is through application of multifaceted interventions. Orientation, mobilization, correcting sensory impairment, maintaining hydration and preventing sleep deprivation were the tenets of the widely disseminated Hospital Elder Life Program (www.hospitalelderlifeprogram.org). Medication review, supporting physiology (such as maintaining oxygenation) and preventing medical complications such as infection, constipation and pain have also shown efficacy.[4,5] The routine assessment of patients (for example, at hospital admission) for risk factors for delirium when exposed to potential delirium precipitants is vital to detect patients who may benefit most from preventative strategies and in whom vigilance for the onset of delirium is particularly important. Assessment of poor cognition indicative of possible dementia or delirium can be done through simple screening tools such as the Abbreviated Mental Test Score.

What measures should be implemented on wards when treating a patient with delirium?

The most important aspect of treating established delirium is to identify and treat the precipitant. In treating patients with delirium, emphasis is placed on ensuring a calming and supportive care environment with family involvement, avoiding restraint, and nursing with familiar staff. Whether there is a clear precipitant or not, risk factors which may aggravate or perpetuate the delirium should be addressed through continuation of the tenets of delirium prevention. Investigations and interventions which are not time-critical may be postponed if they appear to aggravate symptoms. Delirium is a risk factor for falls, and appropriate prevention strategies should be instigated. Agitated patients often respond to calming verbal and non-verbal communication strategies. Although direct evidence of benefit is lacking, there is broad agreement across healthcare professionals and guidelines on this approach.

There is no convincing evidence base for drug treatment for delirium and currently no drugs are directly licensed. Conventional management with low-dose haloperidol is usually reserved for specific indications:

- Patients in significant distress due to their delirium.
- To enable essential investigations and treatments.
- To protect staff or others when other strategies are not feasible or fail.

What are the factors to consider in treating older patients with radioactive iodine who are at risk of delirium?

In our patient's case a cognitive assessment such as the Abbreviated Mental Test Score should have been performed on admission and could have revealed pre-existing cognitive impairment, putting the patient at higher risk of developing delirium. The patient was subsequently due to receive radioactive iodine treatment. Remnant ablation with iodine-131 and subsequent thyroid-stimulating hormone (TSH) suppression commonly follow a total thyroidectomy. Iodine is usually taken up by the thyroid gland in order to synthesize triiodothyronine and thyroxine via the sodium–iodide symporter in the membrane of the follicular cells. This delivery system into the cell is exploited for therapy by administering the isotope iodine-131 with the aim of ablating residual remnants of normal thyroid tissue and any remaining thyroid cancer. Iodine-131 has a half-life of around 8 days and emits mainly beta radiation, which gives it a therapeutic penetration of a few millimetres. It is therefore an extremely targeted method of delivering radiation. However, there is also a component of gamma decay that causes issues with radiation protection, which is why this treatment is given on an inpatient basis, with patients being isolated in appropriately protected rooms until the level of emitted radiation drops sufficiently for the patient to be discharged into the community. In order to maximize uptake of iodine-131, patients are asked to adhere to a low-iodine diet for 2 weeks prior to treatment. A raised TSH level is also recommended on the day of administration to optimize the uptake of iodine-131 into the remaining thyroid and thyroid cancer cells. This can be done by withdrawing a patient's thyroxine for 4 weeks; however, hypothyroidism can precipitate delirium and therefore in our patient's case, and in all cases involving older patients or those with significant comorbidities, it was recommended she receive intramuscular recombinant TSH on 2 consecutive days prior to administration of the iodine-131 rather than stop her thyroxine. As our patient had undergone a total thyroidectomy it was also key to monitor her calcium level, as hypocalcaemia secondary to hypoparathyroidism can precipitate delirium.

Iodine-131 is given orally and the majority of it is excreted in the urine and sweat over 3–5 days. Patients are admitted to the ward for assessment prior to administration. After administration, patients are then isolated in a radioiodine suite which has an individual ensuite toilet and washing facilities. The average duration of admission is 3 days and during that time the nursing staff limit how much time they spend with the patient in order to reduce the radiation dose they receive. Visitors are usually restricted to 30 min on the first day, but visiting times may be longer on days 2 and 3 depending on daily measurements performed by the nuclear medicine or medical physics staff. Visitors should not have physical contact with the patient. As our patient's daughter was already concerned about her mother's management, this should be explained carefully and in detail to relatives prior to treatment.

Patients undergoing radioactive iodine ablation must therefore be independent in terms of their activities of daily living, as the level of nursing support should be minimal. Thus, patients are screened carefully and any comorbidities reviewed in order to optimize the performance status of the patient prior to isolation in order to minimize the risk of having to closely nurse or treat a patient emitting radiation. Patients who have specific risk factors for delirium such as alcohol withdrawal, or diabetic patients who manage their own blood sugars, should be risk-stratified prior to deciding on treatment and a medication review should be performed. Our patient was carefully counselled as to the psychological effect of isolation and the importance of remaining well hydrated, given her history of urinary tract infections. Incontinence presents difficulties with management of radioactive waste and may sometimes prevent a patient receiving therapy, but it can usually be managed for example with temporary catheterization or careful management of incontinence pads. As interventions such as urinary catheters can precipitate delirium, it is essential to screen the patient's urinary function. As iodine-131 is excreted in bodily fluids, the towels and sheets are changed daily by the patient. If a patient develops urinary incontinence it raises concerns over the spread of radioactive material and causes difficulties for nursing and cleaning staff in terms of radiation protection.

Conclusion

 Delirium is a common condition amongst hospital inpatients and is more prevalent amongst older and frail people: a group which encompasses many patients with cancer. It is distressing for both the patient and the family, and it is associated with increased mortality and increased expense from prolonged hospital stay, complications and investigations.

In this chapter we have highlighted certain predisposing factors amongst oncology patients that put them at particular risk of delirium. The emphasis in delirium care should be on prevention, as treatment options have a limited evidence base. In patients with thyroid cancer, particular care should be placed on screening for delirium risk factors prior to admission and regular review for early detection, as delirium development during treatment can lead to complications in patients' ward management and potential risks to the staff involved.

References

1 Ljubisavljevic, V, Kelly, B. Risk factors for development of delirium among oncology patients. *Gen Hosp Psychiatry* 2003; 25: 345–52.

2 Witlox J, Eurelings LS, de Jonghe JF, *et al.* Delirium in elderly patients and the risk of postdischarge mortality, institutionalization, and dementia: a meta-analysis. *JAMA* 2010; 304: 443–51.

3 Inouye SK, van Dyck CH, Alessi CA, *et al.* Clarifying confusion: the confusion assessment method. New method for detection of delirium. *Ann Intern Med* 1990; 113: 941–8.

4 Inouye SK, Bogardus ST Jr, Charpentier PA, *et al.* A multicomponent intervention to prevent delirium in hospitalized older patients. *N Engl J Med* 1999; 340: 669–76.

5 Marcantonio ER, Flacker JM, Wright RJ, *et al.* Reducing delirium after hip fracture: a randomized trial. *J Am Geriatr Soc* 2001; 49: 516–22.

Further reading

• Inouye SK, Westendorp RGJ, Saczynski JS. Delirium in elderly people. *Lancet* 2014; 383: 911–22.

• Maclullich AM, Anand A, Davis DH, *et al.* New horizons in the pathogenesis, assessment and management of delirium. *Age Ageing* 2013; 42: 667–74.

• National Institute for Health and Care Excellence (2010). *Delirium. Diagnosis, prevention and management. NICE clinical guideline 103.* Available from: www.nice.org.uk/guidance/cg103 (accessed 30 April 2015).

• British Thyroid Association (www.british-thyroid-association.org).

16 Pancreatic Cancer in a Patient on More Than 10 Internal Medicine Therapies

Alicia Okines, Ian Chau, Juliet Wright

Case history

Ronald was an 82-year-old retired taxi driver with a past medical history of mild chronic obstructive pulmonary disease (COPD), hypertension and ischaemic heart disease. He had been diagnosed with type 2 diabetes 6 months ago and started on oral hypoglycaemic agents. His medications at that point were salbutamol and tiotropium inhalers, ramipril, simvastatin, bisoprolol, glyceryl trinitrate spray, aspirin, metformin and gliclazide. Ronald developed epigastric pain and anorexia 3 months after the diagnosis of diabetes was made. The pain progressively worsened, and he lost more than 5 kg in weight. He had recently become acutely jaundiced and was admitted to hospital for investigations, which revealed a 3 cm tumour in the head of his pancreas causing common bile duct obstruction and multiple liver metastases. A liver biopsy confirmed the diagnosis of metastatic adenocarcinoma of the pancreas. He underwent endoscopic retrograde cholangiopancreatography and biliary stenting, which resolved the jaundice; his pain was controlled by a combination of paracetamol, modified-release morphine and gabapentin. Ronald's appetite improved considerably after commencing low-dose dexamethasone, which was prescribed with lansoprazole for gastric protection. Despite his comorbidities and resultant polypharmacy, his performance status (PS) was 1.

Ronald was offered palliative chemotherapy with single-agent gemcitabine.

What are the aims of anticancer treatment in this patient?

What is the evidence base for the different treatment options for metastatic pancreatic cancer in older patients?

Is there an evidence base for selecting different treatment options on the basis of age or comorbidities?

What could have been done to improve the patient's tolerance of anticancer treatment?

What are the aims of anticancer treatment in this patient?

Ronald's prognosis was a matter of months and the goals of his treatment were to maximize his quality of life and minimize his disease-related symptoms whilst supporting him and his family with advance care planning. Using the Comprehensive Geriatric Assessment framework, areas where more assessment and intervention were required were identified and the appropriate interventions put in place.[1] In optimizing quality of life and function for Ronald it was important to establish the details of his social circumstances and his hopes and fears for the coming months. As Ronald was independent, review by the community physiotherapists and occupational therapists to maintain his independence and safety in the home were arranged. The aim of such assessments was to identify any visual or hearing deficits and minimize the risk of falls, and it was hoped the measures would reduce social isolation and the risk of depression. These initial assessments formed the basis of the developing care plan for Ronald and served to inform advance care decisions about where he would like to be as his condition deteriorated, and what factors were most important to him in his decision making.

What is the evidence base for the different treatment options for metastatic pancreatic cancer in older patients?

Pancreatic cancer is the third most common cause of cancer death in both sexes, predicted to cause over 85,000 deaths in Europe in 2015.[2] Most patients present with advanced inoperable disease, at which point the only active treatment is palliative chemotherapy. Palliative care alone is associated with a median survival of just 3 months for these patients.[3,4] From 1997 until 2011, the standard chemotherapy was gemcitabine monotherapy, based on improved median overall survival (5.65 vs 4.41 months; $p=0.003$) and clinical benefit (reduced pain and analgesic requirements, improvement in PS and/or weight; 24% vs 5%; $p=0.002$) compared with fluorouracil (5-FU) monotherapy.[5] Common toxicities of this weekly treatment include myelosuppression, fatigue, nausea and vomiting, rash and peripheral oedema. Despite numerous combination chemotherapy studies, gemcitabine monotherapy remained the standard of care until a French study demonstrated a significant survival benefit from a triplet chemotherapy comprising folinic acid, 5-FU, irinotecan and oxaliplatin (FOLFIRINOX). The FOLFIRINOX regimen was evaluated in patients with Eastern Cooperative Oncology Group (ECOG) PS 0–1, with a median age of 61 years. The oldest patient in the study was 76. A significant improvement in overall survival compared with standard gemcitabine was reported (median 11.1 vs 6.8 months; $p<0.001$); however, the regimen is also more toxic, with significantly more grade 3–4 neutropenia and febrile neutropenia, thrombocytopenia, diarrhoea, sensory neuropathy and hepatotoxicity.[6] Despite these toxicities, a quality-of-life analysis favoured the FOLFIRINOX regimen. Age >65 years was an independent predictor of poor prognosis in the study, which changed clinical practice in young, fit patients.[7] More recently, the phase III Albumin-bound Paclitaxel Plus Gemcitabine Versus Gemcitabine Alone in Metastatic Adenocarcinoma of the Pancreas (MPACT) study reported a significant (albeit more modest) survival benefit in a more generalizable combination regimen. This trial demonstrated that adding albumin-bound paclitaxel (nab-paclitaxel) to gemcitabine prolonged median survival from 6.7 to 8.5 months ($p<0.001$). The study included patients with Karnofsky PS ≥70% (equivalent to ECOG 0–2),[8] and, although the median age of the trial participants was 63, patients up to 88 years old were included. Inevitably the combination regimen was associated with more grade 3–4 toxicities (neutropenia, peripheral neuropathy and fatigue),[9] and age >65 years was once more confirmed to predict worse survival.[10]

A phase II study is planned of modified FOLFIRINOX chemotherapy in patients aged >70 years with metastatic pancreatic cancer, to assess both the efficacy and tolerability, measured by preservation of independence in daily living using the Katz Index of Independence in Activities of Daily Living (ClinicalTrial.gov registration no. NCT02143219). However, a precision medicine approach to pancreatic cancer treatment is also of relevance to older patients as a potential strategy to maximize response and minimize unnecessary toxicity. Thus far, studies evaluating targeted agents have done so in molecularly unselected populations, with disappointing results. A small survival benefit was reported from the addition of the anti-EGFR tyrosine kinase inhibitor erlotinib to gemcitabine,[11] but the additional median 0.33 months of life that the targeted agent conferred did not change clinical practice. Of interest, comorbidity using the Charlson Comorbidity Index was evaluated in patients randomized within the study and correlated with clinical outcome. Whilst low pain scores and good PS at baseline were found to be independent predictors of survival, age and comorbidity were not.[12]

Is there an evidence base for selecting different treatment options on the basis of age or comorbidities?

That older patients are experiencing reduced survival despite inclusion in well-conducted clinical trials likely reflects a true phenomenon of worse outcomes in older pancreatic cancer patients, irrespective of treatment. How then should we select patients for gemcitabine monotherapy, a doublet with nab-paclitaxel, gemcitabine monotherapy or palliative care alone? At present, there is no recommended algorithm, and PS is the most commonly used factor to select patients who are suitable for active treatment and more intensive regimens. Although chronological age is not traditionally used to direct treatment, lack of experience with the FOLFIRINOX regimen in patients aged >76 should caution physicians considering this combination in an older patient, particularly given the toxicity involved. By contrast, older patients wishing for a more active regimen could be reasonably recommended the gemcitabine/nab-paclitaxel doublet, if carefully counselled regarding the increased toxicity and unknown relative effect on quality of life. Gemcitabine monotherapy remains an option for patients wishing for active treatment but wanting to avoid additional toxicity; however, the response rate with this drug is less than 10%; therefore, the chance of meaningful benefit is relatively low. A suggested algorithm is shown in Figure 16.1.

What could have been done to improve the patient's tolerance of anticancer treatment?

With respect to managing comorbidities, consideration should be given to acute and chronic issues, with particular focus on the adverse effects associated with the prescribing cascade that often accompanies a new diagnosis.

COPD

Ronald's COPD remains an infection risk whilst he is on immunosuppressive agents. Therefore, his COPD treatment regimen should be continued, particularly given the low likelihood of interactions with his new medications.

Cardiovascular disease

The medical management for symptoms of ischaemic heart disease remains a priority, as these could become more significant in the presence of anaemia or dehydration due to chemotherapy-induced diarrhoea or vomiting. Although coronary artery spasm from 5-FU is not always associated with pre-existing coronary artery disease,[13] its consequence can be more serious in patients with pre-existing cardiac conditions. However, medications for the *secondary* prevention of vascular endpoints should be reviewed. As a result, it would seem reasonable to conclude that the risks of side effects and the additional polypharmacy associated with simvastatin now outweigh the long-term benefits and it should be stopped. A review of BP recordings including postural readings may be of use in considering reducing the medicine burden. In the absence of significant ventricular impairment and presence of symptomatic postural hypotension, stopping ramipril may be of symptomatic benefit. Given the risks of nephrotoxicity with chemotherapy-

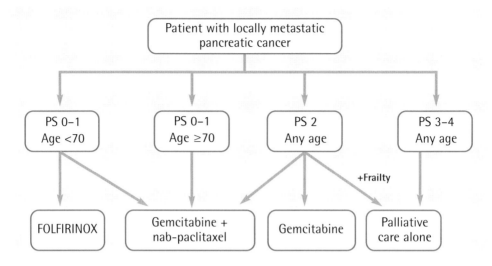

Figure 16.1 Suggested algorithm for first-line treatment decisions.

induced nausea and vomiting, the overall risks of the antihypertensive medication, particularly to renal function, may well now outweigh the benefits.

Diabetes

With respect to diabetes, maintaining nutrition whilst minimizing symptoms of hypo- and hyperglycaemia are the priorities of care. Metformin may be associated with diarrhoea, and gliclazide with hypoglycaemia. Referral to the community diabetes specialist nurses will be key, particularly given the addition of dexamethasone to the prescription, which may increase glucose levels and associated symptoms, and pose an increased risk of infections.

Disease-related symptoms

Medications prescribed for the treatment of cancer-related symptoms may also be a potential source of adverse drug reactions. Lansoprazole is commonly associated with diarrhoea as well as hyponatraemia; therefore, with this and the previously mentioned risks to renal function of the antihypertensives and chemotherapy- and metformin-induced lactic acidosis, regular assessment of electrolyte and kidney function should be arranged. Low-dose dexamethasone may be associated with increased confusion/delirium and difficulty sleeping, particularly in older patients, and is something that should be kept under review by the community palliative care team. Ronald has no reported previous history of mood disturbance, but in the context of his new diagnosis this is something that should be screened for at each review using a tool such as the Geriatric Depression Scale.[14]

Conclusion and learning points

- Metastatic pancreatic cancer has a poor prognosis, and patients aged 65 and over have a worse outcome compared with younger patients.
- Polypharmacy is not unique to older patients but provides another important consideration when discussing treatment with advanced cancer patients.
- Patients' drug histories must be carefully checked prior to commencement of any anticancer agent.

- There are relatively few drug–drug interactions with commonly used cytotoxic agents, but patients with pre-existing organ dysfunction, as a result of comorbidity or its treatment, must be counselled regarding their higher risk of morbidity and mortality should they develop a toxicity which further impacts on organ function.

- Optimization of comorbidities and rationalizing polypharmacy should ideally occur synchronously with referral of an older cancer patient for oncological therapy.

References

1   Rubenstein LZ, Stuck AE, Siu AL, Wieland D. Impacts of geriatric evaluation and management programs on defined outcomes: overview of the evidence. *J Am Geriatr Soc* 1991; 39 (9 part 2): 8–16S.

2   Malvezzi M, Bertuccio P, Rosso T, *et al.* European cancer mortality predictions for the year 2015: does lung cancer have the highest death rate in EU women? *Ann Oncol* 2015; 26: 779–86.

3   Palmer KR, Kerr M, Knowles G, *et al.* Chemotherapy prolongs survival in inoperable pancreatic carcinoma. *Br J Surg* 1994; 81: 882–5.

4   Glimelius B, Hoffman K, Sjödén PO, *et al.* Chemotherapy improves survival and quality of life in advanced pancreatic and biliary cancer. *Ann Oncol* 1996; 7: 593–600.

5   Burris HA 3rd, Moore MJ, Andersen J, *et al.* Improvements in survival and clinical benefit with gemcitabine as first-line therapy for patients with advanced pancreas cancer: a randomized trial. *J Clin Oncol* 1997; 15: 2403–13.

6   Conroy T, Desseigne F, Ychou M, *et al.*; Groupe Tumeurs Digestives of Unicancer; PRODIGE Intergroup. FOLFIRINOX versus gemcitabine for metastatic pancreatic cancer. *N Engl J Med* 2011; 364: 1817–25.

7   Gourgou-Bourgade S, Bascoul-Mollevi C, Desseigne F, *et al.* Impact of FOLFIRINOX compared with gemcitabine on quality of life in patients with metastatic pancreatic cancer: results from the PRODIGE 4/ACCORD 11 randomized trial. *J Clin Oncol* 2013; 31: 23–9.

8   Ma C, Bandukwala S, Burman D, *et al.* Interconversion of three measures of performance status: an empirical analysis. *Eur J Cancer* 2010; 46: 3175–83.

9   Von Hoff DD, Goldstein D, Renschler MF. Albumin-bound paclitaxel plus gemcitabine in pancreatic cancer. *N Engl J Med* 2014; 370: 479–80.

10 Tabernero J, Chiorean EG, Infante JR, *et al.* Prognostic factors of survival in a randomized phase III trial (MPACT) of weekly nab-paclitaxel plus gemcitabine versus gemcitabine alone in patients with metastatic pancreatic cancer. *Oncologist* 2015; 20: 143–50.

11 Moore MJ, Goldstein D, Hamm J, *et al.*; National Cancer Institute of Canada Clinical Trials Group. Erlotinib plus gemcitabine compared with gemcitabine alone in patients with advanced pancreatic cancer: a phase III trial of the National Cancer Institute of Canada Clinical Trials Group. *J Clin Oncol* 2007; 25: 1960–6.

12 Vickers MM, Powell ED, Asmis TR, *et al.* Comorbidity, age and overall survival in patients with advanced pancreatic cancer – results from NCIC CTG PA.3: a phase III trial of gemcitabine plus erlotinib or placebo. *Eur J Cancer* 2012; 48: 1434–42.

13 Ambrosy AP, Kunz PL, Fisher GA, Witteles RM. Capecitabine-induced chest pain relieved by diltiazem. *Am J Cardiol* 2012; 110: 1623–6.

14 Neal RM, Baldwin RC. Screening for anxiety and depression in elderly medical outpatients. *Age Ageing* 1994; 23: 461–4.

17 Advanced Ovarian Cancer in a Patient Who Is Socially Isolated and Deaf

Emily Grist, Lucy Dumas, Jacqueline Gilbert, Susana Banerjee

Case history

An 80-year-old woman presented with a 3 month history of abdominal swelling, pain, breathlessness, fatigue and loss of appetite. Her past medical history included significant hearing impairment, depression since the death of her husband, and osteoarthritis. She lived alone with no close friends or family. She rarely left the house because of increasing abdominal pain, low mood and anxiety in relation to difficulty communicating due to a hearing deficit. She regularly missed meals. Her performance status (PS) was 2.

On abdominal examination, ascites was clinically detectable and confirmed by an ultrasound scan. A right-sided pleural effusion was clinically evident. Blood tests demonstrated normocytic anaemia (Hb 95 g/l), normal renal function and low albumin (27 g/l). A CT chest, abdomen and pelvis scan demonstrated diffuse peritoneal stranding with large-volume ascites, a pelvic mass and a large right pleural effusion. No other visceral disease was noted. CA-125 tumour marker was elevated at 12,672 U/ml.

Ascitic and pleural fluid was drained and sent for cell block examination, which confirmed adenocarcinoma. Biopsy of the pelvic mass confirmed high-grade serous adenocarcinoma. Based on pleural involvement, this patient was diagnosed with stage IV ovarian cancer.

The patient did not attend her first oncology clinic appointment, as she was unable to get to the hospital. The gynaecology cancer specialist nurse was unable to communicate with her over the telephone. The patient attended her rebooked oncology appointment 2 weeks later, unaccompanied.

What are the goals of treatment for this patient?

What is the evidence base to support the patient's treatment options?

What is the role of bevacizumab?

How do the patient's comorbidities affect her cancer treatment options?

How does the patient's social isolation affect her management?

What are the goals of treatment for this patient?

The aim of treatment is to prolong overall survival (OS) and progression-free survival (PFS) whilst improving and maintaining the patient's quality of life. This patient has a high-grade serous ovarian carcinoma and has a good chance of deriving clinical benefit and improved survival with a combination of chemotherapy and debulking surgery.

What is the evidence base to support the patient's treatment options?

Optimal (no residual disease) debulking surgery in specialist gynae-oncology surgical centres has consistently been shown to significantly increase OS and PFS regardless of age.[1,2] A decision had to be made as to whether the patient should proceed directly to primary debulking surgery or whether she should receive neoadjuvant chemotherapy and interval debulking. A randomized trial comparing these strategies showed that the neoadjuvant chemotherapy approach was non-inferior.[3]

Platinum agents have been the backbone of first-line chemotherapy regimens for the last 40 years in advanced ovarian cancer. It has been demonstrated that the addition of paclitaxel to platinum treatment improves OS.[4-6] Results from a phase III trial comparing the efficacy of paclitaxel and carboplatin versus paclitaxel and cisplatin were retrospectively reviewed in patients less than 70 years of age and older than 70 years of age.[7] Early discontinuation of treatment was more frequent in patients older than 70 years, with no significant differences in regard to cycle delays, dose reductions or the use of granulocyte colony-stimulating factor (GCSF) and antibiotics. Toxicities were comparable between older and younger patients, except for febrile neutropenia (5% in patients >70 years of age vs <1% in patients <70 years of age; $p=0.005$). Further evidence for combination chemotherapy in older ovarian cancer patients is limited and often derived from retrospective subgroup analyses of phase II and III clinical trials in which older patients are underrepresented. Such retrospective studies, however, have shown that older patients are prescribed less standard-combination chemotherapy compared with single-agent carboplatin. Furthermore, patients ≥65 years had similar rates of initial response, platinum resistance, PFS and OS to those of younger patients.[8] Therefore, older women who can tolerate it should be considered for combination platinum plus taxane chemotherapy.

This patient's case was discussed at the multidisciplinary team (MDT) meeting. Given her PS of 2, anaemia and hypoalbuminaemia, it was thought unlikely that she would be fit to proceed directly with primary debulking surgery. The time required to optimize her condition to tolerate surgery would lead to deterioration in her cancer-related symptoms. Therefore, it was thought that she should be offered three cycles of neoadjuvant carboplatin (AUC 5) in combination with paclitaxel 175 mg/m^2 administered intravenously every 3 weeks. It was anticipated that during this time the patient would be referred to gynae-oncology surgical and anaesthetic teams for optimization prior to debulking surgery. Geriatric oncological input would be very helpful at this point.

What is the role of bevacizumab?

Bevacizumab is a monoclonal antibody that targets vascular endothelial growth factor, a critical component in angiogenesis. Angiogenesis is an important component of ovarian cancer growth and progression.

Two randomized trials, the Gynaecologic Oncology Group trial 218[9] and the International Collaborative Ovarian Neoplasm (ICON) 7 trial,[10] both reported a PFS advantage for the addition of bevacizumab to carboplatin plus paclitaxel, with subsequent maintenance bevacizumab as front-line therapy. The benefit of bevacizumab is greater in patients defined as being at the highest risk of progression (around 3.6 months). Furthermore, in ICON7, a significant improvement in OS with bevacizumab was seen in the high-risk group, defined as having International Federation of Gynecology and Obstetrics (FIGO) stage IV disease, or FIGO stage III disease and more than 1.0 cm of residual disease after debulking surgery. The demonstration of a survival benefit of almost 8 months in patients with a poor prognosis is very encouraging (28.8 vs 36.6 months; HR 0.64, 95% CI 0.48–0.85, $p<0.002$).

Toxicities associated with bevacizumab include hypertension, bleeding and thrombosis, poor wound healing, proteinuria and bowel perforation/fistula.

The patient discussed in this case had no comorbidities that would contraindicate the use of bevacizumab. Given the greater prevalence of hypertension and renal impairment in the older patient population, however, careful monitoring of BP is important, as is regular urinalysis to test for proteinuria. It should also be considered that with prolonged maintenance treatment there would be an increased number of hospital attendances for the patient.

How do the patient's comorbidities affect her cancer treatment options?

Completing a Comprehensive Geriatric Assessment to determine medical health, mental health, functional capacity, social and environmental challenges, in order to facilitate a holistic treatment plan, is integral to this case.

Paclitaxel and carboplatin combination chemotherapy is myelosuppressive. The patient needs to be aware she must report a fever, as she is at risk of febrile neutropenia. The patient will be given a chemotherapy alert card to inform people in an emergency that she is at risk of neutropenic sepsis. The patient must have access to a home thermometer and will need to be able to communicate the need for medical assistance if she feels unwell or develops a febrile illness. Social services can provide a medical alert system for her home. Should persistent neutropenia become problematic, GCSF or dose reductions of chemotherapy should be considered to minimize the risk of neutropenic sepsis and maintain dose intensity.

Peripheral neuropathy is a toxicity associated with paclitaxel treatment. In older patients it may increase their risk of falls. It is important that the patient is asked about pretreatment peripheral neuropathy. Should she develop worsening peripheral neuropathy secondary to chemotherapy, her paclitaxel should be reduced or omitted.

The patient has hearing loss, and carboplatin can cause ototoxicity. If the patient reports a further decline in her hearing, carboplatin may need to be reduced or omitted. It may be useful to refer the patient for audiology assessment prior to commencing chemotherapy.

Fatigue is a significant problem in older patients receiving chemotherapy and can exacerbate social isolation. Fatigue may be associated with anaemia requiring red blood cell transfusion. A package of care should be considered during chemotherapy if the patient has difficulty with activities of daily living. Social services are also able to advise on the availability of local assistance with food preparation including meals-on-wheels service.

Patients with cancer receiving chemotherapy are at risk of thrombosis, including deep vein thrombosis and arterial thrombosis. Bevacizumab can further increase the risk of thrombosis. Vascular risk factors should always be considered when taking a past medical history in older patients being considered for chemotherapy. The patient is at high risk of a deep vein thrombosis given her poor mobility secondary to osteoarthritis and she should be warned of this risk and the need to keep mobile and hydrated to reduce her risk factors.

How does the patient's social isolation affect her management?

Half of people over 75 years of age live alone and have less than monthly contact with friends, family and neighbours.[11] Cancer specialist nurses and Macmillan teams can assist the patient in contacting local voluntary services such as Age UK and local befriending services for socially isolated older people. The patient's GP should be kept up to date with her progress, as the GP is an integral part of the patient's community team.

The incidence of depression increases with age and can contribute to social isolation, which may be further exacerbated by alopecia associated with paclitaxel. It is important that the patient's mental state is assessed regularly and that she has capacity to make decisions. Should the patient's mood worsen during treatment it would be important to involve psychological services and specifically older persons' mental health teams.

Given the patient's hearing impairment, all efforts need to be made during each consultation to optimize communication with the use of hearing aids, written material and use of body language. Background noise needs to be minimized. It is important the patient can communicate with medical teams.

The patient has abdominal discomfort, which can limit PS, impair quality of life and exacerbate depression. Community palliative care teams should be involved early to offer expertise on symptom management. In addition, the patient's clinical nurse specialist will be very important as a key worker helping her through cancer treatment and beyond. Use of a dosette box should be considered to assist the patient in managing her medication.

Logistical factors need to be considered early on and hospital transport arranged so the patient can attend her frequent appointments. The Next Generation Text service helps people with hearing loss to access the telephone system. A relay assistant acts as an intermediary to convert speech to text and vice versa for the two people in conversation. This means the patient can be contacted about her appointments and she will be enabled to report problems early.

Conclusion and learning points

- Older patients need to be assessed by the MDT for primary debulking surgery or neoadjuvant chemotherapy followed by interval debulking surgery. Combination chemotherapy (carboplatin and paclitaxel), together with surgery, offers the best chance of improving OS.
- Bevacizumab should be considered for patients with high-risk (residual disease/stage IV) ovarian cancer, irrespective of age.
- It is important that the benefits, toxicities and practicalities of chemotherapy are explained in detail to older patients. Treatment should not be withheld because of complex care needs that require specific geriatric assessment and intensive support.

References

1 du Bois A, Reuss A, Pujade-Lauraine E, *et al*. Role of surgical outcome as prognostic factor in advanced epithelial ovarian cancer: a combined exploratory analysis of 3 prospectively randomized phase 3 multicenter trials: by the Arbeitsgemeinschaft Gynäkologische Onkologie Studiengruppe Ovarialkarzinom (AGO-OVAR) and the Groupe d'Investigateurs Nationaux Pour les Etudes des Cancers de l'Ovaire (GINECO). *Cancer* 2009; 115: 1234–44.

2 van der Burg ME, van Lent M, Buyse M, *et al*. The effect of debulking surgery after induction chemotherapy on the prognosis in advanced epithelial ovarian cancer. Gynecological Cancer Cooperative Group of the European Organisation for Research and Treatment of Cancer. *N Engl J Med* 1995; 332: 629–34.

3 Vergote I, Tropé CG, Amant F, *et al*. Neoadjuvant chemotherapy or primary surgery in stage IIIC or IV ovarian cancer. *N Engl J Med* 2010; 363: 943–53.

4 du Bois A, Lueck H, Meier W, *et al*. Cisplatin/paclitaxel vs carboplatin/paclitaxel in ovarian cancer: update of an AGO trial. *Proc Am Soc Clin Oncol* 1999; 18: 356 (abstract 1374).

5 Neijt JP, Engelholm SA, Tuxen MK, *et al.* Exploratory phase III study of paclitaxel and cisplatin versus paclitaxel and carboplatin in advanced ovarian cancer. *J Clin Oncol* 2000; 18: 3084-92.

6 Ozols RF, Bundy BN, Greer BE, *et al.* Phase III trial of carboplatin and paclitaxel compared with cisplatin and paclitaxel in patients with optimally resected stage III ovarian cancer: a Gynecologic Oncology Group Study. *J Clin Oncol* 2003; 21: 3194–200.

7 Hilpert F, du Bois A, Greimel ER, *et al.* Feasibility, toxicity and quality of life of first-line chemotherapy with platinum/paclitaxel in elderly patients aged ≥70 years with advanced ovarian cancer – a study by the AGO OVAR Germany. *Ann Oncol* 2007; 18: 282–7.

8 Eisenhauer EL, Tew WP, Levine DA, *et al.* Response and outcomes in elderly patients with stages IIIC–IV ovarian cancer receiving platinum–taxane chemotherapy. *Gynecol Oncol* 2007; 106: 381–7.

9 Burger RA, Brady MF, Bookman MA, *et al.* Incorporation of bevacizumab in the primary treatment of ovarian cancer. *N Engl J Med* 2011; 365: 2473–83.

10 Perren TJ, Swart AM, Pfisterer J, *et al.* A phase 3 trial of bevacizumab in ovarian cancer. *N Engl J Med* 2011; 365: 2484–96.

11 Age UK. *Loneliness and isolation. Evidence review.* Available from: www.ageuk.org.uk/documents/en-gb/for-professionals/evidence_review_loneliness_and_isolation.pdf?dtrk=true (accessed 25 February 2015).

18 Fitness for Radical Surgery in a Patient with Uterine Cancer, Hypertension, Obesity and Peripheral Vascular Disease

Edward Armstrong, Ingrid Kane, Sonali Kaushik, Kate Lankester

Case history

A 79-year-old woman presented with a 2 month history of intermittent postmenopausal vaginal bleeding. She initially tried topical vaginal oestrogen cream, thinking she had atrophic vaginitis, but there was no improvement. She had no pain, vaginal discharge or weight loss. Her GP referred her urgently for a transvaginal ultrasound scan, which identified endometrial thickening of 9 mm. An endometrial biopsy confirmed a grade 2 endometrioid adenocarcinoma. She had an MRI scan of the abdomen and pelvis, which demonstrated deep myometrial invasion >50%, but no obvious pelvic or para-aortic lymph node involvement. Her chest x-ray was normal.

Her medical history included peripheral vascular disease (PVD) and obesity. Her BP was 168/102 mmHg and her BMI was 34 kg/m². She was able to walk 80 m before developing claudication. She became short of breath ascending one flight of stairs. She was taking aspirin and simvastatin. Her performance status was 2. She had had two children, both with normal vaginal deliveries. She lived alone and had weekly visits from relatives.

Her case was discussed in the gynaecological cancers multidisciplinary team (MDT) meeting. Her cancer was assessed as stage IB (i.e. >50% myometrial invasion) according to the classification of the International Federation of Gynecology and Obstetrics (FIGO) (Table 18.1).[1] It was recommended that she have a laparoscopic hysterectomy and bilateral salpingo-oophorectomy plus pelvic lymph node sampling. The MDT recommended a review by a care of the elderly physician, optimization of medical comorbidities and an assessment in the surgical clinic regarding her suitability for surgery and anaesthetic risk.

What are the goals of treatment for this patient?

What can be done preoperatively to optimize her for surgery?

How is obesity relevant to her management?

What can be done to improve her postoperative recovery?

What adjuvant treatment might be recommended?

If the risk of surgery was deemed to be too high, what alternative treatment could be recommended?

Table 18.1	FIGO staging of endometrial cancer (2009).
Stage I	Confined to the corpus uteri
A B	Less than 50% myometrial invasion More than 50% myometrial invasion
Stage II	Invades cervical stroma but not beyond uterus
Stage III	Local and/or regional spread
A B C1 C2	Invasion of serosa of the corpus uteri and/or adnexae Vaginal and/or parametrial involvement Pelvic node involvement Para-aortic lymph node involvement with or without pelvic lymph node involvement
Stage IV	
A B	Invasion of bladder and/or bowel mucosa Distant metastases including intra-abdominal and or inguinal lymph nodes

What are the goals of treatment for this patient?

For early-stage endometrial cancer, patients should be offered treatment with curative intent. This usually involves primary surgery followed by an evaluation of the potential benefits of adjuvant radiotherapy (external beam radiation therapy [EBRT] or brachytherapy) and adjuvant chemotherapy. There must be a compelling reason to deviate from such a potentially curative pathway. However, in a patient with comorbidities care needs to be taken to ensure that the patient is fit enough for a radical treatment approach. This applies to primary surgery but is equally important when considering adjuvant therapies.

What can be done preoperatively to optimize her for surgery?

An assessment of the patient's anaesthetic and complication risk and prompt optimization of comorbidities are necessary. Preoperative identification of risks pertinent to the individual patient may allow interventions to be made to modify such risks and plan for postoperative recovery and rehabilitation. The patient was reviewed by the care of the elderly team. They performed a Comprehensive Geriatric Assessment to enable a coordinated and integrated plan for her treatment.

Uncontrolled hypertension is a risk factor for anaesthetic complications such as stroke and cardiac events. The patient's BP was managed in accordance with British Hypertension Society Guidelines 2011 (Figure 18.1).[2] These recommend checking BP twice in the clinic and recording the lower reading (which in this patient's case was 168/102 mmHg) before arranging ambulatory BP monitoring to confirm the diagnosis. The target clinic BP in a patient under 80 years of age is 140/90 mmHg and in those over 80 years, 150/90 mmHg. Depending on the urgency of surgery, the geriatrician may take the decision to start treatment based on clinic BP readings, the initial drug of choice in this patient being a calcium channel blocker. In view of her hypertension and PVD she was advised to continue her simvastatin and aspirin along with the addition of her new antihypertensive. An assessment for end-organ damage (including checking for proteinuria) was also performed.

PVD is common in the older population: it is estimated that 20% of people aged above 60 have some degree of peripheral arterial disease.[3] The patient was examined for evidence of peripheral

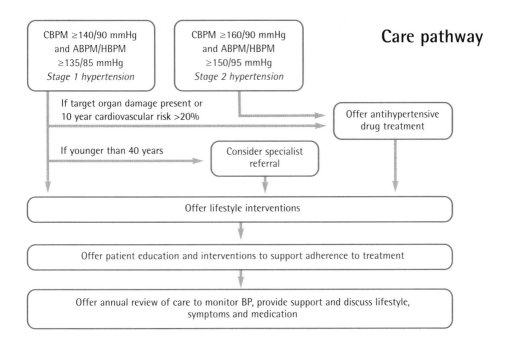

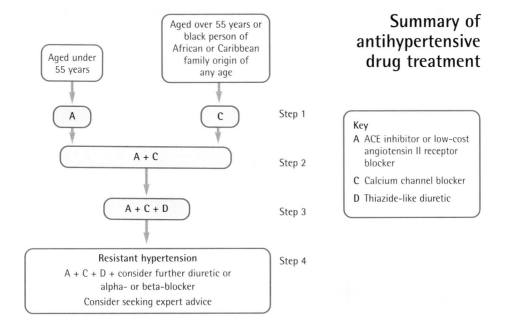

Figure 18.1 British Hypertension Guidelines (adapted from NICE guidelines[2]). ABPM, ambulatory BP measurement; CBPM, clinic BP measurement; HBPM, home BP measurement.

ischaemia and was found to have weak but present dorsalis pedis and posterior tibial pulses. Her ankle–brachial pressure index was measured with a Doppler probe and was calculated to be 0.8, suggesting mild-to-moderate arterial disease. In view of her PVD and newly diagnosed hypertension, a preoperative assessment of cardiac function was required to exclude undiagnosed cardiac disease. This included an ECG, and, depending on other clinical findings, an echocardiogram and myocardial perfusion scan (since she was unable to perform an exercise tolerance test due to her PVD) may be indicated. If aspirin must be discontinued for the operation, it should be recommenced as soon as possible.[4] PVD has further relevance if a patient requires lower limb elevation whilst placed in the lithotomy surgical position.

Postoperative care should be planned and communicated to ward teams prior to surgery. For this patient this includes early mobilization (increased risk of postoperative pneumonia, venous thromboembolism and physical deconditioning if delayed), early catheter removal (risks of catheter-associated infections and exacerbating/precipitating urinary incontinence, which is more common in obese individuals) and discharge planning (rehabilitation plans, arranging necessary equipment and social services input ahead of surgery).

How is obesity relevant to her management?

Owing to the increased oestrogen production by adipose tissue, obesity is an independent risk factor for the development of endometrial cancer and is associated with approximately 50% of all UK cases of endometrial cancer.[5]

MRI is used for preoperative staging, as tumour extent within the uterus cannot be seen accurately on CT scans. Many MR scanners, however, have a weight and circumference limit, prohibiting imaging of patients with gross or morbid obesity, thus compromising accurate staging where it is most needed.

Significant obesity also increases anaesthetic and surgical risk, both in terms of the systemic comorbidities associated with obesity (diabetes, cardiovascular disease, dyslipidaemia and obstructive sleep apnoea) and also in terms of the technical challenge at the time of intubation and extubation. There is a higher conversion rate from laparoscopic to open hysterectomy in obese patients undergoing endometrial cancer surgery. This may lead to increased wound infection, analgesic requirements, longer postoperative recovery and length of hospitalization. It is also technically more challenging to remove pelvic lymph nodes in an obese patient: a pragmatic decision not to proceed with lymphadenectomy may have to be made, particularly if preoperative imaging does not identify any lymph node enlargement. In patients deemed unfit for general anaesthesia, a total abdominal hysterectomy and bilateral salpingo-oophorectomy via a Pfannensteil (transverse) incision under spinal anaesthesia is an alternative surgical option.

What can be done to improve her postoperative recovery?

Extra consideration may be necessary to improve postoperative recovery in older patients. The care of the elderly team reviewed her preoperatively and she was put on the enhanced recovery programme.[6]

She was regularly reviewed by the acute pain team to enable pain-free early mobilization. Her supervising physiotherapist implemented a planned recovery programme. She was prescribed nutritional high-calorie supplement drinks preoperatively and then encouraged to recommence a normal diet when allowed following surgery.

In advance of her surgery, pre-emptive discharge planning was implemented including liaison with an intermediate care facility to arrange a period of rehabilitation. This also included early assessment by the occupational therapy team and social services to arrange a package of care and ongoing rehabilitation at home for when she was discharged.

The patient's rehabilitation needs were explained to her next of kin, and her GP was informed of the changes to her medication and her personal rehabilitation goals.

What adjuvant treatment might be recommended?

Stage I endometrial cancer has an excellent prognosis, with relative 5 year survival of 95%.[7] In the earliest stages (stage IA grade 1–2), no further treatment is recommended following surgical resection. The Postoperative Radiation Therapy in Endometrial Carcinoma (PORTEC) 1 trial compared surgery alone with surgery followed by postoperative radiotherapy in women with stage I endometrial cancer.[8] Thirty-four percent of the trial population were aged 70 or over: at 15 years' follow-up the local recurrence rate was 6% in those who received postoperative EBRT and 15.5% in those who did not.[9] However, the absolute benefit that an individual older patient derives from radiotherapy will be influenced by the risk of death from competing causes, particularly when considering 15 year outcomes. Moreover, pelvic radiotherapy involves 5 weeks of daily treatment and can cause bowel and bladder toxicity. These side effects may be more difficult for an older patient to manage or tolerate, especially in the presence of medical comorbidities. The most likely site of recurrence is at the vaginal vault. A more recent trial has shown that high-dose-rate brachytherapy to the vaginal vault provides equivalent control rates to those of pelvic EBRT, with significantly fewer gastrointestinal side effects.[10] For brachytherapy, the patient needs to be able to lie flat comfortably and get into the lithotomy position. In selected older patients this approach may be a suitable alternative to EBRT. There is currently no consensus regarding the role for adjuvant chemotherapy in high-risk stage I endometrial cancer, although trials evaluating this question are ongoing.

If the risk of surgery was deemed to be too high, what alternative treatment could be recommended?

In older patients who are too frail for surgery, it is unlikely that they would be fit for prolonged courses of radical radiotherapy. However, short courses of palliative radiotherapy (e.g. 20 Gy in five fractions) can help reduce bleeding and pain. Hormonal therapy using progestogens or aromatase inhibitors can also be used to for palliation, particularly for low-grade tumours.

Conclusion and learning points

- Early-stage (stage I) endometrial cancer should be treated with curative intent, assuming the patient is deemed fit enough for radical treatment.

- Obesity is a risk factor for endometrial cancer and its recurrence, and it is associated with higher operative complications.

- Comorbidities should be reviewed and optimized in the preoperative setting to maximize the chance of treating a patient with curative intent, and to minimize the risks of complications. This requires close collaboration between geriatricians and gynaecological oncology surgeons.

- The presence of obesity should alert the clinician to proactively exclude associated significant comorbidities such as cardiac disease and diabetes.

- Adjuvant EBRT has a potential role in stage I endometrial cancer in reducing rates of local recurrence. But the absolute benefits are modest at 15 years of follow-up, and the influences of competing mortality risk and acute radiotherapy toxicity need to be borne in mind.

- Palliative radiotherapy and hormone therapy can be considered in the older patient unfit for surgery.

References

1 The new FIGO staging system for cancers of the vulva, cervix, endometrium, and sarcomas. *Gynecol Oncol* 2009; 115: 325–8.

2 National Institute for Health and Care Excellence (2011). *Hypertension. Clinical management of primary hypertension in adults. NICE clinical guideline 127.* Available from: www.nice.org.uk/guidance/cg127/resources/guidance-hypertension-pdf (accessed 30 April 2015).

3 National Institute for Health and Care Excellence (2014). *Lower limb peripheral arterial disease: diagnosis and management.* Available from: http://pathways.nice.org.uk/pathways/lower-limb-peripheral-arterial-disease (accessed 30 April 2015).

4 Fleisher LA, Beckman JA, Brown KA, *et al.* ACC/AHA 2007 guidelines on perioperative cardiovascular evaluation and care for noncardiac surgery: a report of the American College of Cardiology/American Heart Association Task Force on Practice Guidelines (Writing Committee to Revise the 2002 Guidelines on Perioperative Cardiovascular Evaluation for Noncardiac Surgery) developed in collaboration with the American Society of Echocardiography, American Society of Nuclear Cardiology, Heart Rhythm Society, Society of Cardiovascular Anesthesiologists, Society for Cardiovascular Angiography and Interventions, Society for Vascular Medicine and Biology, and Society for Vascular Surgery. *J Am Coll Cardiol* 2007; 50: e159–241.

5 Reeves GK, Pirie K, Beral V, *et al.*; Million Women Study Collaboration. Cancer incidence and mortality in relation to body mass index in the Million Women Study. *BMJ* 2007; 335: 1134.

6 NHS Institute for Innovation and Improvement. *Quality and service improvement tools. Enhanced recovery programme.* Available from: www.institute.nhs.uk/quality_and_service_improvement_tools/quality_and_service_improvement_tools/enhanced_recovery_programme.html (accessed 30 April 2015).

7 Cancer Research UK. *Cancer statistics for the UK.* Available from: www.cancerresearchuk.org/health-professional/cancer-statistics (accessed 30 April 2015).

8 Creutzberg CL, van Putten WL, Koper PC, *et al.* Surgery and postoperative radiotherapy versus surgery alone for patients with stage-1 endometrial carcinoma: multicentre randomised trial. PORTEC Study Group. *Lancet* 2000; 355: 1404–11.

9 Creutzberg CL, Nout RA, Lybeert ML, *et al.* Fifteen-year radiotherapy outcomes of the randomized PORTEC-1 trial for endometrial carcinoma. *Int J Radiat Oncol Biol Phys* 2011; 81: e631–8.

10 Nout RA, Smit VT, Putter H, *et al.*; PORTEC Study Group. Vaginal brachytherapy versus pelvic external beam radiotherapy for patients with endometrial cancer of high-intermediate risk (PORTEC-2): an open-label, non-inferiority, randomised trial. *Lancet* 2010; 375: 816–23.

Further reading

- Colombo N, Preti E, Landoni F, *et al.*; ESMO Guidelines Working Group. Endometrial cancer: ESMO clinical practice guidelines for diagnosis, treatment and follow-up. *Ann Oncol* 2013; 24 (suppl 6): vi33–8.

19 A Patient with Head and Neck Cancer Who Is a Heavy Smoker with Emphysema and Poor Nutrition

Kee Howe Wong, Fionna Martin, Peter Diem, Shree Bhide

Case history

An 82-year-old man presented with a 2 month history of sore throat and a neck lump. He was a heavy smoker with a 60 pack-year history. His past medical history included emphysema, hypertension, hypothyroidism and alcohol misuse. His repeat prescription list detailed inhalers, furosemide, losartan, amlodipine, levothyroxine, thiamine and vitamin B complex. He admitted not taking his medications regularly. At a slow pace, he could walk about 150 m on the flat before stopping and had been hospitalized once in the last year with pneumonia. He lived alone in a two-storey maisonette without carers, but his nephew visited him weekly.

Examination revealed a man wearing trousers two sizes too large with a BMI of 18 kg/m². His chest was barrel-shaped and peripheral oedema was evident. Blood tests revealed macrocytic anaemia, low creatinine, and albumin 27 g/l. The right-sided cervical lymph nodes were palpable. Imaging of his head and neck demonstrated a right tonsillar tumour with ipsilateral level II pathological lymph nodes. Ultrasound-guided fine needle aspiration from the node confirmed p16-negative moderately differentiated squamous cell carcinoma. Following MRI and PET/CT, he was staged as T2N2bM0 and referred on to the local preoperative assessment clinic for further evaluation of his cardiorespiratory and nutritional status.

A detailed assessment at the clinic identified:

- Multifactorial malnutrition (dysphagia, poor dentition, alcoholism, financial hardship and difficulties shopping).

- Stage III airflow obstruction (FEV$_1$ 45%) with grade 3 dyspnoea (MRC scale) and poor inhaler technique.

- An unwillingness to alter his smoking habit.

- Functional decline, with difficulty getting to shops and bank.

At the subsequent joint head and neck clinic, the risks and benefits of surgical and radiotherapy interventions as well as palliative options were discussed in detail alongside exploration of the patient's personal goals for treatment. A decision was made to proceed with radical radiotherapy after a short period of medical and nutritional optimization.

What is the evidence base for his treatment options?

What treatment factors influenced decision making in this case?

What patient factors influenced decision making in this case?

Why is the finding of malnutrition so important?

How can this patient's comorbidities be optimized prior to treatment?

What is the evidence base for his treatment options?

This patient had locally advanced head and neck cancer, for which the primary treatment modalities are surgery and external beam radiotherapy. Aggressive surgical management in the older population has been shown to be effective but poses a higher risk of systemic complications.[1] On the other hand, radical radiotherapy offers the benefit of functional organ preservation. There are no large randomized controlled trials comparing chemoradiation versus a surgical approach in patients with locally advanced oropharyngeal cancer. Nevertheless, excellent overall survival (OS) and swallowing results have been reported with chemoradiation approaches for advanced oropharyngeal cancer,[2] which increasingly have become the preferred treatment modality.

Concomitant platinum-based chemotherapy with radiotherapy improves 5 year OS by 6.5%, but subgroup analyses demonstrated harm in those over 70, in part due to chemotoxicity resulting in delayed or prevented completion of radiotherapy.[3] There is currently no evidence to support the use of other radiosensitizers, e.g. cetuximab, in the over-70s. Therefore, the recommended curative treatment was radical radiotherapy alone.

What treatment factors influenced decision making in this case?

Surgical considerations

Surgery for this patient would involve right pharyngectomy and selective neck dissection under general anaesthesia requiring a postoperative HDU/ITU stay and possibly a temporary tracheostomy. In older patients, the duration and extent of the operative procedure are important parameters of concern, in addition to preoperative comorbidities.[4] This patient had a significant risk of postoperative pneumonia – both immediate (ventilator-associated) and late (due to impaired cough and sputum clearance with microaspiration). His continued cigarette smoking and emphysema added to his pulmonary complication risk. Other potential complications were failure to wean from respiratory support, tracheostomy-related complications, delirium, worsened nutritional status and functional dependence. Moreover, he might require adjuvant radiotherapy due to potential close or involved surgical margin, which made primary surgery a less attractive treatment option.

Radiotherapy considerations

Radical radiotherapy consists of daily weekday treatments over 6 weeks. This patient required bilateral neck radiotherapy due to the risk of contralateral lymphatic spread, and he was able to lie flat for the 15 min treatment time. The incidence of acute and late toxicities from radiotherapy is independent of age, but older patients tolerate acute toxicity less well.[5] Active support during treatment is therefore crucial, and this patient was fortunate to have a nephew who was able to support him. His emphysema was not considered to be a risk factor for head and neck radiotherapy, but acute pharyngeal mucositis with inflammation and oedema of muscles involved in swallowing during radiotherapy predisposes patients to aspiration pneumonia. This risk was mitigated to some degree with prophylactic enteral feeding and regular clinical review. Overall, radiotherapy offered him the best chance of long-term control with the least morbidity.

What patient factors influenced decision making in this case?

A problem-seeking approach using Comprehensive Geriatric Assessment at his initial oncology clinic appointment allowed rapid identification of the patient's complex health needs and risk factors for treatment.

- Malnutrition is a well-recognized risk factor for postoperative complications and is a common preoperative finding in head and neck cancer patients, attributable to poor dietary habits, excess alcohol consumption and local tumour effects. Patients are at severe nutritional risk if they have any one of the following: BMI <18.5 kg/m^2, serum albumin <30 g/l, or unintentional weight loss >10% in the preceding 6 months. This patient's nutritional status needed to be carefully considered in the decision whether to proceed with any active treatment.

- Emphysema with a significantly reduced exercise capacity engenders increased morbidity and mortality risk from surgery.[6] Continued smoking also increases the risk of treatment failure.[7] Overall, his stage III airflow obstruction on spirometry strongly favoured the radiotherapy treatment option, avoiding the high risks associated with a general anaesthetic and postoperative complications.

- Peripheral oedema could have been due to a number of possible causes, including amlodipine therapy, malnutrition, likely chronic venous insufficiency and a mildly raised urinary protein:creatinine ratio. Importantly, alcoholic liver disease was excluded. Echocardiography demonstrated a mean pulmonary arterial pressure of 30 mmHg, excluding clinically significant pulmonary hypertension.

- Functional ability was assessed by a domiciliary occupational therapy visit, which identified difficulties with food shopping, meal preparation and stair mobility. A decline in physical function was anticipated during radiotherapy largely due to fatigue, but radiotherapy remained the more tolerable treatment.

- The patient's goals were to pursue curative treatment but avoid surgery: he disliked the prospect of hospital admission, as he was concerned about losing his independence and having restricted freedom to smoke. Although realistic about the potential toxicity of radiotherapy, the patient felt this modality gave him the best chance of gaining additional years of quality life.

Why is the finding of malnutrition so important?

A low BMI is a red flag warranting further investigation. Although not always associated with malnutrition (including vitamin deficiencies), evidence of the latter should be sought. Head and neck cancer contributes to malnutrition through increased energy expenditure, skeletal muscle wasting and abnormal metabolism, and directly impacts swallowing function. Nevertheless, it would be wrong always to assume that low weight is all cancer-related. Many causes of low BMI are potentially modifiable, e.g. malabsorption, chronic inflammatory states, mood disorders, hyperthyroidism and poor dentition, as are social contributors such as financial hardship and difficulties shopping/cooking. Other causes may not be reversible (alcoholic cirrhosis, cognitive impairment, cardiac and respiratory cachexia) but can be supported once identified. The use of nutritional screening tools (e.g. MUST, the Malnutrition Universal Screening Tool) in the oncology clinic can quickly identify at-risk patients for assessment and intervention. Low BMI is associated with poor intensive care outcomes; low pretreatment serum albumin indicates worse cancer survival outcomes regardless of treatment modality chosen.[8] Enteral feeding is widely accepted to be necessary prior to surgical or radiotherapy treatment of head and neck cancer, but the optimal feeding route remains unclear.[9]

How can this patient's comorbidities be optimized prior to treatment?

Malnutrition

Once identified, malnutrition is best addressed through a multidisciplinary approach.

- Identify the cause (as described in the case above) and treat commonly associated vitamin deficiencies. The patient's blood tests revealed macrocytosis secondary to vitamin B_{12} and folate deficiency and alcoholism. Vitamin replacement was organized by his GP. As regards alcohol history, the patient consumed three cans of strong lager daily. He reported prioritizing the purchase of lager over food in the last few years. A referral to local alcohol misuse services was made and he was started on B vitamins and vitamin C supplements (Pabrinex) to reduce the risk of Wernicke–Korsakoff syndrome. A focused clinical history, stool analysis and calcified appearance of the pancreas on abdominal x-ray excluded chronic pancreatitis, which is an important cause of malabsorption in heavy drinkers.

- Social factors: address financial hardship and emerging difficulty in managing food shopping.

- Head and neck cancer-related causes: dysphagia to solids secondary to his tumour was identified. The patient had a feeding tube inserted prior to radiotherapy to improve calorie and protein intake. The patient and his nephew were given training on how to manage the feeding tube and pump at home.

- Dental review: the patient had poor dentition and his remaining teeth had to be extracted before radiotherapy, due to the risk of osteoradionecrosis. He would require new dentures following recovery from his radiotherapy.

- Consider re-feeding syndrome: the patient was at high risk of electrolyte derangement with resumption of regular nutrition. Routine measurements of phosphate, magnesium, calcium and potassium were paramount.

Emphysema

The following should be carefully assessed and optimized where possible.

- Review medical therapy: the patient described being increasingly wheezy and breathless, so his inhaler therapy was optimized according to Global Initiative for Chronic Obstructive Lung Disease guidelines (stepwise approach to treatment of chronic obstructive pulmonary disease depending on the severity of underlying disease). Mucolytic therapy was commenced before radiotherapy to assist with mucus clearance.

- Assess inhaler technique: an airways nurse specialist review was organized for education, and a volumizer was provided.

- Treat infection: if a productive cough is present, obtain sputum samples for microbiology and prescribe antibiotics if indicated.

- Address smoking cessation by providing cessation advice, nicotine replacement, and referral to local smoking cessation services for support.

Functional impairment
- The occupational therapist found that the patient struggled with coming downstairs overnight to use the toilet. Extra banisters, bath-rails and an upstairs commode were installed.
- A meal delivery service was organized and a new microwave purchased.
- Daily hospital transport for radiotherapy was arranged.

Medication review
- The amlodipine was stopped in view of the ankle oedema.
- There were no signs of heart failure and the patient was at risk of dehydration, due to radiation mucositis. His losartan and furosemide were stopped.
- An endocrine opinion suggested that his raised level of thyroid-stimulating hormone on levothyroxine was related to poor medication compliance, resulting in undertreated hypothyroidism.
- Medication compliance issues prompted creation of a dosette box, delivered by his local pharmacy.

Conclusion and learning points

- There is no benefit of adding concomitant chemotherapy or cetuximab to radical head and neck cancer radiotherapy in patients above 70 years old.
- Active support is mandatory in older head and neck cancer patients due to lower ability to tolerate acute toxicity of radiotherapy.
- Be wary of increased risk of aspiration pneumonia for patients undergoing radical radiotherapy, especially in those with compromised respiratory reserve.
- Low BMI is a red flag sign which indicates malnutrition and is associated with poorer outcomes. It may not be just cancer-related and requires a thorough work-up to identify potential causes.
- Treat vitamin deficiencies and be wary of re-feeding syndrome.

References

1 Clayman GL, Eicher SA, Sicard MW, *et al.* Surgical outcomes in head and neck cancer patients 80 years of age and older. *Head Neck* 1998; 20: 216–23.

2 Feng FY, Kim HM, Lyden TH, *et al.* Intensity-modulated chemoradiotherapy aiming to reduce dysphagia in patients with oropharyngeal cancer: clinical and functional results. *J Clin Oncol* 2010; 28: 2732.

3 Pignon J, Le Maitre A, Maillard E, *et al.* Meta-analysis of chemotherapy in head and neck cancer (MACH-NC): an update on 93 randomised trials and 17,346 patients. *Radiother Oncol* 2009: 92: 4–14.

4 Sanabria A, Carvalho AL, Melo RL, *et al.* Predictive factors for complications in elderly patients who underwent head and neck oncologic surgery. *Head Neck* 2008; 30: 170–7.

5 Pignon T, Horiot JC, Van den Bogaert W, *et al.* No age limit for radical radiotherapy in head and neck tumours. *Eur J Cancer* 1996; 32A: 2075–81.

6 Chow WB, Rosenthal RA, Merkow RP, *et al.* Optimal preoperative assessment of the geriatric surgical patient: a best practices guideline from the American College of Surgeons National Surgical Quality Improvement Program and the American Geriatrics Society. *J Am Coll Surg* 2012; 215: 453–66.

7 Browman GP, Wong G, Hodson I, *et al.* Influence of cigarette smoking on the efficacy of radiation therapy in head and neck cancer. *N Engl J Med* 1993; 328: 159–63.

8 Gupta D, Lis CG. Pretreatment serum albumin as a predictor of cancer survival: a systematic review of the epidemiological literature. *Nutr J* 2010; 9: 69.

9 Nugent B, Lewis S, O'Sullivan JS. Enteral feeding methods for nutritional management in patients with head and neck cancers being treated with radiotherapy and/or chemotherapy. *Cochrane Database Syst Rev* 2010; 3: CD007904.

Further reading

• Global Initiative for Chronic Obstructive Lung Disease (2015). *Pocket guide to COPD diagnosis, management and prevention.* Available from: www.goldcopd.org/uploads/users/files/GOLD_Pocket_2015_Feb18.pdf (accessed 15 July 2015).

• Harari D, Hopper A, Dhesi J, *et al.* Proactive care of older people undergoing surgery ('POPS'): designing, embedding, evaluating and funding a comprehensive geriatric assessment service for older elective surgical patients. *Age Ageing* 2007; 36: 190–6.

• National Confidential Enquiry into Patient Outcome and Death (2010). *An age old problem. A review of the care received by elderly patients undergoing surgery.* Available from: www.ncepod.org.uk/2010report3/downloads/EESE_fullReport.pdf (accessed 15 July 2015).

• Kondrup J, Rasmussen HH, Hamberg O, *et al.* Nutritional risk screening (NRS 2002): a new method based on an analysis of controlled clinical trials. *Clin Nutr* 2003; 22: 321–6.

• Sarris EG, Harrington KJ, Saif MW, Syrigos KN. Multimodal treatment strategies for elderly patients with head and neck cancer. *Cancer Treat Rev* 2014; 40: 465–75.

20 Fitness of a Patient with Advanced Melanoma for Therapy with Checkpoint Inhibitors

Lucy Dumas, Joanna Hampton, James Larkin

Case history

A 77-year-old man was referred to the oncology clinic by the acute medical team following admission with shortness of breath on exertion. He informed the team that he had had a suspicious mole removed from his back a few years ago. He had grown up in South Africa. A full systems review elicited a further history of a 3–4 month gradual decline with fatigue, loss of appetite and weight loss of 3 kg in the last 6 months. He lived with his wife, who was in good health. Both were independent for personal and extended activities of daily living, although he admitted he was less active in recent months, leaving the house less and spending more of his day in a chair due to his breathlessness and fatigue. His Eastern Cooperative Oncology Group (ECOG) performance status (PS) was 2.

His past medical history included atrial fibrillation, for which he was receiving anticoagulation medication, type 2 diabetes mellitus, hypertension and angina. He did not regularly monitor his glucose levels but was under the care of his GP practice nurse who undertook regular cardiovascular and diabetes health checks. He had no known drug allergies and was taking digoxin, warfarin, metformin, ramipril and bisoprolol.

The acute medical team had organized a chest x-ray, which demonstrated a right-sided pleural effusion. A subsequent CT scan demonstrated widespread lymphadenopathy above and below the diaphragm, multiple lung metastases, liver metastases and a moderate right-sided pleural effusion. An ultrasound-guided liver biopsy revealed findings consistent with metastatic melanoma: molecular analysis did not demonstrate a *BRAF* V600 mutation.

What is the evidence for the use of contemporary treatments for metastatic melanoma in older patients?

What potential toxicities should physicians be aware of and what resources are available to guide their management?

What factors in our patient would influence treatment decision making and how should these be addressed?

What therapies are currently in development and is there any evolving evidence to support their use in older patients?

What is the evidence for the use of contemporary treatments for metastatic melanoma in older patients?

Malignant melanoma mortality rates have been rising since the 1970s, with the largest rise seen in those over the age of 75.[1] Metastatic melanoma is an aggressive disease which historically has been associated with poor outcomes. Chemotherapy in the form of dacarbazine or biological agents such as interferon-alpha or interleukin-2 had little impact on the natural history of the disease.[1–3] However, the advent of immunotherapy and targeted treatments has changed the therapeutic landscape for patients with metastatic melanoma. Ipilimumab is a fully human monoclonal antibody against cytotoxic T-lymphocyte-associated protein 4, an immune checkpoint molecule that downregulates T-cell activation. Inhibiting this crucial checkpoint mechanism increases T-cell activation and T-cell-mediated cell death. In 2010, a large phase III study of ipilimumab demonstrated for the first time an improvement in overall survival (OS) in patients with metastatic, previously treated melanoma.[2] Patients who were aged 65 and over appeared to derive benefits from ipilimumab, compared with active control (glycoprotein 100 peptide vaccine), that were similar to those seen in younger patients: HR for OS 0.61 (95% CI 0.38–0.99) for those aged ≥65 years compared with 0.65 (95% CI 0.47–0.90) for younger patients.[4] Responses to ipilimumab are typically durable: the 5 year survival for advanced melanoma is reported to be just under 20%.[3,4]

Vemurafenib is an orally available BRAF kinase inhibitor, which compared with dacarbazine shows improved response rates and OS in patients with metastatic melanoma with a *BRAF* V600 mutation.[5] In a large multicentre safety study evaluating vemurafenib in *BRAF* V600 mutant patients, predefined subgroups of age ≥75 and age <75 were assessed.[5] Progression-free survival (PFS) and response rates were comparable for the two age groups, although ECOG PS ≥2 (not infrequently reported in older patients) was associated with a worse PFS.[5] Toxicity leading to treatment discontinuation was more common in patients over the age of 75. There is, therefore, relevant experience of contemporary therapies to treat metastatic melanoma in older patients, although caution should be exercised in extrapolating these data to less fit, older patients with multiple comorbidities and polypharmacy.

What potential toxicities should physicians be aware of and what resources are available to guide their management?

The toxicities of ipilimumab include diarrhoea, nausea, vomiting, pruritus, rash and fatigue, as well as the immune-generated toxicities of colitis, endocrinopathies and hepatotoxicity.[2–4] An Italian group, using data from an ipilimumab expanded access programme, demonstrated a comparable safety profile (at the licensed 3 mg/kg dose): the commonest toxicities in those over the age of 70 were rash, pruritus, nausea, vomiting, diarrhoea and hepatotoxicity.[6] Six percent of patients experienced a grade 3 or 4 toxicity attributable to ipilimumab. The majority of patients received the full four doses and response rates were comparable to those in patients under the age of 70. There are clear guidelines for the management of immune-mediated colitis and hepatitis,[7] and prompt recognition and proactive management are key. The impact on quality of life of systemic therapies for older patients with advanced disease is particularly relevant. Revicki *et al.*[5] published quality-of-life data collected from just under two-thirds of patients in the landmark MDX010-20 study.[5] Ipilimumab resulted in little to no impairment of health-related quality-of-life outcomes in patients with advanced melanoma. However, subset analysis of those over the age of 65 reported more symptom-related effects, from diarrhoea to breathlessness, despite similar responses.

What factors in our patient would influence treatment decision making and how should these be addressed?

Our patient, who was aged 77 and had a PS of 2, had a number of medical issues that had to be considered prior to treatment. Although currently these are well managed, there is a risk of decompensation either from therapy or disease. Further background information from his GP and previous cardiologist should be sought and an echocardiogram carried out to assess baseline ventricular function if no recent data are available. Warfarin should be switched to low-molecular-weight heparin. If he were to suffer a severe episode of ipilimumab-mediated colitis, gastrointestinal bleeding would be a serious concern. The risk–benefit ratio of ongoing anticoagulation medication should be considered and he should be informed of the additional risk. His diabetic control will need to be carefully monitored throughout treatment.

It is crucial to have an honest conversation with the patient and his family to explain that the side effects of treatment are harder to predict in his case and that, although the majority of ipilimumab toxicities respond to treatment interruption, supportive care and potentially the use of corticosteroids or other immunosuppressive agents, a small proportion of these may be serious and potentially life threatening.

He would benefit from a Comprehensive Geriatric Assessment (CGA), undertaken by a multidisciplinary team that includes a geriatrician, an oncologist and an oncology clinical nurse specialist, as well as potential involvement from the district nursing team, community palliative care team, social workers, occupational therapist and physiotherapist, depending on the needs identified.[8] A formal functional assessment, using, for example, the Barthel Index, may more sensitively evaluate his current level of fitness than the standard ECOG PS used in clinical trials. Although there is no overt cognitive impairment, a brief assessment using the abbreviated mental test score would be prudent prior to requesting his consent for potentially toxic therapy.

What therapies are currently in development and is there any evolving evidence to support their use in older patients?

Since the approval of ipilimumab in 2011, the field of immunotherapy has rapidly progressed with the development of two newer agents: nivolumab and pembrolizumab.

Nivolumab, a fully human immunoglobulin G4 anti-programmed cell death protein 1 (PD-1) monoclonal antibody, confers a significant survival benefit compared with chemotherapy in both first-line use and in pretreated patients.[9,10] In two large phase III studies, an improved toxicity profile was seen compared with chemotherapy: the main severe (grade 3 or 4) side effects reported were itch, rash, diarrhoea and vomiting. Although patients up to the age of 87 were included, the PS of these patients was extremely good, with 99% of patients being PS 0 or 1. More recently a large phase III study evaluating nivolumab and ipilimumab in combination versus either as a monotherapy demonstrated a very significant PFS advantage for the combination:[11] 112 (12.5%) patients were over the age of 75 and, except for one patient, PS 0 or 1. The toxicities seen were similar to those previously described, with a clearly increased toxicity profile in the combination arm: over a third of patients in the combination arm stopped treatment due to an adverse event compared with 5.1% in the nivolumab arm and 13.2% in the ipilimumab arm. Our patient, however, was less fit than the patients included in these studies, and the toxicity of treatment in a less fit group, particularly with combination therapy, remains unclear.

Pembrolizumab (previously known as lambrolizumab), a humanized monoclonal antibody against PD-1, has demonstrated impressive efficacy in a phase I study, including in patients with prior ipilimumab treatment.[12] The Keynote-006 study[13] demonstrated marked superiority of pembrolizumab compared with ipilimumab in patients regardless of *BRAF* mutational status. In line with previous studies, there was no upper age limit: patients up to the age of 89 were included, although all were PS 0 or 1. In addition to a significant survival advantage, pembrolizumab also was better tolerated with notably less diarrhoea and colitis of any grade. Although thyroid dysfunction and fatigue did occur more frequently, on the whole these are more manageable and less debilitating issues, which may have relevance for treating older, frailer patients.

Conclusion and learning points

- Metastatic melanoma is an aggressive malignancy with a rapidly rising incidence and mortality in older people.
- Advanced disease can progress rapidly and cause significant symptomatic burden.
- Immune checkpoint inhibitors and BRAF kinase inhibitors have markedly improved treatment outcomes. However, older, less fit patients are markedly underrepresented in the evidence base.
- Treatment decision making should be informed by a thorough CGA, and patients and their families require careful and honest counselling, as the risk–benefit ratio in older patients is less clear.

References

1 Cancer Research UK. *Skin cancer incidence trends over time.* Available from: www.cancerresearchuk.org/health-professional/cancer-statistics/statistics-by-cancer-type/skin-cancer/incidence#heading-Two (accessed 20 April 2015).

2 Hodi FS, O'Day SJ, McDermott DF, *et al.* Improved survival with ipilimumab in patients with metastatic melanoma. *N Engl J Med* 2010; 363: 711–23.

3 Maio M, Grob JJ, Aamdal S, *et al.* Five-year survival rates for treatment-naive patients with advanced melanoma who received ipilimumab plus dacarbazine in a phase III trial. *J Clin Oncol* 2015; 33: 1191–6.

4 Schadendorf D, Hodi FS, Robert C, *et al.* Pooled analysis of long-term survival data from phase II and phase III trials of ipilimumab in unresectable or metastatic melanoma. *J Clin Oncol* 2015; 33: 1889–94.

5 Revicki DA, van den Eertwegh AJ, Lorigan P, *et al.* Health related quality of life outcomes for unresectable stage III or IV melanoma patients receiving ipilimumab treatment. *Health Qual Life Outcomes* 2012; 10: 66.

6 Chiarion Sileni V, Pigozzo J, Ascierto PA, *et al.* Efficacy and safety of ipilimumab in elderly patients with pretreated advanced melanoma treated at Italian centres through the expanded access programme. *J Exp Clin Cancer Res* 2014; 33: 30.

7 *Yervoy (ipilumumab). Immune-mediated adverse reaction management guide.* Available from: www.hcp.yervoy.com/pdf/rems-management-guide.pdf (accessed 21 April 2015)

8 British Geriatrics Society (2010). *Comprehensive assessment of the frail older patient.* Available from: www.bgs.org.uk/index.php/topresources/publicationfind/goodpractice/195-gpgcgassessment (accessed 21 April 2015).

9 Weber JS, Minor D, D'Angelo SP, *et al.* A phase 3 randomized, open-label study of nivolumab (anti-PD-1; BMS-936558; ONO 4538) versus investigator's choice of chemotherapy (ICC) in patients with advanced melanoma with prior anti-CLTA-4 therapy [abstract]. Presented at: European Society for Medical Oncology, Madrid, 26–30 September 2014.

10 Robert C, Long GV, Brady B, *et al.* Nivolumab in previously untreated melanoma without *BRAF* mutation. *N Engl J Med* 2015; 372: 320–30.

11 Larkin J, Chiarion-Sileni V, Gonzalez R, *et al.* Combined nivolumab and ipilimumab or monotherapy in untreated melanoma. *N Engl J Med* 2015; 373: 23–34.

12 Hamid O, Robert C, Daud A, *et al.* Safety and tumor responses with lambrolizumab (anti-PD-1) in melanoma. *N Engl J Med* 2013; 369: 134–44.

13 Robert C, Schachter J, Long GV, *et al.*; KEYNOTE-006 Investigators. Pembrolizumab versus ipilimumab in advanced melanoma. *N Engl J Med* doi: 10.1056/NEJMoa1503093.

21 A Patient with Parkinson's Disease and Oesophageal Cancer Exhibiting Significant Upper Gastrointestinal Toxicity, Nausea and Vomiting from Chemotherapy

Adam Sharp, Pamela Seenan, David Watkins

Case history

A 79-year-old man presented with retrosternal discomfort and progressive dysphagia to solids. Endoscopy revealed a tumour at the gastro-oesophageal junction. Biopsy showed human epidermal growth factor receptor 2 (HER2)-negative adenocarcinoma. CT staging demonstrated multiple liver metastases and he was referred to oncology for consideration of palliative chemotherapy. At his appointment he was noted to have a past medical history of hypertension, hypercholesterolaemia, osteoarthritis and well-controlled Parkinson's disease. He denied any baseline hearing impairment. His medications were amlodipine, paracetamol, simvastatin and co-beneldopa. He lived with his wife (aged 83) in a single-storey house. His Eastern Cooperative Oncology Group performance status (PS) was 1 and he mobilized with no walking aids. His gait was parkinsonian, but not unsteady, with a timed up-and-go test of 12 s. He was functionally independent and continued to drive. He was managing a soft diet and maintaining his weight (60 kg). His BP was controlled on amlodipine (135/85 mmHg) and there was no postural drop. Investigations demonstrated his left ventricular ejection fraction (MUGA scan) and glomerular filtration rate (EDTA) to be normal.

Palliative epirubicin, cisplatin and capecitabine (ECX) chemotherapy was discussed and administered with standard antiemetic prophylaxis. He was admitted to hospital 3 days after his chemotherapy with a 24 h history of nausea and vomiting with associated dehydration and hypotension. He was unable to keep his Parkinson's medications down, resulting in his mobility slowing. Capecitabine and amlodipine were withheld and he improved with intravenous ondansetron and fluids. The oncology team discussed his medications with the Parkinson's nurse on his arrival at hospital. Co-beneldopa was immediately substituted with a rotigotine patch until the vomiting improved, when the co-beneldopa was recommenced. He remained normotensive throughout the 48 h admission, and the amlodipine was permanently discontinued. He was discharged and recommenced capecitabine.

He returned to clinic prior to the second cycle of ECX and described tinnitus for 5 days following his first cycle. Taken together with the admission for nausea and vomiting, his treatment was switched from ECX to carboplatin + capecitabine to minimize the risk of nausea, vomiting and ototoxicity. Carboplatin + capecitabine was well tolerated; however, at the time of his third cycle he reported worsening dysphagia (only managing fluids and medications), increased fatigue and weight loss (5 kg). CT imaging demonstrated progressive disease at all sites. The options of best supportive care (BSC) or second-line docetaxel were discussed.

What are the challenges in treating metastatic oesophageal cancer in older patients and how do they influence the choice of first-line treatment?

How should the patient's nausea and vomiting be managed?

What are the potential complications of this admission?

What are the second-line treatment options in this patient?

What are the challenges in treating metastatic oesophageal cancer in older patients and how do they influence the choice of first–line treatment?

Around 8000 people were diagnosed with oesophageal cancer and 7700 people died from oesophageal cancer in 2012 in the UK.[1] The average age of patients diagnosed with oesophageal cancer is 72. Older patients (≥65 years) with metastatic oesophageal cancer derive similar benefits from chemotherapy to those in younger patients (<65 years), but they experience increased treatment-related toxicities.[2] The risk of treatment-associated morbidity may be reduced by optimization of nutritional status and social circumstances, as well as management of the patient's comorbidities and concurrent medications.[3]

The patient was maintaining his weight with a soft diet and, importantly, he was able to swallow his Parkinson's medications. His BP was normal and not over controlled. On his current medications, the Parkinson's disease and osteoarthritis were not causing significant functional impairment. He therefore proceeded to chemotherapy. The patient, his wife and his daughter were given written information on the common side effects of ECX and the telephone numbers of his clinical nurse specialist and the acute oncology unit so they could contact his oncology team in the event of any toxicities in order to reduce associated morbidity by seeking urgent advice.

The patient initially received ECX chemotherapy but was switched to carboplatin + capecitabine due to toxicities (nausea, vomiting and tinnitus). A variety of chemotherapy regimens have been studied in the first-line treatment of HER2-negative oesophageal cancer.[4] Accepted alternative first-line options include: epirubicin, oxaliplatin and capecitabine; fluorouracil (5-FU), folinic acid and oxaliplatin; and folinic acid, 5-FU and irinotecan (FOLFIRI). Guimbaud and colleagues[5] investigated the efficacy of FOLFIRI and ECX in metastatic adenocarcinoma of the stomach and gastro-oesophageal junction in a phase III study. FOLFIRI improved time-to-treatment failure when compared with ECX (5.1 vs 4.2 months; $p=0.008$). There was no difference in response rate (39.2% and 37.8%) and overall survival (OS) (9.5 vs 9.7 months; $p=0.95$). There were significantly fewer grade 3–4 toxicities with FOLFIRI compared with ECX (38% vs 64.5%; $p≤0.001$).[5] The activity and toxicity profile of FOLFIRI offers a useful alternative first-line treatment regimen for older patients, particularly those unsuitable for platinum-based regimens.

The choice of first-line chemotherapy should be personalized to avoid exacerbating pre-existing medical conditions. Cisplatin should be avoided in patients with hearing loss, tinnitus, renal dysfunction or cardiac failure, as its use may be associated with ototoxicity and renal impairment, and the associated fluid loading may exacerbate cardiac failure. Anthracyclines (epirubicin) should be avoided in cardiac failure, as they are associated with a risk of cardiac toxicity and worsening left ventricular function. Capecitabine and 5-FU should be used with caution or avoided in patients with active angina, as they are associated with a risk of coronary artery spasm. Oxaliplatin, and to a lesser extent cisplatin, can cause peripheral neuropathy and should be used with caution in patients in whom development of neuropathy may worsen mobility (e.g. pre-existing gait and balance disorders, neurological deficits/disorders, quadriceps muscle weakness), and should be avoided in those who already have recurrent falls.

How should the patient's nausea and vomiting be managed?

The risk of emesis from individual chemotherapies may be graded high, moderate, low or minimal, and appropriate antiemetic prophylaxis should be given accordingly (Figure 21.1). Written information and verbal explanations, as well as telephone contacts, should be given to patients and their families to ensure that medication is taken appropriately. Despite taking appropriate antiemetics (ondansetron, dexamethasone and fosaprepitant), the patient called his clinical nurse specialist on day 3 of the first cycle to say he had been vomiting over the past 24 h and was not opening his bowels. She arranged for him to be reviewed. As he was unable to maintain his oral intake and was clinically dehydrated, he was admitted to hospital (Figure 21.2).

The patient received intravenous fluids, ondansetron and regular laxatives. In choosing an antiemetic regimen it is important to recognize both cautions and side effects of antiemetic therapy, as these can exacerbate pre-existing medical conditions (especially Parkinson's disease) and potentiate/interact with concomitant medications (Figure 21.3). Many of the antiemetics summarized in Figure 21.1 are contraindicated in Parkinson's disease, as they may worsen extrapyramidal symptoms. These are dopamine antagonists that cross the blood–brain barrier (metoclopramide, haloperidol, prochlorperazine and cyclizine). Safe antiemetics to use are domperidone (as it exerts no central dopamine antagonism) and ondansetron. This patient received appropriate antiemetics with his chemotherapy and during his hospital admission. Caution is required to review the standard antiemetic protocol with a planned chemotherapy regimen for patients with Parkinson's disease and to substitute antiemetics with a safer alternative where required. In patients with persistent nausea and vomiting, other causes should be investigated and managed appropriately, including gastric outflow obstruction, constipation, hypercalcaemia and raised intracranial pressure (Figure 21.2).

The patient's nausea, vomiting and constipation improved within 48 h, he was able to restart the Parkinson's medications and he was discharged. As his amlodipine was stopped on admission and he remained normotensive, it was not restarted on discharge. His statin was also discontinued, as it had unlikely prognostic benefit in the context of his cancer. Cisplatin was changed to the less emetogenic carboplatin for his second cycle to reduce the risk of recurrent nausea and vomiting. Epirubicin was omitted to minimize the risk of significant haematological toxicity and fatigue. In addition, he was given laxatives to prevent further constipation. Constipation is a common non-motor symptom of patients with Parkinson's disease and is also a common side effect of ondansetron. Where constipation is an anticipated toxicity of chemotherapy, clinical history around baseline bowel habit should be elicited in Parkinson's patients and treated as needed prior to commencing chemotherapy.

What are the potential complications of this admission?

Hospital admissions can be associated with functional decline in the older population.[6] This

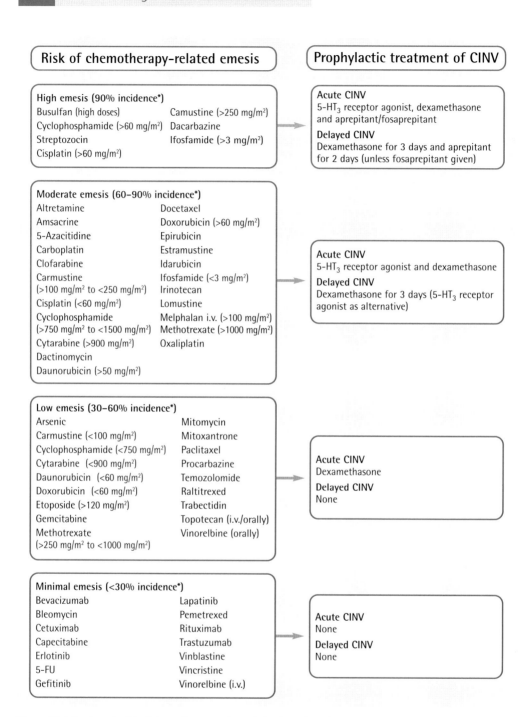

Risk of chemotherapy-related emesis

Prophylactic treatment of CINV

High emesis (90% incidence*)
Busulfan (high doses)	Camustine (>250 mg/m²)
Cyclophosphamide (>60 mg/m²)	Dacarbazine
Streptozocin	Ifosfamide (>3 mg/m²)
Cisplatin (>60 mg/m²)	

Acute CINV
5-HT₃ receptor agonist, dexamethasone and aprepitant/fosaprepitant
Delayed CINV
Dexamethasone for 3 days and aprepitant for 2 days (unless fosaprepitant given)

Moderate emesis (60–90% incidence*)
Altretamine	Docetaxel
Amsacrine	Doxorubicin (>60 mg/m²)
5-Azacitidine	Epirubicin
Carboplatin	Estramustine
Clofarabine	Idarubicin
Carmustine (>100 mg/m² to <250 mg/m²)	Ifosfamide (<3 mg/m²)
	Irinotecan
Cisplatin (<60 mg/m²)	Lomustine
Cyclophosphamide (>750 mg/m² to <1500 mg/m²)	Melphalan i.v. (>100 mg/m²)
	Methotrexate (>1000 mg/m²)
Cytarabine (>900 mg/m²)	Oxaliplatin
Dactinomycin	
Daunorubicin (>50 mg/m²)	

Acute CINV
5-HT₃ receptor agonist and dexamethasone
Delayed CINV
Dexamethasone for 3 days (5-HT₃ receptor agonist as alternative)

Low emesis (30–60% incidence*)
Arsenic	Mitomycin
Carmustine (<100 mg/m²)	Mitoxantrone
Cyclophosphamide (<750 mg/m²)	Paclitaxel
Cytarabine (<900 mg/m²)	Procarbazine
Daunorubicin (<60 mg/m²)	Temozolomide
Doxorubicin (<60 mg/m²)	Raltitrexed
Etoposide (>120 mg/m²)	Trabectidin
Gemcitabine	Topotecan (i.v./orally)
Methotrexate (>250 mg/m² to <1000 mg/m²)	Vinorelbine (orally)

Acute CINV
Dexamethasone
Delayed CINV
None

Minimal emesis (<30% incidence*)
Bevacizumab	Lapatinib
Bleomycin	Pemetrexed
Cetuximab	Rituximab
Capecitabine	Trastuzumab
Erlotinib	Vinblastine
5-FU	Vincristine
Gefitinib	Vinorelbine (i.v.)

Acute CINV
None
Delayed CINV
None

Figure 21.1 Emetogenic risk of chemotherapy and prophylactic antiemetic guidelines. The figure identifies the risk of chemotherapy-induced nausea and vomiting (CINV). Chemotherapy agents are divided into high, moderate, low and minimal emesis depending on the number of patients who would experience emesis without prophylactic antiemetics (*). Prophylactic treatment regimens from guidelines of the European Society of Medical Oncology and the American Society of Clinical Oncology are shown for acute and delayed CINV.

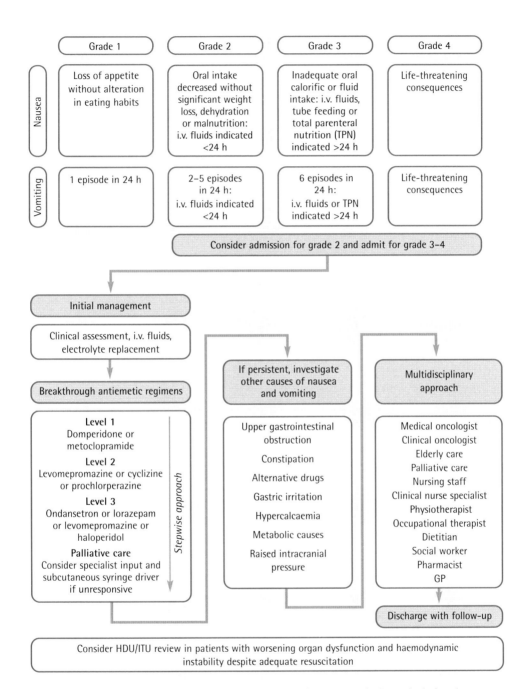

Figure 21.2 Grading of nausea and vomiting and its management. Common terminology criteria for adverse events (version 4, the most recent) are shown. Patients with grade 2 (consider) and grade 3–4 nausea and vomiting should be admitted to hospital. They should be appropriately resuscitated and antiemetics commenced. Patients with persistent nausea and vomiting should be investigated for alternative causes of their symptoms. Appropriate follow-up should be arranged on discharge. Patients with worsening organ function and haemodynamic stability despite appropriate treatment should be discussed with HDU/ITU.

Drug	Cautions/side effects	Interactions
Dexamethasone	Gastrointestinal side effects Sleep disturbances Glycaemic control	Fosaprepitant Cytochrome P450 3A4 (CYP3A4) inducers increase clearance Dexamethasone reduces plasma concentration of certain retrovirals
Ondansetron	Constipation QT prolongation Caution in hepatic dysfunction	CYP3A4 inducers increase clearance Exacerbate other QT-prolonging drugs
Fosaprepitant	Hiccups Fatigue Raised alanine aminotransferase Constipation Reduced appetite Caution in hepatic dysfunction	Multiple interactions
Metoclopramide	Extrapyramidal side effects Caution in older patients Avoid in Parkinson's disease Avoid in young patients Avoid in gastrointestinal obstruction	Increased risk of extrapyramidal side effects when given with antipsychotics
Cyclizine	Urticarial rash Drowsiness Headache Tachycardia Dry mouth Constipation Caution in glaucoma, hepatic dysfunction, epilepsy and gastrointestinal obstruction	Enhanced by alcohol and hypnotics Enhances other anticholinergic drugs Counteracts prokinetic effect of metoclopramide
Domperidone	Avoid in gastrointestinal obstruction Avoid in prolactinoma Ventricular arrhythmias/sudden cardiac death	CYP3A4 inhibitors that prolong QT interval should be avoided
Levomepromazine	Drowsiness Confusion Disorientation Dry mouth Hypotension QT prolongation Hyperglycaemia	Increased risk of arrhythmias when used with other drugs that prolong QT interval Enhances other anticholinergic drugs
Lorazepam	Drowsiness Confusion Caution in pulmonary insufficiency Caution in hepatic dysfunction	Increased sedative effect with alcohol or opioids Enhanced hypotensive effect with antihypertensives

Figure 21.3 Cautions and side effects of commonly used antiemetics in chemotherapy-induced nausea and vomiting. Common antiemetic therapies are shown. Cautions, side effects and interactions of each antiemetic are shown.

decline is multifactorial and includes immobility, malnutrition, delirium, sensory deprivation, isolation and low mood.[6] Functional decline is a particular risk in older people with Parkinson's disease, in whom it may be exacerbated by changes to the administration of medications. These include medications not being given at the usual times because they do not coincide with routine drug rounds, delayed administration due to ward stock availability, and omissions due to current symptomology (nausea, vomiting and inability to swallow) or medical direction (e.g. nil by mouth). Significant efforts should be made to ensure medications are available and given on time. If the patient's Parkinson's medications cannot be taken orally despite antiemetics (or for other reasons: for instance, if he is unable to swallow), same day urgent expert advice should be sought to discuss the temporary conversion of his levodopa to alternative routes of administration (usually via rotigotine patches). Co-beneldopa may be administered in a dispersible formulation (at the same dose) in patients who have dysphagia of solids but who can manage liquids. Most hospitals have a Parkinson's specialist nurse, Parkinson's specialist neurologist/geriatrician, pharmacist or general geriatrician whose advice may be sought. Parkinson's disease symptoms deteriorate very quickly (within hours) without medications and may result in a significant decline in mobility, function and swallowing (with resulting risk of aspiration pneumonia).

A multidisciplinary team (MDT) approach should be taken to caring for older oncology patients admitted to hospital (Figure 21.2). Patients should be encouraged to remain independent and physically active during admission to maintain mobility for discharge, as deconditioning in older people can occur, sometimes quickly. In addition, admission provides the opportunity to reassess their regular medications and social circumstances to ensure these have not contributed to the admission.

What are the second-line treatment options in this patient?

When progression occurs after first-line treatment, median OS with BSC is 3–4 months.[7] Second-line treatment with either irinotecan or docetaxel has been shown to improve OS when compared with BSC.[7-9] However, patients who have a poor PS are less likely to benefit from second-line chemotherapy and in this scenario consideration of alternative strategies to help with symptom control, including oesophageal stenting or radiotherapy, and palliative care support alone should be considered.[10]

Conclusion and learning points

- A thorough assessment taking into account comorbidities, social circumstances and patient preferences is required to inform decision making and the optimal choice of first-line chemotherapy in older patients with oesophageal cancer.
- Older patients should be considered for standard systemic therapy for oesophageal cancer with an awareness of the increased risk of treatment toxicities.
- A stepwise approach to antiemetics can be used to manage treatment-related nausea and vomiting, but particular care is required in the choice of antiemetics in patients with Parkinson's disease.
- Proactive MDT treatment plans are required for older patients with cancer at risk of functional decline during inpatient hospital stays.

References

1 Cancer Research UK. *Cancer mortality statistics.* Available from: www.cancerresearchuk.org/cancer-info/cancerstats/mortality/cancerdeaths/ (accessed 28 May 2015).

2 Jatoi A, Foster NR, Egner JR, *et al.* Older versus younger patients with metastatic adenocarcinoma of the esophagus, gastroesophageal junction, and stomach: a pooled analysis of eight consecutive North Central Cancer Treatment Group (NCCTG) trials. *Int J Oncol* 2010; 36: 601–6.

3 Balducci L. Systemic treatment of gastric and esophageal adenocarcinoma in elderly patients. *J Gastrointestinal Oncol* 2015; 6: 75–8.

4 Wiedmann MW, Mossner J. New and emerging combination therapies for esophageal cancer. *Cancer Manage Res* 2013; 5: 133–46.

5 Guimbaud R, Louvet C, Ries P, *et al.* Prospective, randomized, multicenter, phase III study of fluorouracil, leucovorin, and irinotecan versus epirubicin, cisplatin, and capecitabine in advanced gastric adenocarcinoma: a French intergroup (Fédération Francophone de Cancérologie Digestive, Fédération Nationale des Centres de Lutte Contre le Cancer, and Groupe Coopérateur Multidisciplinaire en Oncologie) study. *J Clin Oncol* 2014; 32: 3520–6.

6 Kleinpell RM, Fletcher K, Jennings BM. Reducing functional decline in hospitalized elderly. In: Hughes RG, ed. *Patient safety and quality: an evidence-based handbook for nurses.* Rockville, MD: Agency for Healthcare Research and Quality, 2008.

7 Kang JH, Lee SI, Lim do H, *et al.* Salvage chemotherapy for pretreated gastric cancer: a randomized phase III trial comparing chemotherapy plus best supportive care with best supportive care alone. *J Clin Oncol* 2012; 30: 1513–18.

8 Ford HE, Marshall A, Bridgewater JA, *et al.* Docetaxel versus active symptom control for refractory oesophagogastric adenocarcinoma (COUGAR-02): an open-label, phase 3 randomised controlled trial. *Lancet Oncol* 2014; 15: 78–86.

9 Thallinger CM, Raderer M, Hejna M. Esophageal cancer: a critical evaluation of systemic second-line therapy. *J Clin Oncol* 2011; 29: 4709–14.

10 Dai Y, Li C, Xie Y, *et al.* Interventions for dysphagia in oesophageal cancer. *Cochrane Database Syst Rev* 2014; 10: CD005048.

22 Diarrhoea in a Patient on Chemotherapy for Colorectal Cancer

Alexandra Pender, James Fleet, Danielle Harari, Naureen Starling

Case history

A 70-year-old man presented as an emergency admission requiring a right hemicolectomy for an obstructive caecal mass. He had a medical history of type 1 diabetes with grade 1 peripheral neuropathy, gastrointestinal reflux disease, hearing impairment, mild mitral regurgitation and benign essential tremor. The postoperative histological findings were a pT4N2 poorly differentiated *KRAS*-mutant adenocarcinoma with neuroendocrine differentiation. Further imaging revealed tumour recurrence at the surgical anastomosis, extensive liver metastases with no segmental sparing, and peritoneal disease. On assessment for palliative chemotherapy, the patient's Eastern Cooperative Oncology Group performance status (PS) was 2. Chemotherapy with fluorouracil (5-FU; de Gramont regimen), folinic acid (400 mg/m^2/day) and irinotecan (180 mg/m^2/day) every 2 weeks (FOLFIRI) was commenced 7 weeks postoperatively. Bevacizumab 5 mg/kg was added with the second cycle of chemotherapy 9 weeks after surgery.

Following 3 weeks of chemotherapy, the patient reported anorexia, more frequent yellow stool and weight loss of 19% of his original body weight. Dietary changes were advised. A week later, he reported grade 2 diarrhoea despite regular use of low-dose loperamide. A week after his third cycle of chemotherapy, the patient was admitted with faecal incontinence and grade 3 diarrhoea secondary to *Clostridium difficile*. He received a 5 day course of oral fidaxomicin and supportive care. His diarrhoea improved but due to persistent grade 2 diarrhoea he completed a further 5 day course of fidaxomicin. Three days after completion of the second course of antibiotics, the patient was readmitted to hospital with non-neutropenic sepsis of unknown source which responded to broad spectrum intravenous antibiotics. Restaging performed during this admission 8 weeks after commencing chemotherapy demonstrated disease progression with multi-site colonic stenosis and progressive liver, nodal and peritoneal disease.

What palliative chemotherapy regimens are recommended in older patients with metastatic colorectal cancer?

What is the risk of diarrhoea with these treatments and what are the mechanisms?

What other causes of diarrhoea need to be considered and what investigations may be required?

How is *C. difficile* diagnosed and managed?

How can faecal incontinence be best managed?

What palliative chemotherapy regimens are recommended in older patients with metastatic colorectal cancer?

Colorectal cancer is one of the commonest cancers diagnosed worldwide[1] and approximately 60% of diagnoses are in individuals aged 70 years or older.[2] Older patients are underrepresented in the clinical trial population evaluating treatment strategies in metastatic colorectal cancer,[3] but pooled retrospective analyses of patients <70 years and ≥70 years have reported similar response rates, progression-free survival (PFS) and overall survival with oxaliplatin and irinotecan combined with 5-FU/folinic acid.[4,5] 5-FU can also be administered as an oral pro-drug, capecitabine, in combination with irinotecan (XELIRI). A meta-analysis of six phase II and III randomized controlled trials of FOLFIRI and XELIRI concluded that the efficacy of both regimens was comparable, although the median age of participants in the trials included in the meta-analysis was less than 67 years.[6]

Older patients considered unfit for doublet chemotherapy may be considered for 5-FU-based treatment alone. Capecitabine has been investigated in the over-75s at a 20% reduction of the licensed dose (2000 mg/m^2). In some patients, this was due to dosing limitations secondary to creatinine clearance, but in one study subgroup, where investigators could reduce the dose at their discretion, 78% of patients over 75 years received a dose of 2000 mg/m^2 due to investigator choice alone.[7] The benefit of adding bevacizumab to capecitabine (PFS 5.8 months capecitabine alone vs 10.8 months capecitabine plus bevacizumab) in the over-75s was demonstrated in a subgroup analysis of 99 patients in the MAX study, although 88% of these patients were of PS 0 or 1.[8] Toxicity profiles and dose administered were similar in the 75–84 years and under 75 years cohorts. Similar efficacy was seen in a prospective study of capecitabine vs capecitabine plus bevacizumab in 280 patients aged 70 years or older (median PFS 5.1 months [95% CI 4.2–6.3] vs 9.1 months [95% CI 7.3–11.4]; HR 0.53 [0.41–0.69]; $p<0.0001$).[9] There are therefore a number of chemotherapy options for older patients with colorectal cancer. The older patients enrolled in the trials described were, however, generally of good PS (0 or 1) and were not necessarily representative of patients seen in routine clinical practice such as the patient described in this case study.

What is the risk of diarrhoea with these treatments and what are the mechanisms?

Given the reported frequency of grade 3/4 diarrhoea with FOLFIRI chemotherapy in various studies (11–15%),[10–12] and with the other regimens described above, it would not be unreasonable to consider chemotherapy-related diarrhoea as a differential diagnosis in this case. 5-FU can cause diarrhoea due to lactose intolerance in up to 10% of patients and is reversible on discontinuation of chemotherapy.[13] Chemotherapy can also cause secretory diarrhoea, due to damage to the usual homeostatic mechanisms of fluid absorption from the bowel; and osmotic diarrhoea, due to mucosal damage and poor absorption of carbohydrates or fat secondary to bile acid malabsorption or small bowel bacterial overgrowth.[14] Limited evidence suggests that changes in gut microflora following chemotherapy may contribute to mucositis,[15,16] which can respond to antibiotic therapy.[14]

What other causes of diarrhoea need to be considered and what investigations may be required?

Older people may have other contributors to diarrhoea that should be considered (Table 22.1). This patient has diabetes and had recently been started on vildagliptin, an oral hypoglycaemic drug that can cause loose stool. A bowel history prior to his cancer revealed that he had chronic constipation (also associated with diabetes).

Initial supportive measures with regular loperamide and codeine were commenced (advising the patient to titrate the doses down if stools became too hard), the vildagliptin was stopped and a SeHCAT (23-seleno-25-homo-tauro-cholic acid) test was arranged to investigate bile acid malabsorption.

Immunosuppression following chemotherapy may result in infection or inflammation of the bowel, as likely occurred in this case. A variety of other pathogens such as cytomegalovirus, other viruses, fungi and bacteria may cause colitis and may only be detected on appropriate stool examination, including polymerase chain reaction, biopsy or later serology.[17]

Table 22.1 Non-oncological causes of diarrhoea that need to be considered in older people.

Aetiology	Diagnosis and treatment
Drugs	Trial of discontinuation
Antibiotics	Substitute other agents without this adverse effect (e.g. gliclazide in diabetes, i.v. vs oral iron)
Caffeine	
Oral hypoglycaemic agents: metformin, gliptins, glitazones	
Antidepressants: selective serotonin reuptake inhibitors	
Cholinesterase inhibitors	
Laxatives	
Iron supplements	
Alcohol	
Impaction and overflow	Passive leakage of non-offensive liquid stool
Drugs: anticholinergics, opiates, iron supplements, calcium channel antagonists	DRE will show distal impaction: if present clear with enema
Dehydration	Abdominal x-ray will show colonic impaction
Immobility	Disimpaction regimen: polyethylene glycol sachets (Movicol) and enemas followed by maintenance laxatives
Neurological disease: Parkinson's disease, stroke, dementia	
Inflammatory bowel disease	Colonoscopy and biopsy
Ulcerative colitis	Small bowel barium follow-through
Microscopic colitis	
Crohn's disease	
Malabsorption	Coeliac antibodies
Coeliac disease	Abdominal imaging, e.g. MR cholangiography; faecal elastase
Chronic pancreatitis	
Small bowel bacterial overgrowth from slow transit	Glucose hydrogen breath test
Diabetes	Treat with prokinetic (e.g. metoclopramide) and broad spectrum antibiotic
Scleroderma	
Lactose intolerance	Lactose hydrogen breath test
Can be acquired in older people; increased risk with chemotherapy	Dietary trial
Hyperthyroidism	Thyroid function tests

How is *C. difficile* diagnosed and managed?

C. difficile infection (CDI) is the most frequent serious cause of diarrhoea seen in hospital, and older inpatients comprise the group most affected. It represents a significant morbidity and mortality risk: up to 13% of affected patients die in hospital.[18]

The diagnosis is made in the presence of appropriate clinical features and microbiological confirmation of a toxin-producing *C. difficile* strain.[19,20] CDI can be diagnosed in the absence of microbiological evidence if colonoscopy shows that pseudomembranous colitis and other clinical features are present. CDI can be toxin-negative in up to 10% of neutropenic patients, and appearances on endoscopy can be atypical.[14] Any of the following features suggest severe CDI: fever, rigors, peritonitis or bowel perforation, haemodynamic instability, toxic megacolon, ileus, elevated serum lactate, white cell count $>15\times10^9$/l of which <20% are neutrophils, hypoalbuminaemia (<25 mg/l), serum creatinine elevation of at least 50% over baseline, and imaging or colonoscopic appearances consistent with CDI.[19] Age over 70 years has been suggested as an independent risk factor for severe complications of CDI.[17]

Metronidazole is routinely used as first-line treatment in non-severe CDI, with oral vancomycin for severe or recurrent CDI.[21] Fidaxomicin treatment can also be used against CDI and has demonstrated a significantly higher cure rate and lower rate of recurrent infection than treatment with vancomycin,[22] although cost may limit its use to recurrent disease. Supportive therapy includes adequate hydration and nutrition and prevention of complications such as pressure sores and deep vein thrombosis (heparin prophylaxis). The development of peritonitis, severe colitis, megacolon or shock should initiate prompt surgical consultation.

This patient had gastrointestinal reflux disease and was taking a proton pump inhibitor. Proton pump inhibitors increase the risk of CDI. The necessity of this treatment should be reviewed and discontinued where possible to reduce the risk.

How can faecal incontinence be best managed?

Faecal incontinence is generally defined as the inability to voluntarily control the passage of stool through the anal canal. It is increasingly more common with advancing age and its prevalence ranges from 12% to 22% in those over 80 years of age.[23] It is particularly prevalent in hospitals and care homes.

Although both distressing and socially isolating, it is often a hidden condition, as only one in eight people seek help, often misinterpreting a condition they view as embarrassing as part of the ageing process. Faecal incontinence is, however, very often treatable once the cause has been established. It is therefore important to sensitively enquire about disturbance of bowel function.

Continence is maintained by integrity of the two anal sphincters. The internal sphincter, under autonomic control, is in the anal canal (tone reduced in diabetes and other neurological diseases). The external sphincter, innervated by the pudendal nerve, is under voluntary control. The main causes of faecal incontinence in older people are anorectal (due to weak sphincters or rectal prolapse), colorectal disease, constipation with overflow, and functional (not reaching the toilet in time). Age itself plays a relatively small role; therefore, diagnosis and treatment should always be sought. In common with other geriatric syndromes, often more than one contributing factor is found. An important step in managing faecal incontinence is to aim for a stool that is neither too hard nor too loose. Possible causes of loose stool should be addressed (Table 22.1). Digital rectal examination is mandatory to exclude impaction, and, importantly, external sphincter tone can also be assessed by asking the patient to 'squeeze as if holding on'. This will simultaneously instruct the patient in pelvic floor strengthening exercises, which are effective in muscular weakness. Patients should be asked how easy it is to access their toilet at home (refer them to occupational therapy as required) and a GP request should be made to supply continence pads if needed (no NHS charge).

Conclusion and learning points

Older patients with metastatic colorectal cancer can be treated with the same chemotherapy regimens as younger patients subject to PS, renal function, comorbidities and cognitive function. The efficacy of these treatments reported in older patients enrolled in clinical trials is similar to that seen in younger patients. As with younger patients, treatments can be adjusted according to comorbidities.

- Diarrhoea is a common complication of chemotherapy for colorectal cancer.

- Other causes of diarrhoea (including overflow from faecal impaction) need to be considered in older people with cancer who report this symptom.

- Faecal incontinence is demoralizing and debilitating and needs to be managed supportively especially during cancer treatment.

References

1 Ferlay J, Shin H-R, Bray F, *et al.* Estimates of worldwide burden of cancer in 2008: GLOBOCAN 2008. *Int J Cancer* 2010; 127: 2893–917.

2 Papamichael D, Audisio RA, Glimelius B, *et al.* Treatment of colorectal cancer in older patients: International Society of Geriatric Oncology (SIOG) consensus recommendations 2013. *Ann Oncol* 2015; 26: 463–76.

3 Lewis JH, Kilgore ML, Goldman DP, *et al.* Participation of patients 65 years of age or older in cancer clinical trials. *J Clin Oncol* 2003; 21: 1383–9.

4 Goldberg RM, Tabah-Fisch I, Bleiberg H, *et al.* Pooled analysis of safety and efficacy of oxaliplatin plus fluorouracil/leucovorin administered bimonthly in elderly patients with colorectal cancer. *J Clin Oncol* 2006; 24: 4085–91.

5 Folprecht G, Seymour MT, Saltz L, *et al.* Irinotecan/fluorouracil combination in first-line therapy of older and younger patients with metastatic colorectal cancer: combined analysis of 2,691 patients in randomized controlled trials. *J Clin Oncol* 2008; 26: 1443–51.

6 Guo Y, Shi M, Shen X, *et al.* Capecitabine plus irinotecan versus 5-FU/leucovorin plus irinotecan in the treatment of colorectal cancer: a meta-analysis. *Clin Colorectal Cancer* 2014; 13: 110–18.

7 Tebbutt NC, Wilson K, Gebski VJ, *et al.* Capecitabine, bevacizumab, and mitomycin in first-line treatment of metastatic colorectal cancer: results of the Australasian Gastrointestinal Trials Group Randomized Phase III MAX Study. *J Clin Oncol* 2010; 28: 3191–8.

8 Price TJ, Zannino D, Wilson K, *et al.* Bevacizumab is equally effective and no more toxic in elderly patients with advanced colorectal cancer: a subgroup analysis from the AGITG MAX trial: an international randomized controlled trial of capecitabine, bevacizumab and mitomycin C. *Ann Oncol* 2012; 23: 1531–6.

9 Cunningham D, Lang I, Marcuello E, *et al.* Bevacizumab plus capecitabine versus capecitabine alone in elderly patients with previously untreated metastatic colorectal cancer (AVEX): an open-label, randomised phase 3 trial. *Lancet Oncol* 2013; 14: 1077–85.

10 Saltz LB, Douillard JY, Pirotta N, *et al.* Irinotecan plus fluorouracil/leucovorin for metastatic colorectal cancer: a new survival standard. *Oncologist* 2001; 6: 81–91.

11 Falcone A, Ricci S, Brunetti I, *et al.* Phase III trial of infusional fluorouracil, leucovorin, oxaliplatin, and irinotecan (FOLFOXIRI) compared with infusional fluorouracil, leucovorin, and irinotecan (FOLFIRI) as first-line treatment for metastatic colorectal cancer: the Gruppo Oncologico Nord Ovest. *J Clin Oncol* 2007; 25: 1670–6.

12 Van Cutsem E, Köhne C-H, Lang I, *et al.* Cetuximab plus irinotecan, fluorouracil, and leucovorin as first-line treatment for metastatic colorectal cancer: updated analysis of overall survival according to tumor *KRAS* and *BRAF* mutation status. *J Clin Oncol* 2011; 29: 2011–19.

13 Osterlund P, Ruotsalainen T, Peuhkuri K, *et al.* Lactose intolerance associated with adjuvant 5-fluorouracil-based chemotherapy for colorectal cancer. *Clin Gastroenterol Hepatol* 2004; 2: 696–703.

14 Andreyev J, Ross P, Donnellan C, Lennan E. Guidance on the management of diarrhoea during cancer chemotherapy. *Lancet Oncol* 2014; 15: e447–60.

15 Stringer AM, Gibson RJ, Logan RM, *et al.* Gastrointestinal microflora and mucins may play a critical role in the development of 5-fluorouracil-induced gastrointestinal mucositis. *Exp Biol Med (Maywood)* 2009; 234: 430–41.

16 Bustillo I, Larson H, Saif MW. Small intestine bacterial overgrowth: an underdiagnosed cause of diarrhea in patients with pancreatic cancer. *JOP* 2009; 10: 576–8.

17 Andreyev HJN, Davidson SE, Gillespie C, *et al.* Practice guidance on the management of acute and chronic gastrointestinal problems arising as a result of treatment for cancer. *Gut* 2012; 61: 179–92.

18 Wenisch JM, Schmid D, Tucek G, *et al.* A prospective cohort study on hospital mortality due to *Clostridium difficile* infection. *Infection* 2012; 40: 479–84.

19 Cheng AC, Ferguson JK, Richards MJ, *et al.* Australasian Society for Infectious Diseases guidelines for the diagnosis and treatment of *Clostridium difficile* infection. *Med J Aust* 2011; 194: 353–8.

20 Department of Health, HCAI (2012). *Updated guidance on the diagnosis and reporting of Clostridium difficile.* Available from: www.gov.uk/government/uploads/system/uploads/attachment_data/file/215135/dh_133016.pdf (accessed 23 February 2015).

21 Joshi NM, Macken L, Rampton DS. Inpatient diarrhoea and *Clostridium difficile. Clin Med Roy Coll Phys* 2012; 12: 583–8.

22 Cornely OA, Nathwani D, Ivanescu C, *et al.* Clinical efficacy of fidaxomicin compared with vancomycin and metronidazole in *Clostridium difficile* infections: a meta-analysis and indirect treatment comparison. *J Antimicrob Chemother* 2014; 69: 2892–900.

23 Harari D. Faecal incontinence in older people. *Rev Clin Gerontol* 2009; 19: 87–101.

23 A Patient with Breast Cancer Experiencing Cardiac Toxicity on Chemotherapy

M.H. Ruhe Chowdhury, Joanna Hardwick, Mark Kinirons, Mark Harries

Case history

A 76-year-old woman had a right-side wide local excision with axillary nodal clearance for early breast cancer. Histology showed a pT2 32 mm grade 2 ductal carcinoma, oestrogen receptor-positive (7/8), progesterone receptor-positive (7/8) and human epidermal growth factor receptor 2-positive (3+) with 4/22 lymph node involvement. At the multidisciplinary team (MDT) meeting it was decided that she should be offered chemotherapy and trastuzumab, followed by radiotherapy and an aromatase inhibitor.

An essential cardiac history was taken: she had had angina 10 years previously and undergone coronary stent insertion. She had not had chest pain since, but she did describe a 2 year history of fatigue on moderate exertion, no shortness of breath and occasional ankle swelling. ECG showed poor R wave progression. Other comorbidities were hypertension. Clinically, she appeared anxious, BP 150/80 mmHg, with no drop in lying to standing, jugular venous pressure not raised, no heart murmurs, clear lungs, and mild pitting oedema on both ankles. Medications included bisoprolol, aspirin 75 mg, and simvastatin. An echocardiogram showed apical dyskinesia (consistent with ECG) and an ejection fraction of 50%.

Optimal adjuvant systemic therapy guidance in the absence of comorbidities would suggest that she should be offered an anthracycline, taxane and trastuzumab-based regimen. Cardiac optimization prior to treatment was undertaken, including increasing the dose of bisoprolol, starting an ACE inhibitor (ramipril), and instituting strategies to reduce anxiety levels.

The patient's ejection fraction decreased during treatment and she was managed according to Figure 23.1, with an increase in the dose of ramipril from 1.25 to 3.75 mg. Her ejection fraction increased to 52% and she was able to resume trastuzumab and complete the standard 18 cycles.

What is the patient's risk of cardiotoxicity from chemotherapy?

How would cardiotoxicity present itself?

How can cardiac risk be assessed and monitored?

How can the patient's cardiac status be optimized medically?

Can alternative chemotherapy regimens be considered to reduce the risk?

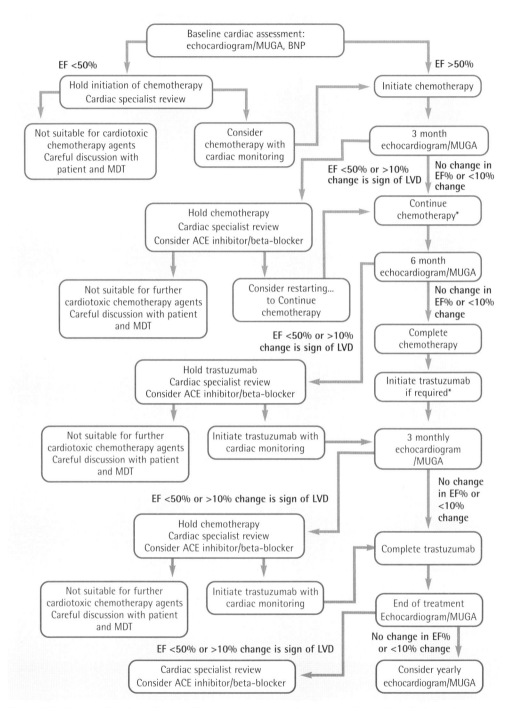

Figure 23.1 Summary flowchart of the cardiac management of patients undergoing cardiotoxic chemotherapy.
*Depending on chemotherapy regimen, trastuzumab may be initiated mid-chemotherapy treatment. During each
cycle, monitor BNP, carry out full cardiac exam and consider further investigations if warranted. EF, ejection fraction;
LVD, left ventricular dysfunction.

What is the patient's risk of cardiotoxicity from chemotherapy?

The degree of cardiotoxicity depends upon the cytotoxic agent and whether it causes irreversible cardiac damage (type 1), typically due to cellular loss, or reversible cardiac damage (type 2), from cellular dysfunction.[1] Cardiotoxicity can present in an acute or chronic setting. Acute and subacute cardiotoxicity occur at any time from the initiation of treatment up to 6 weeks after completion. Late and chronic cardiotoxicity can occur within the first year of completion of treatment, or can present many years thereafter. Anthracyclines and trastuzumab are widely acknowledged to cause cardiotoxicity; however, other agents can also play a part, particularly when in combination (Table 23.1).

Table 23.1 Summary of chemotherapy agents and their cardiac risks.

Chemotherapy class	Agent	Mechanism of cardiotoxicity and risk
Anthracycline	Doxorubicin Epirubicin	• Proportional to cumulative dosage: maximum doxorubicin dosage 550 mg/m^2, but increasing risk >350 mg/m^2; maximum epirubicin dosage 900 mg/m^2 • Cardiac risk: doxorubicin 4–36%; epirubicin is less cardiotoxic • Early-onset chronic progressive form occurs in 1.6–2.1% of patients • Late-onset chronic progressive form occurs in 1.6–5% of patients • Pathophysiology: myocyte death through the release of free radicals resulting in loss of myofibrils, dilation of the sarcoplasmic reticulum, cytoplasmic vacuolization, swelling of mitochondria, and increased number of lysosomes • Long term and irreversible
Taxanes	Paclitaxel Docetaxel	• Pro-arrhythmic effects, either directly affecting the Purkinje fibres or through the release of histamine, leading to bradycardia • Cardiac risk: 0.5–1.6% • Ventricular dysfunction is relatively low compared with anthracyclines: rates vary from 0.7% to 1.6% if treated in combination with other cytotoxic drugs, particularly docetaxel, doxorubicin, 5-FU and cyclophosphamide
Fluoropyrimidines	5-FU Capecitabine	• Within 72 h of administration, although can be seen in later cycles depending on the regimen • Cardiac risk: 1–68%, particularly in high-dose 5-FU • Angina-like chest pain, arrhythmias, heart failure, cardiogenic shock and sudden death • Pathophysiology: coronary vasospasm, myocardial toxicity, coronary artery thrombus, autoimmune response or activation of the coagulation pathway
Alkylating agents	Cyclophosphamide	• Associated with cardiomyopathy at high doses ($\geq$150 mg/kg and 1.5 g/m^2/day) used in haematological cancers
Aromatase inhibitors		• A meta-analysis of aromatase inhibitors with tamoxifen[5] suggested a relative risk of 1.31 (95% CI 1.01–1.60, p=0.007) and a low absolute risk of ~0.5%

Trastuzumab

Cardiotoxicity related to trastuzumab typically presents as an asymptomatic decrease in left ventricular function. It is reversible with cessation of trastuzumab and many patients can be re-challenged after optimization of cardiac function. Increased cardiac events are found in patients who receive concomitant or prior anthracycline therapy. In a pivotal clinical trial,[2] cardiac events were reported in 27% of patients who received trastuzumab in combination with anthracyclines and cyclophosphamide compared with 8% in those who received only anthracycline and cyclophosphamide. In women with prior anthracycline therapy, cardiac events were reported in 13% of patients who received trastuzumab with paclitaxel compared with 1% in those who received paclitaxel alone.[3] A meta-analysis of trial data showed that severe left ventricular function (New York Heart Association III and IV) was recorded in 2.4% of patients compared with 0.4% who did not receive trastuzumab.[4] The mechanism of this cardiac dysfunction is much debated and remains unclear.

How would cardiotoxicity present itself?

The incidence of cardiovascular disease increases with age, and undiagnosed heart disease is common in older patients. Heart failure is commonly an insidious presentation in older people, with an average age at diagnosis of 76 years, and it carries a 30–40% 1 year mortality.[6] Acute and chronic heart failure may be part of a more complex cardiorenal syndrome, in which cardiac and renal failure progress in synchrony. Common causes of heart failure in older people include ischaemic heart disease or previous myocardial infarction, hypertension, arrhythmias and valve disease. Presenting symptoms of acute myocardial infarction change with ageing: 20% of patients have no symptoms, 35% have dyspnoea only, and only 20% have chest pain. Ongoing ischaemic heart disease can present with exertional symptoms other than chest pain, such as fatigue, as in this case.

How can cardiac risk be assessed and monitored?

Objective assessment of cardiac disease is essential, especially prior to cancer treatment (chemotherapy or surgery), and should include a full assessment of any related conditions (e.g. renal impairment, or in this case significant anxiety). The oncology clinic is well placed to identify cardiac disease.

The risk of cardiotoxicity increases with cardiovascular risk factors (smoking, hyperlipidaemia, hypertension, diabetes, obesity), which should be identified and addressed (smoking cessation, BP, glucose control, appropriate exercise programmes). Symptom enquiry for heart failure includes screening questions for syncope, chest pain and breathlessness, and other exertional symptoms such as fatigue (Table 23.2).

A resting 12-lead ECG is a useful 'rule out' test for heart failure in older people, as left ventricular dysfunction is rare in the presence of a completely normal ECG, and generally only an abnormal ECG would prompt an echocardiogram. However, patients receiving potentially cardiotoxic chemotherapy should have a baseline echocardiogram and a chest radiograph to look for cardiomegaly, enlarged atria or signs of pulmonary congestion.

The 2010 NICE guideline for management of heart failure[6] suggests that B-type natriuretic peptide (BNP) be the first method of diagnosis: serum BNP or serum N-terminal pro-BNP (NTproBNP) should be measured in patients with no previous myocardial infarction. Patients with a BNP level between 100 and 400 pg/ml (29–116 pmol/l) or an NTproBNP level between 400 and 2000 pg/ml (47–236 pmol/l) should be referred for an echocardiogram and specialist assessment (within 6 weeks).[6] Patients with a previous myocardial infarction should be referred

Table 23.2 Symptoms and signs of heart failure.

Symptom	Sign
Shortness of breath	Oedema
(Cardiac) wheeze or cough	Tachycardia
Ankle oedema	Gallop rhythm (third heart sound)
Fatigue	Elevated jugular venous pressure/hepatojugular reflex
Weight loss (cardiac cachexia)	Laterally displaced apex beat
Pallor (anaemia)	Pulmonary crackles, pleural effusion
Reduced exercise tolerance	Heart murmur
Palpitations	Tachypnoea
Chest pain	Hepatomegaly, ascites
Orthopnoea	
Paroxysmal nocturnal dyspnoea	
Depression, loss of appetite	
Syncope	

straight for specialist assessment and echocardiogram within 2 weeks.[6]

There is a group of patients who present with a clinical syndrome of heart failure but have preserved left ventricular function on the echocardiogram (heart failure with preserved ejection fraction). This is predominantly seen in older women and should be managed in the same way as left ventricular function (heart failure with reduced ejection fraction). The diagnostic criteria are summarized in Table 23.3.[7]

How can the patient's cardiac status be optimized medically?

Most UK hospitals have a heart failure service (usually inpatient with community outreach) with a cardiologist and a nurse specialist. Nurse-led intervention has been shown to reduce mortality and reduce readmissions in heart failure patients. An initial review by the heart failure team should be sought for patients with risk factors for cardiotoxicity. Further decisions regarding whether the patient needs revascularization or investigation for other causes of heart failure (e.g. valvular disease, arrhythmias, amyloidosis or other cardiomyopathies) should be carried out and optimization provided. The mainstay of treatment is the initiation of an ACE inhibitor and a beta-blocker, and modification of risk factors. Our patient presented mainly with exertional fatigue;

Table 23.3 Diagnostic criteria for heart failure.[7]

Heart failure with reduced ejection fraction	Heart failure with preserved ejection fraction
Typical symptoms of heart failure	Typical symptoms of heart failure
Signs typical of heart failure	Signs typical of heart failure
Reduced left ventricular ejection fraction	Normal or mildly reduced left ventricular ejection fraction and left ventricle not dilated
	Presence of left ventricular hypertrophy, left atrial enlargement and/or diastolic dysfunction

therefore, a geriatrician review is well placed to assess multifactorial causes of symptoms and to interpret investigations according to the patient's age and frailty. Anxiety is known to drive up heart rate, and cognitive behavioural therapy and advice on gentle exercise programmes can be helpful. Anaemia, renal impairment and hyponatraemia can all contribute to cardiotoxicity and can be measured with a baseline blood test.

The monitoring of patients and their cardiac risk throughout chemotherapy is of great importance and is summarized in Figure 23.1.

Can alternative chemotherapy regimens be considered to reduce the risk?

Our patient's risk factors for cardiotoxicity included her age, sex and history of hypertensive ischaemic heart disease (Table 23.4). The predicted prognosis for 10 year survival (using Predict, an online statistical analysis tool at www.predict.nhs.uk) for breast cancer, without any further adjuvant treatment, is 39.5%. Adjuvant hormonal therapy would add an additional 8.7%, and third-generation chemotherapy with trastuzumab an additional 10.7%. Therefore, given the magnitude of these benefits she should be considered for adjuvant cytotoxic therapy.

Typically the chemotherapy would be fluorouracil (5-FU), epirubicin and cyclophosphamide for three cycles, followed by three cycles of docetaxel or a similar regimen with trastuzumab given concomitantly with the taxane. A clear assessment of her baseline cardiac function needs to be undertaken, and, depending on its outcome, the above regimen could be given (with careful monitoring) or an alternative chemotherapy regimen such as docetaxel and cyclophosphamide with trastuzumab, or weekly paclitaxel with trastuzumab should be considered.

If the baseline ejection fraction is less than 45%, either on echocardiography or MUGA scanning, the patient should be referred to a cardiologist. A reassessment of cardiac function should be undertaken after cardiac optimization by a cardiologist or geriatrician, with or without prior administration of a non-anthracycline-based chemotherapy. All cardiac optimization needs to take place within the recommended timeframe for initiation of adjuvant therapy. Prophylactic therapies to prevent cardiotoxicity are available. Dexrazoxane, an inhibitor of topoisomerase IIB and an intracellular iron chelator, has been shown to prevent anthracycline cardiotoxicity,[8] although it is rarely used. ACE inhibitors and beta-blockers have been shown to improve survival in patients

Table 23.4 Risk factors for developing cardiotoxicity after chemotherapy.

Patient-related risk	Agent-related risk
Age	Chemotherapy agent
Valvular disease	Accumulative dose
Coronary disease	Dose schedule/administration rate
Myocardial infarction	Concurrent administration with other chemotherapy agents
Previous chemotherapy/left chest wall/breast or mantle radiotherapy	
Hypertension	
Female sex	
Ethnicity	
Chromosomal abnormalities, e.g. inherited hypertrophic cardiomyopathy	
Liver disease	

with congestive heart failure, cardiac hypertrophy and reperfusion abnormalities:[9] ACE inhibitors are routinely used to improve the ejection fraction on trastuzumab.

Conclusion and learning points

- When considering cardiotoxic chemotherapy, oncologists should identify cardiac risk factors, symptoms and related comorbidities in older people by clinical assessment, baseline ECG, echocardiogram, BNP measurement and baseline blood tests.

- If risk factors are identified, an initial cardiologist/heart failure service review should be sought for further risk assessment and cardiac optimization.

- Geriatric input can help with optimization of other related symptoms and needs, and with follow-through during treatment.

- All appropriate optimization should take place within a timely interval to initiate adjuvant therapy.

- Optimal cancer therapy should be the aim, together with appropriate medical, social and psychological support.

References

1 Curigliano G, Cardinale D, Suter T, *et al.* Cardiovascular toxicity induced by chemotherapy, targeted agents and radiotherapy: ESMO clinical practice guidelines. *Ann Oncol* 2012; 23 (suppl 7): vii155–66.

2 Seidman A, Hudis C, Pierri MK, *et al.* Cardiac dysfunction in the trastuzumab clinical trials experience. *J Clin Oncol* 2002; 20: 1215–21.

3 Slamon D, Leyland-Jones B, Shak S, *et al.* Addition of Herceptin (humanized anti-HER2 antibody) to first line chemotherapy for HER2 overexpressing metastatic breast cancer (HER2+/MBC) markedly increases anticancer activity: a randomized, multinational controlled phase III trial. *Proc Am Soc Clin Oncol* 1998; 17: 98a.

4 Moja L, Tagliabue L, Balduzzi S, *et al.* Trastuzumab containing regimens for early breast cancer. *Cochrane Database Syst Rev* 2012; 4: CD006243.

5 Cuppone F, Bria E, Verma S, *et al.* Do adjuvant aromatase inhibitors increase the cardiovascular risk in postmenopausal women with early breast cancer? Meta-analysis of randomized trials. *Cancer* 2008; 112: 260–7.

6 National Institute for Health and Care Excellence (2010). *Chronic heart failure. Management of chronic heart failure in adults in primary and secondary care. NICE clinical guideline 108.* Available from: www.nice.org.uk/guidance/cg108/resources/guidance-chronic-heart-failure-pdf (accessed 12 March 2015).

7 McMurray JJV, Adamopoulos S, Anker SD, *et al.* ESC guidelines for the diagnosis and treatment of acute and chronic heart failure. *Eur Heart J* 2012; 33: 1787–847.

8 Huh W, Jaffe N, Durand J, *et al.* Comparison of doxorubicin cardiotoxicity in pediatric sarcoma patients when given with dexrazoxane versus continuous infusion. *J Pediatr Hematol Oncol* 2010; 27: 546–57.

9 Jones AL, Barlow M, Barrett-Lee PJ, *et al.* Management of cardiac health in trastuzumab-treated patients with breast cancer: updated United Kingdom National Cancer Research Institute recommendations for monitoring. *Br J Cancer* 2009; 100: 684–92.

24 Chemotherapy Resulting in Acute Kidney Injury in a Patient with Bladder Cancer

Iva Damyanova, Vidhya Nair, Christy Ralph

Case history

A 77-year-old man presented with a 1 week history of haematuria. His past medical history included hypertension, type 2 diabetes, mild mitral regurgitation, hiatus hernia, diverticulosis and hypercholesterolaemia. His drug history included bendroflumethiazide, ramipril, metformin and simvastatin. He lived alone and was independent in his activities of daily living. Investigations revealed a muscle-invasive bladder cancer with pelvic nodal metastases.

The oncologist requested isotopic measurement of the patient's glomerular filtration rate (GFR) and recommended full-dose palliative chemotherapy with gemcitabine and cisplatin. Serum creatinine was 77 µmol/l and isotope GFR was 65 ml/min.

Following cycle 1, the patient developed dizziness on standing, grade 2 vomiting and grade 2 fatigue. He was admitted to hospital and his vital signs were: temperature 37.0°C, pulse 115 bpm, BP 96/55 mmHg. His blood tests revealed: Na 140 mmol/l, K 5.7 mmol/l, urea 16.2 mmol/l, creatinine 252 µmol/l. White blood cell count, C-reactive protein and calcium were normal. Serum glucose was 10 mmol/l.

The management of his acute kidney injury involved fluid resuscitation, antiemetics, and stopping bendroflumethiazide, ramipril and metformin. A bedside bladder scan performed on admission excluded post-renal acute kidney injury from urinary retention. Urine analysis excluded infection. Ultrasonography of the kidneys was performed within 24 h and also ruled out upper urinary tract obstruction.

His acute kidney injury improved with conservative measures; a repeat isotope GFR was 55 ml/min. The cause was ascribed to dehydration secondary to chemotherapy-related vomiting and an element of cisplatin-related nephrotoxicity, all exacerbated by his medications. Post-discharge performance status (PS) was 1.

The oncologist discussed the risks and benefits of further palliative chemotherapy. In light of his renal impairment he was offered gemcitabine/carboplatin, instead of continuing with gemcitabine/cisplatin, and a reassessment CT scan after his next treatment. He decided to proceed with the chemotherapy but to retain the option to stop his treatment if the fatigue had a significant impact on his quality of life.

How should this patient be managed?

What were the goals of cancer treatment in this patient?

Are there challenges specific to older patients?

What could be done to reduce his risk of acute kidney injury as he underwent cancer treatment?

What is the evidence base for his treatment options?

How should this patient be managed?

The patient should be admitted to an acute oncology unit, where initial investigations should include: immediate bedside bladder scan to exclude post-renal acute kidney injury, urinalysis (for infection and presence of protein and/or blood), arterial/venous blood gases to exclude metabolic acidosis, and an ECG if the patient is hyperkalaemic. NICE guidelines recommend that renal ultrasound is performed within 24 h if no cause of acute kidney injury is identified or if renal tract obstruction is a possibility.[1] In this patient's case, the bladder tumour put him at risk of renal obstruction; therefore, renal ultrasound was performed. Prompt fluid replacement may reverse acute kidney injury secondary to hypovolaemia and/or limit kidney injury due to acute tubular necrosis. Intravenous fluids should be prescribed following assessment of the patient's volume status. The optimal infusion rate varies depending on clinical status and comorbidities. The patient's vital signs (BP, heart rate, respiratory rate) should be monitored along with repeated clinical examination (capillary refill, jugular venous pressure, chest examination for presence of crackles) to ensure that volume overload does not occur. A urine output of at least 0.5 ml/kg/h should be maintained. Bladder catheterization is not essential but it does enable measurement of hourly urine output (indicated if there is significant renal impairment with persistent hypotension). Where hourly measurements are not required, daily urine output can be effectively measured using urine bottles or convenes.

Neutropenic and non-neutropenic sepsis should be considered at initial presentation. The possibility of sepsis should continue to be monitored, even if it was not evident on admission. Septic acute kidney injury is independently associated with higher odds of death and longer duration of hospitalization.[2]

If fluid resuscitation is unsuccessful in maintaining adequate urine output, or if hypotension and/or metabolic acidosis or significant hyperkalaemia persists despite adequate hydration, early referral to critical care and renal specialists is advised. Renal function should be repeated regularly, daily in the first instance, until an improving trend is clear.

Some of the patient's medications should be discontinued. Metformin is associated with an increased risk of lactic acidosis in the context of renal impairment and therefore should be stopped. If blood glucose levels are high without metformin, alternative agents should be considered in consultation with the patient's diabetologist. His ACE inhibitor should also be stopped (nephrotoxic: may worsen hypotension and contribute to organ hypoperfusion including kidney). Bendroflumethiazide should also be discontinued, as it may also worsen hypovolaemia, hypotension and electrolyte imbalance. Any new medication dosing must be adapted to altered kinetics in acute kidney injury. Improved control of emesis can be achieved by using alternative antiemetics or using alternative routes of administration intravenously, subcutaneously or via a syringe driver.

Malnutrition (which is more common in older people) is associated with in-hospital mortality in patients with acute kidney injury independently of complications and comorbidities;[3,4] therefore, a dietetics referral should be considered. Patients with acute kidney injury should receive 25–35 kcal/kg/day. Trace elements and water-soluble vitamins should be supplemented as required.

What were the goals of cancer treatment in this patient?

The goals of treatment for metastatic bladder cancer should be driven by a balance of improvement in survival with improvement in quality of life, including symptom control and preserved functional status regardless of age. Of note, patients with good PS and lymph node-only disease have a low but significant rate of achieving a durable long-term remission with primary gemcitabine/cisplatin chemotherapy.

Are there challenges specific to older patients?

The gradual decline in GFR that is seen with advancing age results in a prolonged half-life and a higher concentration of renally excreted drugs. Structural kidney changes occur with ageing, including nephrosclerosis, decline in nephron number, decreased kidney cortical volume and development of renal cysts. Age-related loss of muscle mass makes the estimation of GFR based on serum creatinine unreliable as a marker of GFR. Older individuals are at increased risk of dehydration because their bodies have lower water content. Decrease in total body water leads to a much smaller volume of distribution for water-soluble drugs. Comorbidities such as diabetes and hypertension are also more common in older people.

The renal system undergoes loss of functional reserve with age, due to a variable and progressive loss of acute parenchymal cells and their subsequent replacement by interstitial, inactive cells. The loss of renal functional reserve makes the renal system vulnerable to stress. This problem is further compounded if the renal system also has pre-existing pathological degenerative changes.

What could be done to reduce his risk of acute kidney injury as he underwent cancer treatment?

This patient had a number of risk factors for acute kidney injury (Table 24.1) that were evident at his initial oncology assessment but that could be modified prior to commencing treatment. Where possible, his diuretics and ACE inhibitor should be discontinued prior to chemotherapy in discussion with the patient and his GP. The prevention of longer term complications from poorly controlled hypertension is no longer relevant in light of his poor cancer prognosis. If his BP was significantly raised without these medications, alternatives such as amlodipine could be considered.

Regular antiemetics were prescribed to reduce the risk of chemotherapy-induced emesis. Earlier identification of poorly controlled symptoms might, however, have led to earlier adjustments to his supportive medications and/or early intravenous/subcutaneous hydration.

Table 24.1 Risk factors for acute kidney injury summarized from the NICE guidelines.[1]

- Chronic kidney disease (or history of)
- Diabetes
- Heart failure
- Sepsis
- Hypovolaemia
- Age 65 years or over
- Use of drugs with nephrotoxic potential (for example, NSAIDs, ACE inhibitors)
- Use of iodinated contrast agents within past week
- Oliguria
- Liver disease
- Limited access to fluids, e.g. due to neurological impairment
- Deteriorating early warning scores
- Symptoms or history of urological obstruction

This might have mitigated the impact of vomiting on his volume status and resulting acute kidney injury. Enhanced monitoring or early telephone follow-up calls for those deemed to be at higher risk of such toxicities may be useful, at least during the first cycle. Diabetic control should be checked with HbA_{1c} measurement. Metformin was stopped, as creatinine clearance was <60 ml/min, and he was started on glimepiride. Plans were made for mid-cycle creatinine clearance monitoring in the community during chemotherapy and he was advised to increase his oral fluid intake. Fluid diaries may help the patient and clinical staff assess how well his fluid intake is being maintained.

What is the evidence base for his treatment options?

Bladder cancer mostly occurs in men. Transitional cell carcinoma is the most predominant histological type. Despite bladder cancer being sensitive to chemotherapy, the prognosis of patients with metastatic disease remains poor. Five year survival for stage IV bladder cancer in men was 9% for patients diagnosed during 2002–2006 in the former Anglia Cancer Network. In women, 5 year survival was 11%.[5] A phase III randomized trial of 405 patients was conducted to compare gemcitabine/cisplatin with methotrexate/vinblastine/doxorubicin/cisplatin.[6,7] The median age of the patients was 63 years. The respective response rates (49% vs 46%), time to progression (median 7.4 vs 7.4 months) and overall survival (OS; median 13.8 vs 14.8 months) were similar in each arm. More importantly, doublet gemcitabine/cisplatin was better tolerated than the four drug regimen: 63% of cycles in the gemcitabine/cisplatin arm were administered with no dose modifications compared with 37% in the four drug arm.

One randomized phase II study of 140 patients compared gemcitabine/cisplatin with gemcitabine/carboplatin as first-line therapy for advanced transitional cell carcinoma.[8] No differences between arms were noted in the overall toxicity profiles or any parameter of toxicity. Overall response, evaluated in 80 patients, was 49.1% for gemcitabine/cisplatin and 40.0% for gemcitabine/carboplatin. Median time to progression was 8.3 months for gemcitabine/cisplatin and 7.7 months for gemcitabine/carboplatin. Median survival was 12.8 months for gemcitabine/cisplatin and 9.8 months for gemcitabine/carboplatin. These data suggest that the carboplatin doublet is active in metastatic bladder cancer and has a similar toxicity profile to that of gemcitabine/cisplatin. The European Organisation for Research and Treatment of Cancer conducted a phase III trial in patients with metastatic transitional cell carcinoma who were deemed unfit for gemcitabine/cisplatin therapy.[9] The study compared gemcitabine/carboplatin with methotrexate, carboplatin and vinblastine, repeated every 28 days. The median age of the patients was 71 years. The results, presented at the American Society of Clinical Oncology meeting in 2010, demonstrated equivalent OS between the two treatments, with a better toxicity profile in favour of gemcitabine/carboplatin.[9]

Conclusion and learning points

- Gemcitabine/cisplatin should be considered first-line treatment in fit, older patients with metastatic bladder cancer.
- Gemcitabine/carboplatin has similar outcomes to gemcitabine/cisplatin and should be offered to those in whom cisplatin is not suitable.
- Identify risk factors for acute kidney injury (summarized in Table 24.1) prior to administering potentially nephrotoxic chemotherapies. Modify such risk factors where possible.
- Avoid co-administration of nephrotoxic drugs, e.g. ACE inhibitors and non-steroidal anti-inflammatory drugs (NSAIDs), when using cisplatin-based regimens. Discuss the potential to withhold or stop such medications with the patient and GP.

- Consider enhanced monitoring and/or early follow-up of those deemed to be at high risk of expected toxicities.
- Consider formal assessment of renal function with isotope GFR prior to platinum-based chemotherapy, especially in patients with diabetes or in those receiving diuretic treatment.

References

1 National Institute for Health and Care Excellence (2013). *Acute kidney injury. NICE clinical guideline 169.* Available from: www.nice.org.uk/guidance/cg169/resources (accessed 15 June 2015).

2 Bagshaw SM, Uchino S, Bellomo R, *et al.* Septic acute kidney injury in critically ill patients: clinical characteristics and outcomes. *Clin J Am Soc Nephrol* 2007; 2: 431–9.

3 Druml W. Nutritional management of acute renal failure. *J Ren Nutr* 2005; 5: 63–70.

4 Abdel-Kader K, Palevsky P. Acute kidney injury in the elderly. *Clin Geriatr Med* 2009; 25: 331–58.

5 Cancer Research UK. *Bladder cancer survival statistics.* Available from: www.cancerresearchuk. org/health-professional/cancer-statistics/statistics-by-cancer-type/bladder-cancer/survival# heading-Three (accessed 20 July 2015).

6 von der Maase H, Hansen SW, Roberts JT, *et al.* Gemcitabine and cisplatin versus methotrexate, vinblastine, doxorubicin, and cisplatin in advanced or metastatic bladder cancer: results of a large, randomized, multinational, multicenter, phase III study. *J Clin Oncol* 2000; 18: 3068–77.

7 von der Maase H, Sengelov L, Roberts JT, *et al.* Long-term survival results of a randomized trial comparing gemcitabine plus cisplatin, with methotrexate, vinblastine, doxorubicin, plus cisplatin in patients with bladder cancer. *J Clin Oncol* 2005; 23: 4602–8.

8 Dogliotti L, Cartenì G, Siena S, *et al.* Gemcitabine plus cisplatin versus gemcitabine plus carboplatin as first-line chemotherapy in advanced transitional cell carcinoma of the urothelium: results of a randomized phase 2 trial. *Eur Urol* 2007; 52: 134–41.

9 De Santis M, Bellmunt J, Mead G, *et al.* Randomized phase II/III trial comparing gemcitabine/carboplatin (GC) and methotrexate/carboplatin/vinblastine (M-CAVI) in patients (pts) with advanced urothelial cancer (UC) unfit for cisplatin-based chemotherapy (CHT): phase III results of EORTC study 30986. *J Clin Oncol* 2009; 27: 5634–9.

Further reading

- Sawhney R, Sehl M, Naeim A. Physiologic aspects of aging: impact on cancer management and decision making, part I. *Cancer J* 2005; 11: 449–60.
- Launay-Vacher V, Chatelut E, Lichtman SM, *et al.* Renal insufficiency in elderly cancer patients: International Society of Geriatric Oncology clinical practice recommendations. *Ann Oncol* 2007; 18: 1314–21.
- Hurria A, Togawa K, Mohile SG, *et al.* Predicting chemotherapy toxicity in older adults with cancer: a prospective multicenter study. *J Clin Oncol* 2011; 29: 3457–65.
- Ramjaun A, Nassif MO, Krotneva S, *et al.* Improved targeting of cancer care for older patients: a systematic review of the utility of comprehensive geriatric assessment. *J Geriatr Oncol* 2013; 4: 271–81.
- Jerkic M, Vojvodic S, Lopez-Novoa JM. The mechanism of increased renal susceptibility to toxic substances in the elderly. Part I. The role of increased vasoconstriction. *Int Urol Nephrol* 2001; 32: 539–47.

25 Partial Nephrectomy Followed by Hand–Foot Syndrome in a Patient with Renal Cancer Receiving Tyrosine Kinase Inhibitor Therapy

Nicola Hughes, Vidhya Nair, Naveen Vasudev

Case history

A 76-year-old man presented to his GP with haematuria. Investigations demonstrated a 5 cm primary renal tumour in the upper pole of the kidney. Biopsy of the primary revealed a clear cell renal cell carcinoma, grade 3. Prior to his cancer diagnosis he had lived alone and managed his activities of daily living (ADL) with the help of his family, who visited once weekly to assist with shopping and cleaning. He left the house on a daily basis and liked to attend the local social club to catch up with friends. His past medical history included high cholesterol and hypertension controlled with atorvastatin and ramipril, respectively, and marginal chronic renal failure (glomerular filtration rate 58 ml/min). The discussion at the multidisciplinary team (MDT) meeting proposed that a radical nephrectomy was not appropriate because of his impaired renal function, but that alternative methods of controlling the tumour locally should be considered. The interventional radiologist felt that the tumour was too large for radiofrequency ablation (RFA), and the urological surgeon recommended partial nephrectomy. This was carried out laparoscopically 1 week later and, after an overnight stay in the HDU for meticulous attention to fluid balance and BP, he mobilized and went home 5 days later.

Eighteen months later he re-presented with cough, weight loss and fatigue, and a CT scan showed multiple bilateral lung metastases. He was seen in the oncology outpatient clinic and discussed the options of a tyrosine kinase inhibitor (TKI) or best supportive care. He chose a TKI and commenced sunitinib. He did not require changes to medications prior to commencing sunitinib, as his BP was normal (125/75 mmHg) on ramipril.

Eight weeks into treatment he presented with a significant decline in function secondary to painful hands and feet. His daughter had called the renal clinical nurse specialist to express her concerns regarding her father. Over the last week his hands and feet had become increasingly painful and he was struggling to mobilize around the house. He had not been seen in the social club for 5 days and his oral intake had declined, as he was finding it easier to stay in bed due to the pain and feeling generally unwell. His daughter stated that her father had not wanted to bother anyone and she felt he was becoming low in mood. A recent CT scan had shown stable disease.

He was reviewed on the oncology assessment unit and found to have erythematous swollen areas on the pressure points of his hands and feet, consistent with sunitinib-induced hand-foot syndrome. His BP was 115/60 mmHg. Routine blood tests showed a mild acute kidney injury, urea 14 mmol/l, creatinine 120 μmol/l.

What are the options for the treatment of a renal primary in patients with reduced renal function?

What is the place of sunitinib in metastatic disease in older patients?

What is the side effect profile of sunitinib in older patients?

What is hand–foot syndrome?

How should this patient be managed?

What are the options for the treatment of a renal primary in patients with reduced renal function?

Although radical nephrectomy has been standard therapy for the management of patients with a diagnosis of primary renal cancer for many decades, there is now good evidence that partial nephrectomy has a similar long-term oncological outcome and it may be safely and effectively performed laparoscopically.[1–4] Retrospective analysis suggests that the overall survival of patients is at least as good following partial nephrectomy compared with radical nephrectomy, irrespective of the age of the patient.[5] In addition to urological surgeons with expertise in both radical and partial nephrectomy, a modern renal cancer MDT should have access to interventional oncologists, usually radiologists, who are able to deploy an appropriate option for image-guided thermal ablation of the tumour. This is most commonly RFA or cryoablation. Tumour size and location, in particular proximity to the renal pelvis, are factors considered in MDT discussions by urologists and oncologists. Smaller tumours (<4 cm) more than 1 cm away from a relevant vital structure may be commonly treated by thermal ablation. Larger tumours may be successfully treated by partial nephrectomy. For smaller tumours, both RFA and cryoablation are associated with over 90% cancer-specific survival.[6,7] A meta-analysis of results to date suggest that thermal ablation of small renal primary tumours is associated with disease control that is comparable to surgical nephrectomy and has significantly lower complication rates and less decline in renal function.[8] Our patient's tumour was deemed too large for thermal ablation, but a laparoscopic partial nephrectomy was successful. He tolerated this treatment well; careful attention was paid to postoperative fluid balance and BP control.

What is the place of sunitinib in metastatic disease in older patients?

Patients who have metastatic disease but are asymptomatic may be observed without detriment and some have many months or even a few years of excellent quality of life without treatment.[9] In the presence of significant symptoms, however, the patient chose to have systemic therapy. Sunitinib is a multi-targeted TKI that attacks a number of cellular processes including the vascular endothelial growth factor pathway involved in angiogenesis.[10] Other targets include platelet-derived growth factor receptors, stem cell growth factor receptor and fms-related tyrosine kinase 3.[10,11] Sunitinib is taken orally, typically on a 4 weeks on/2 weeks off schedule. The full dose is 50 mg daily, although many patients require dose reductions for toxicity to either 37.5 mg or 25 mg. Current NICE guidelines recommend sunitinib as the first-line treatment for patients with advanced or metastatic renal cell carcinoma and an Eastern Cooperative Oncology

Group performance status (PS) of 0–1. It is also licensed in the treatment of gastrointestinal stromal tumours and pancreatic neuroendocrine tumours. The clinical trials which support the recommendations are summarized in Case 13.

What is the side effect profile of sunitinib in older patients?

Patients taking sunitinib are exposed to an array of potential side effects including fatigue, dysgeusia, mucositis, disruption of wound healing, hypertension, gastrointestinal toxicities, endocrinopathies and skin changes.

A number of retrospective reviews and studies have been carried out to aid treatment decisions regarding the use of sunitinib in older patients.[10,12-14] These indicate that the side effect profiles of patients taking sunitinib are similar at all ages but that those experienced by older people tend to be of a higher grade.[12] As a result, older people are more likely to have their treatment discontinued due to toxicity rather than disease progression.[12,13] One reason for the apparently poor tolerance of sunitinib by some older patients may be the increased prevalence of comorbidities such as hypertension which may be exacerbated by the treatment. It is also possible that differences in drug metabolism (as a result of decreased end-organ function with age or concurrent medications) contribute.

What is hand–foot syndrome?

Hand-foot syndrome, also called palmar-plantar erythrodysaesthesia, is a recognized side effect of a number of systemic therapies used to treat cancer. Recognized causes include conventional cytotoxic chemotherapies (capecitabine, fluorouracil and liposomal anthracyclines), as well as novel targeted agents (including sunitinib, sorafenib, pazopanib and vemurafenib). Hand-foot syndrome of all National Cancer Institute Common Terminology Criteria for Adverse Events version 3.0 grades has been found to occur in 24% of patients older than 70 years taking sunitinib[3] and can occur as soon as 5 days after starting treatment.[15]

Patients develop painful symmetrical erythematous and oedematous areas on the palms and soles of their feet. Periungual areas and the sides of the fingers can also be affected and desquamation may be seen. Paraesthesia, aggravated by warmth, is often associated and may precede any noticeable skin changes. The greatest effect on function is felt when these skin changes occur on pressure points. It is distinguishable from the classic hand-foot changes seen with chemotherapy agents, as affected skin areas tend to be more localized and hyperkeratotic.[16] Stevens–Johnson syndrome associated with sunitinib has been reported.[17]

How should this patient be managed?

The first step in management of this patient is to stop the sunitinib and ramipril. Intravenous rehydration should be administered depending on the degree of renal dysfunction; clinical assessment should be carried out; and it should be ascertained whether he is capable of increasing his oral intake. His serum calcium level should be checked to investigate for hypercalcaemia, which may be contributing to his low mood. Referral to a dietitian for nutritional supplementation should be considered. The majority of cases of hand-foot syndrome are reversible and will resolve once sunitinib is withheld.[16,18] Symptomatic management in the meantime is important. Table 25.1 outlines ways in which this can be achieved.

This man had previously managed independently and enjoyed getting out of the house and socializing. Loss of ability to do this may have a psychological impact on the patient and result in low mood. He should therefore be screened for signs of depression using the Geriatric Depression Scale (GDS), which is quick and easy to perform and has high sensitivity and specificity. If positive, a clinical assessment for depression is required. Psychological input can be provided via support groups or referral to a clinical psychologist if needed. If a baseline Abbreviated Mental Test Score (AMTS) was abnormal, it should be repeated following improvement of mood, as depression may affect memory and present as pseudodementia. A referral to the physiotherapy team is important to assess his mobility, provide any walking aids if needed and to set rehabilitation goals if required. He should also be reviewed by the occupational therapy team who can assess for functional deficits, set functional rehabilitation goals and carry out necessary adaptations to his home to aid him with his ADL. His decline in function is likely to be transient but he will need increased social support in the meantime. This could involve increased family support or the use of intermediate care services. Intermediate care services aim to promote independence by providing a bridge of care (if needed) and by providing rehabilitation with the goal of improving mobility and function (back to premorbid abilities where possible). Home-based intermediate care is usually available to patients for a maximum of a few weeks and is not means-tested. It includes providing necessary temporary social care as well as home-based rehabilitation (physiotherapy for mobility goals, occupational therapy for functional goals). Bed-based rehabilitation (also not means-tested) is available in some but not all areas of the UK. It provides similar care and rehabilitation to home-based services. It is most commonly used for those with complex rehabilitation needs and where the severity of impairments precludes the provision at home. If care is required at the end of home/bed-based rehabilitation, it is provided via social services if the family is unable or unwilling to provide care. Social care is means-tested.

In a situation, such as this, where sunitinib is currently controlling his disease, there is the option of restarting sunitinib at a lower dose once the skin toxicity has resolved. If the decision is made to restart sunitinib, the patient should continue to be closely monitored in a treatment review clinic for signs of toxicity and changes in his PS. The presenting episode may provide the opportunity to explore his wishes regarding increased care needs in the future should his health decline.

Table 25.1 Management, prevention and treatment of hand–foot syndrome.[18]

Management and prevention	Treatment
• Limit exposure to hot water and other sources of heat	• Simple analgesia; non-steroidal anti-inflammatory drugs should be avoided in older patients and those with acute kidney injury
• Avoid exposing skin to strong sunlight	
• Have a manicure and pedicure prior to starting treatment	• Urea-based moisturizing creams
• Avoid contact with irritants such as household chemicals	• If skin becomes broken or blistered, bathe affected areas in Epsom salts; continue to use urea-based creams but stop using moisturizers
• Wear soft, loose-fitting clothes and shoes	• Topical anaesthetics such as lidocaine patches or cream
• Go barefoot in the house if possible	
• Gel pads may help sore feet	
• If symptoms develop, avoid activities that cause excess pressure and friction to the affected areas	
• Keep skin well moisturized with aqueous cream, unscented moisturizers or aloe vera gel	

This patient's sunitinib was withheld and his hand-foot syndrome improved to grade 1 severity. He managed to increase his fluid intake and his acute kidney injury improved. Following review by the dietitian, he was started on nutritional supplements. His daughter was agreeable to increasing her support and so there was no need for a care package to be put in place at this time. The patient accepted that this may be necessary if his health declined and he wished to remain at home. He underwent home-based rehabilitation and his physical function returned to baseline. He returned to the outpatient oncology clinic 4 weeks later and agreed to restart his sunitinib treatment at the reduced dose of 25 mg, which he tolerated well. His BP was monitored regularly with a view to restarting an appropriate antihypertensive if required. His mood had improved and he returned to meeting his friends at the social club. He was agreeable to attending the day centre at the local hospice to get him out of the house.

Conclusion and learning points

- Primary renal cancer with impaired renal function can be managed by a variety of effective treatments which avoid the need for radical nephrectomy.

- Close monitoring and effective management of side effects in older patients are crucial in order to enable them to get the maximum benefit from treatment.

- This case highlights the need to emphasize to patients the importance of reporting side effects whilst on treatment. Treatment-specific patient information leaflets are particularly useful and provide patients with a resource to refer back to, should side effects occur.

- Routinely ask patients whether side effects are affecting their mobility and/or function and identify what the specific difficulties are. Refer to physiotherapy and occupational therapy for further assessment and ongoing rehabilitation where required.

References

1 Fergany AF, Hafez KS, Novick AC. Long-term results of nephron sparing surgery for localized renal cell carcinoma: 10-year followup. *J Urol* 2000; 163: 442–5.

2 Springer C, Hoda MR, Fajkovic H, *et al.* Laparoscopic vs open partial nephrectomy for T1 renal tumours: evaluation of long-term oncological and functional outcomes in 340 patients. *BJU Int* 2013; 111: 281–8.

3 Lam JS, Shvarts O, Pantuck AJ. Changing concepts in the surgical management of renal cell carcinoma. *Eur Urol* 2004; 45: 692–705.

4 Lane BR, Campbell SC, Gill IS. 10-year oncologic outcomes after laparoscopic and open partial nephrectomy. *J Urol* 2013; 190: 44–9.

5 Roos FC, Steffens S, Junker K, *et al.*; German Renal Cell Cancer Network. Survival advantage of partial over radical nephrectomy in patients presenting with localized renal cell carcinoma. *BMC Cancer* 2014; 14: 372.

6 Chapman SJ, Wah TM, Sourbron SP, *et al.* The effects of cryoablation on renal cell carcinoma perfusion and glomerular filtration rate measured using dynamic contrast-enhanced MRI: a feasibility study. *Clin Radiol* 2013; 68: 887–94.

7 Zargar H, Atwell TD, Cadeddu JA, *et al.* Cryoablation for small renal masses: selection criteria, complications, and functional and oncologic results. *Eur Urol* 2015; pii: S0302-2838(15)00246-8.

8 Katsanos K, Mailli L, Krokidis M, *et al.* Systematic review and meta-analysis of thermal ablation versus surgical nephrectomy for small renal tumours. *Cardiovasc Intervent Radiol* 2014; 37: 427–37.

9 Rini B, Dorff T, Elson P, *et al.* A prospective observational study of metastatic renal cell carcinoma (mRCC) prior to initiation of systemic therapy (abstract). *J Clin Oncol* 2014; 32 (suppl 5): 4520.

10 Chen HX, Cleck JN. Adverse effects of anticancer agents that target the VEGF pathway. *Nat Rev Clin Oncol* 2009; 6: 465–77.

11 Verheaul HMW, Pinedo HM. Possible molecular mechanisms involved in the toxicity of angiogenesis inhibition. *Nat Rev Cancer* 2007; 7: 475–85.

12 Hutson T, Bukowski R, Rini B, *et al.* Efficacy and safety of sunitinib in elderly patients with metastatic renal cell carcinoma. *Br J Cancer* 2014; 110: 1125–32.

13 Pal SK, Hsu J, Hsu S, *et al.* Impact of age on treatment trends and clinical outcome in patients with metastatic renal cell carcinoma. *J Geriatr Oncol* 2013; 4: 128–33.

14 Brunello A, Basso U, Sacco T, *et al.* Safety and activity of sunitinib in elderly patients (≥70 years) with metastatic renal cell carcinoma: a multicentre study. *Ann Oncol* 2013; 24: 336–32.

15 Lee WJ, Lee JL, Chang SE, *et al.* Cutaneous adverse effects in patients treated with the multitargeted kinase inhibitors sorafenib and sunitinib. *Br J Dermatol* 2009; 161: 1045–51.

16 Robert C, Soria JC, Spatz A, *et al.* Cutaneous side-effects of kinase inhibitors and blocking antibodies. *Lancet Oncol* 2005; 6: 491–500.

17 Lee JH, Lee JH, Lee JH, *et al.* Case of sunitinib-induced Stevens–Johnson syndrome. *J Dermatol* 2013; 40: 753–4.

18 American Society of Clinical Oncology (2014). *Hand-foot syndrome or palmar-plantar erythrodysesthesia.* Available from: www.cancer.net/navigating-cancer-care/side-effects/hand-foot-syndrome-or-palmar-plantar-erythrodysesthesia (accessed 20 April 2015).

Further reading

• Lacouture ME, Reilly LM, Gerami P, Guitart J. Hand foot skin reaction in cancer patients treated with the multikinase inhibitors sorafenib and sunitinib. *Ann Oncol* 2008; 19: 1955–61.

• National Institute for Health and Care Excellence (2013). *Intravenous fluid therapy in adults in hospital. NICE clinical guideline 174.* Available from: www.nice.org.uk/guidance/cg174 (accessed 19 April 2015).

26 They Disagree! Choice of Therapy by a Patient with Cholangiocarcinoma and His Family

Adel Jebar, Nicola Turner, Daniel Swinson

Case history

A 79-year-old widower, living independently in a ground-floor flat, was suffering from osteoarthritis of the knees and hips that limited his mobility. He had one daughter, who lived abroad. On a recent visit to the UK she was concerned that he had become fatigued, developed pruritus and lost significant weight. Investigations revealed obstructive jaundice due to a solid mass, closely associated with the pancreas and duodenum, with dilated intrahepatic bile ducts and appearance consistent with a T3N1M0 extrahepatic cholangiocarcinoma. The cancer was technically operable, but the patient was malnourished and his fitness precluded pancreatoduodenectomy.

The patient's jaundice was relieved by endoscopic retrograde cholangiopancreatography with stent insertion, and a biopsy confirmed adenocarcinoma. Following discharge, he attended outpatients with his daughter, where chemotherapy and best supportive care (BSC) treatment options were discussed. Initially, he accepted BSC, but a week later he requested a further consultation and asked to be considered for chemotherapy. The patient was assessed to have the capacity to make this decision and was offered cisplatin and gemcitabine. The oncologist was worried that the patient lived alone, and discussions included whether neighbours/friends could visit during treatment. The patient's daughter was able to arrange for a private carer to visit him at his home each morning.

Using oral nutritional supplements, the patient's condition improved to performance status (PS) 1, and he gained 2 kg over 4 weeks. A baseline CT scan was repeated and he received two cycles (repeated every 21 days) of full-dose cisplatin 25 mg/m^2 (days 1 and 8), and dose-reduced gemcitabine 750 mg/m^2 (days 1 and 8) because of concerns about the risk of neutropenia, with additional telephone support from the clinical nurse specialist. He then attended outpatients accompanied by his carer. He explained that he suffered significant fatigue that limited his normal activity. The carer mentioned that the patient questioned the value of chemotherapy but was worried that he may disappoint his daughter. A full blood count revealed significant myelosuppression.

The third cycle was put on hold and an early restaging CT was booked. Two weeks later, he attended outpatients with his daughter. The CT scan showed stable disease. The daughter encouraged her father to persevere with chemotherapy. The oncologist explained that her father's wishes were paramount. The patient explained that he felt much better prior to the chemotherapy. The oncologist revisited the rationale, potential benefits and drawbacks of chemotherapy. The patient asked for cessation of chemotherapy and was given BSC until his death 18 months later.

How should the patient be supported in the decision-making process?

How should the patient's condition be optimized ahead of potential chemotherapy?

What is the evidence behind the treatment options that the patient was offered?

What are the challenges of the Advanced Biliary Cancer (ABC)-02 trial combination chemotherapy regimen in older patients?

In the UK, approximately 2000 people are diagnosed each year with cholangiocarcinoma, and the typical age of presentation is the seventh decade of life. Cholangiocarcinomas are divided by anatomical site; older patients with extrahepatic cholangiocarcinoma, like their younger counterparts, present with jaundice, whilst those with intrahepatic cholangiocarcinoma are more likely to present with non-specific symptoms such as unintentional weight loss and abdominal pain.

How should the patient be supported in the decision-making process?

For consent to be valid, it must be voluntary and informed, based on the likely benefits and risks of treatment. A systematic review of published literature on informed consent revealed evidence of impaired understanding of information in older adults.[1] It can be helpful to summarize the risks and benefits in written form without medical jargon. It is useful to be very specific when discussing the risks and benefits of proposed treatments. For example, if the benefit of palliative chemotherapy is largely symptom control rather than survival time, then this should be clearly explained to enable informed decision making. Not all patients and/or carers, however, feel ready or able to hear prognostic information;[2] therefore, it is necessary to carefully elicit their individual wishes for information. Sufficient time must be provided to enable patients to make up their mind, and multiple discussions may be necessary. Consent forms should be signed during a follow-up visit rather than at the initial visit. This patient was fully entitled to change his mind regarding the initial treatment approach following further discussions with his daughter.

It is normal for patients to consult family members about treatment decisions, and it is often useful to the decision-making process. Sometimes, however, patients may feel pressurized or obliged to make certain decisions (potentially invalidating consent). Family disagreements about cancer treatment decisions are common: one study reported that they occurred in 65% of cases.[3] Steps should be taken to ensure that the patient's will is not overborne. This is best done during consultations when both the patient and family are present. Patients and their family often discuss medical information between themselves during a clinic appointment, often when the clinician leaves the room, but family discussions may also occur in the clinician's presence.[4] Observing family discussions may enable an understanding of the dynamics of the relationship and identify differing views. The treating team has a role in acting as the patient's advocate, speaking up for the patient where necessary. Eliciting the patient's goals in the presence of family members can be effective, but it may be necessary to discuss the patient's wishes alone if undue pressure is sensed. It may be necessary to encourage the family to understand the patient's wishes and goals whilst remaining sympathetic to their concerns. Following this, if there is suspicion that the patient's own views are not being voiced, a follow-up telephone call to the patient or an appointment in the family's absence may be helpful. In the present case, the daughter was more keen than the father for chemotherapy. The opposite may also occur, when an older patient wishes to have treatment but feels pressurized by concerned relatives not to accept it.

Carers are not usually present in consultations such as these, and professional carers are very expensive and not the norm. Nonetheless, if available, carers can help to report patient symptoms, and their views should be taken into account, especially if they have known the patient for a long time.

How should the patient's condition be optimized ahead of potential chemotherapy?

The initial clinical priority for the patient is restoration of effective biliary drainage. The two approaches are cholangiopancreatography and percutaneous transhepatic biliary drainage. The latter requires puncturing the liver and inserting a temporary external drain. Stent insertion is performed in both procedures. Which approach to take should be discussed with the gastroenterology team and interventional radiologist. For the older patient, important considerations are the potential need for repeated procedures, pain necessitating higher doses of opioid analgesia, the risk of precipitating infections with/without associated delirium, and the risk of external drain removal by a delirious patient.

Malnutrition is more common in older patients and is associated with poorer prognosis in those with gastrointestinal tumours receiving chemotherapy.[5] Patients with cholangiocarcinoma frequently lose both their appetite and weight. It is important to exclude proximal bowel obstruction secondary to duodenal involvement, occult peritoneal disease, or pancreatic insufficiency in case of pancreatic involvement. To screen for malnutrition, a reliable and validated screening tool such as the Malnutrition Universal Screening Tool (MUST) has been recommended by NICE. The risk of refeeding syndrome should be considered following acute resolution of feeding problems by duodenal stenting or enteral feeding; appropriate replacement of vitamins as well as monitoring of serum electrolytes should be undertaken. Further complications in the jaundiced patient are poor absorption of fat and fat-soluble vitamins. These complex needs are best managed with the support of a dietitian and a gastroenterologist.

It is also important to investigate and treat underlying conditions: both primary sclerosing cholangitis and hepatitis C virus infection can follow a long, asymptomatic course and present in older patients with advanced hepatobiliary diseases such as cholangiocarcinoma.[6]

The patient's comorbidities should also be reviewed. In the present case, osteoarthritis was limiting his mobility. There may be scope to improve this by adjusting analgesia and/or involving community physiotherapy and occupational health services. Care should be taken to review any non-steroidal anti-inflammatory drugs (NSAIDs), as they are potentially nephrotoxic. In the context of delivering potentially nephrotoxic chemotherapy, it would be sensible to discontinue NSAIDs. The effect of the patient's osteoarthritis on walking and functional tasks should also be actively enquired about prior to commencing treatment, to ensure chemotherapy is delivered in the context of adequate support. His arthritis mainly affected his hips and knees; thus, questions regarding his abilities with stairs, toilet and bed transfers, and getting in and out of the bath are useful. Given that his daughter lives abroad, eliciting whether the osteoarthritis affected his ability to get to the shops for food is pertinent to his nutrition during treatment.

What is the evidence behind the treatment options that the patient was offered?

Recent clinical trials have proven that cholangiocarcinoma is reasonably sensitive to chemotherapy and has a prognosis similar to that of other solid organ cancers. In a recent pooled analysis of 104 trials of patients with advanced biliary tract cancers, the subgroup of patients who received a combination of gemcitabine and platinum-based agents had the greatest benefit.[7] Most importantly, the recently published randomized phase II and III ABC-01 and ABC-02 trials demonstrated that the combination of gemcitabine 1000 mg/m^2 (days 1 and 8) and cisplatin 25 mg/m^2 (days 1 and 8) every 21 days for a maximum of eight cycles improved overall survival (OS) to 11.7 months, compared with 8.1 months with gemcitabine monotherapy (1000 mg/m^2 on days 1, 8 and 15, every 4 weeks for up to six cycles).[8,9] By comparison, an observational study of 1377 patients with advanced unresectable cholangiocarcinoma who received BSC only reported a median OS of 3.9 months.[10]

Although no subgroup analysis based on participant age was undertaken, the oldest participants included were 84 years in both studies. A subgroup analysis of the ABC-02 trial suggested that less fit patients (Eastern Cooperative Oncology Group PS 2) derived no additional benefit from combination chemotherapy, but this subgroup only consisted of 52 patients. Careful consideration should be given before offering such patients chemotherapy. If the deterioration in fitness is disease-related, the best treatment, i.e. combination chemotherapy, should be used in an attempt to reverse the decline. If the lack of fitness is chronic and due to other comorbid conditions, then BSC may be more appropriate. The ABC cisplatin and gemcitabine regimen lends itself to treatment of potentially vulnerable patients, as it permits initial exposure to a low dose of cisplatin and subsequent review prior to day 8 before continuing chemotherapy. Monotherapy with gemcitabine can be considered but is poorly evidence-based, as patients unfit for combination chemotherapy would have been excluded from the original trials and are likely to have an inferior outcome to that of the group who received single-agent chemotherapy in the ABC trials. The risks of toxicity and failure to return to independent living, in return for a probable modest benefit, should be reflected in the consent process.

What are the challenges of the ABC-02 trial combination chemotherapy regimen in older patients?

Two of the most important challenges of delivering combination cisplatin-based therapy to older patients are their reduced renal and bone marrow reserves. In the ABC-02 trial, whilst 32% of patients treated with cisplatin and gemcitabine experienced grade 3 or 4 haematological toxicity, there was no increase in the rate of neutropenic infections. Carers and family members of older patients should be made aware of these possibilities. Similarly, in the ABC-02 trial, impaired renal function was experienced by only 1% and 1.5% of patients taking gemcitabine monotherapy, or cisplatin and gemcitabine, respectively. The ABC-02 trial used an outpatient cisplatin regimen with a shortened hydration period. There is no need for a different approach for older patients. The treating team should be mindful of the fluid load if there is a history of left ventricular dysfunction, and co-medications should be reviewed to stop or change any nephrotoxic drugs.

Another factor to consider is the risk of deep vein thrombosis and thromboembolic events. In ABC-02, these complications were experienced by a higher percentage of patients who received doublet chemotherapy. Particular risk factors for the older patient are a sedentary lifestyle and reduced mobility: in our case, as a result of osteoarthritis. Patients should be advised to maintain hydration and mobilize regularly if possible.

Conclusion and learning points

- Informed consent is an ongoing process that should be regularly revisited, especially if circumstances during treatment change.

- Sufficient time must be provided to enable all patients to make up their mind, and multiple discussions may be necessary.

- Where the views of the patient and relatives differ, the treating team has a role in acting as the patient's advocate, speaking up for the patient where necessary. Eliciting the patient's goals in the presence of family members can be effective, but it may be necessary to discuss the patient's wishes alone if undue pressure is sensed.

- For older patients with advanced cholangiocarcinoma and a good PS, the combination of cisplatin and gemcitabine is superior to gemcitabine monotherapy. The ABC-02 cisplatin/gemcitabine combination regimen lends itself well to the careful treatment of older patients when consideration is given to comorbidity and appropriate supportive strategies.

References

1 Sugarman J, McCrory DC, Hubal RC. Getting meaningful informed consent from older adults: a structured literature review of empirical research. *J Am Geriatr Soc* 1998; 46: 517–24.

2 Fried TR, Bradley EH, O'Leary J. Prognosis communication in serious illness: perceptions of older patients, caregivers and clinicians. *J Am Geriatr Soc* 2003; 51: 1398–403.

3 Zhang AY, Siminoff LA. The role of the family in treatment decision making by patients with cancer. *Oncol Nurs Forum* 2003; 30: 1022–8.

4 Korfage IJ, Audrey S, Hak T, *et al.* Recognising the importance of 'family time-out' in consultations: an exploratory qualitative study. *BMJ Open* 2013; 3: e002144.

5 Attar A, Malka D, Sabaté JM, *et al.* Malnutrition is high and underestimated during chemotherapy in gastrointestinal cancer: an AGEO prospective cross-sectional multicenter study. *Nutr Cancer* 2012; 64: 535–42.

6 Tyson GL, El-Serag HB. Risk factors for cholangiocarcinoma. *Hepatology* 2011; 54: 173–84.

7 Eckel F, Schmid RM. Chemotherapy in advanced biliary tract carcinoma: a pooled analysis of clinical trials. *Br J Cancer* 2007; 96: 896–902.

8 Valle JW, Wasan H, Johnson P, *et al.* Gemcitabine alone or in combination with cisplatin in patients with advanced or metastatic cholangiocarcinomas or other biliary tract tumours: a multicentre randomised phase II study – The UK ABC-01 Study. *Br J Cancer* 2009; 101: 621–7.

9 Valle J, Wasan H, Palmer DH, *et al.* Cisplatin plus gemcitabine versus gemcitabine for biliary tract cancer. *N Engl J Med* 2010; 362: 1273–81.

10 Park J, Kim M-H, Kim K-P, *et al.* Natural history and prognostic factors of advanced cholangiocarcinoma without surgery, chemotherapy, or radiotherapy: a large-scale observational study. *Gut Liver* 2009; 3: 298–305.

27 A Patient with Muscle-Invasive Bladder Cancer for Radiotherapy or Surgery Who Experiences Falls

Daniel Lee, Naveen Vasudev, William Cross, Zuzanna Sawicka, Ann Henry

Case history

A 77-year-old man presented with a history of painless, visible haematuria to his GP. He was fast-track referred to his local urology team and underwent diagnostic cystoscopy and upper urinary tract imaging. A bladder tumour was diagnosed and biopsied and was staged with a CT scan of the chest, abdomen and pelvis. His case was discussed at the urology multidisciplinary team (MDT) meeting. His disease was confirmed as G3T3N0M0 transitional cell carcinoma of the bladder. Curative surgery or radiotherapy was recommended.

He had a past medical history of tablet-controlled type 2 diabetes mellitus, hypertension and hypercholesterolaemia. Current medications included metformin, simvastatin, amlodipine and ramipril. He was a current smoker with a history of 30 packs/year. He had no family history of cancer. He was retired, having previously worked in the manufacturing of industrial dyes. He was widowed but had close family support. He was independent in basic activities of daily living but required assistance with laundry, shopping and cleaning.

At his oncology appointment, a Comprehensive Geriatric Assessment screening tool identified a history of three falls within the last year. He was referred to the falls clinic for urgent assessment. The falls clinic identified the following contributing factors:

- Postural hypotension with pre-syncope (BP drop 115/70 mmHg to 95/60 mmHg) secondary to medications.

- Lower urinary tract symptoms: urgency, frequency and nocturia secondary to bladder cancer, high caffeine intake and detrusor instability. A bladder scan excluded high post-void residual volumes (can occur with anti-muscarinics, obstructing bladder tumours or haematuria-related clots).

- Environmental factors: low night-time lighting, not wearing glasses and clutter on the bedroom floor were identified by occupational therapy.

- Fear of falling: identified by physiotherapy resulting in his no longer going out.

The patient discussed his options with the urologist and specialist stoma nurse and underwent cardiopulmonary exercise testing. He opted against radical cystectomy and proceeded with radical radiotherapy.

What was the goal of cancer treatment for this patient?

What could be done to reduce his risk of falls as he underwent cancer treatment?

What is the evidence base for his treatment options?

What factors would affect the decision to deliver chemotherapy?

What factors influence the choice of surgery versus radiotherapy in older patients with muscle–invasive bladder cancer (MIBC)?

What was the goal of cancer treatment for this patient?

The goal of therapy in this patient with MIBC is cure. Potential treatment strategies include radical cystectomy, radiotherapy or concurrent chemoradiotherapy. Approximately 10% of patients have MIBC at diagnosis. The 3 year survival rates for T2 and T3 disease are 50% and 25%, respectively. Treatment counselling should take into consideration the patient's individual goals, independence, estimated longevity and social support to enable a shared medical decision.

What could be done to reduce his risk of falls as he underwent cancer treatment?

Falls are often multifactorial and can be divided into those with and without syncope.[1] It is estimated that 30% of adults over the age of 65 will experience at least one fall a year.[1] NICE therefore recommends that older people in contact with healthcare professionals be routinely asked about falls risk. Having identified a history of falls, it is important to establish the frequency, context and pattern to enable causes and contributors to be identified. It is equally important to identify the consequences of falls including fractures (for osteoporosis risk) and fear of falling.

As his postural hypotension was medication-related, his amlodipine was discontinued. Further medication reductions were required: management was dependent on the planned cancer treatment. In the context of cystectomy, solifenacin should be discontinued (can cause postural hypotension, no longer required without a bladder). The patient opted, however, for radiotherapy, where lower urinary tract symptoms would likely worsen during treatment; therefore, solifenacin was continued and ramipril was stopped. On completion of radiotherapy and after acute toxicities settle, this should be revisited. If urinary symptoms allow, ramipril could be reconsidered in favour of solifenacin for its prognostic benefits related to diabetes (such as uncontrolled hypertension, microalbuminuria and cardiovascular disease associated with diabetes).

To manage lower urinary tract symptoms, the patient reduced his caffeine intake (caffeine increases urinary frequency and exacerbates detrusor instability). Bedside urine bottles were provided for night-time use. He commenced bladder retraining exercises for detrusor instability. The treatment of his bladder cancer would also reduce lower urinary tract symptoms in the longer term.

Fear of falling is an important consequence of falls and is associated with reduced quality of life and social isolation[2] (in this patient's case, he stopped going out). He underwent physiotherapy to increase confidence and improve strength and balance.[3] Environmental factors were modified by occupational therapy (family removed bedroom clutter, night lighting was improved, patient was encouraged to wear glasses at night).[4]

What is the evidence base for his treatment options?

Bladder cancer most commonly occurs after the 70th year of life.[5] The treatment options for MIBC are outlined below, and evidence for older patients is detailed where available.

Radical cystectomy

Radical cystectomy with pelvic lymphadenectomy and urinary diversion remains the standard treatment for clinically localized MIBC. In men, surgery includes resection of the prostate and seminal vesicles. In women, *en bloc* resection often includes removal of the cervix, uterus, fallopian tubes, ovaries and anterior vaginal wall. The majority of older patients opt for an ileal conduit (urostomy) for urinary drainage rather than a more complex neobladder constructed from bowel.

The complications, morbidity and mortality associated with surgery can be significant, irrespective of age. Due to varied reporting criteria, it is difficult to compare outcomes grouped by age. However, multiple studies have demonstrated a significant relationship between age and postsurgical complication rate.[6] In a large series of octogenarians ($n=117$) from the Memorial Sloan Kettering Cancer Center in the USA, there was a non-significant trend towards an increased overall rate of complications compared with younger patients (72% vs 64%, $p=0.08$), but major complication rates were similar (17% vs 13%, $p=0.3$).[5] Reported 90 day mortality rates were 5.5% in patients aged >65 years, 7.5% in patients aged >75 years, and 11% in patients aged >80 years.[5] Complications and mortality rates are significantly reduced if surgery is performed by high-volume surgeons working in centres of excellence that offer excellent perioperative care which extends to the early period after hospital discharge.

Radiotherapy

Radical radiotherapy is an alternative choice to a surgical approach with radical cystectomy. Radical radiotherapy is usually chosen for those who are not medically suitable for cystectomy or through patient choice. It is associated with a 5 year overall survival (OS) of 30–40%.[7] There are no prospective randomized comparisons between radical radiotherapy and cystectomy. It is therefore difficult to directly compare outcomes from surgery and radiotherapy, as they often do not reflect the same population group. However, a retrospective audit of 458 patients receiving either radical radiotherapy or radical cystectomy in Yorkshire demonstrated equivalent survival.[8]

Radical radiotherapy is associated with palliation of lower urinary tract symptoms and symptoms such as haematuria. Toxicities include gastrointestinal and genitourinary side effects;[9] the burden of multiple daily visits for treatment should also be considered. Radiotherapy schedules vary between cancer centres: treatment is typically delivered over 4 weeks (20 visits) or 6.5 weeks (33 visits).

This patient lived far away from the tertiary centre. It would be difficult for him to attend daily appointments using public transport, especially with urinary symptoms and fear of falling. However, transport arrangements should not preclude treatment choices and should be planned prior to treatment. Cancer teams should assist patients who have difficulties with transport by engaging relatives where able (this patient had family who were able to drive him), arranging hospital transport if eligible and directing to voluntary sector drivers if needed. If treatment can be delivered closer to home, this should be explored if the patient wishes.

Chemoradiotherapy

Concurrent chemoradiotherapy has not demonstrated a statistically significant increase in 5 year OS against radiotherapy alone. However, there is a lower local recurrence rate which supports its use. Regimens include fluorouracil and mitomycin C[9] or concurrent cisplatin.[8]

Neoadjuvant chemotherapy with methotrexate, cisplatin and vinblastine prior to concurrent chemoradiotherapy has shown no significant benefit and carries the cost of additional toxicity.[10] It is therefore not recommended.

Perioperative chemotherapy

Neoadjuvant cisplatin-based chemotherapy is associated with improved outcomes in both randomized controlled trials and meta-analyses. There is an associated 5% increase in 5 year OS (from 45% to 50%), irrespective of the modality of local treatment.[10,11] There are, however, a number of contraindications to the use of cisplatin chemotherapy, including impaired hearing, cardiovascular disease, poor performance status (PS) and renal impairment, which may make safe delivery to older patients difficult. It is currently estimated that only 13% of patients in the USA who are in their 70s receive neoadjuvant chemotherapy.[12]

Adjuvant chemotherapy has not been conclusively proven to demonstrate benefit after either radical cystectomy or radiotherapy.

What factors would affect the decision to deliver chemotherapy?

A large proportion of patients with urothelial cancer have impaired renal function. Risk factors for renal dysfunction include age-related decline in glomerular filtration rate (GFR), ureteral obstruction and comorbidities such as diabetes, hypertension and smoking[13] (which is also associated with bladder cancer). If the patient had decided upon surgery, his renal function was not adequate for neoadjuvant cisplatin. Reversible contributors to renal impairment were excluded: there was no urinary retention; no ureteric obstruction; his renal toxic medications were reviewed, and his GP confirmed there was no reduction in estimated GFR on starting ramipril; there was no known diabetic nephropathy. This patient decided on radiotherapy. Concurrent chemotherapy schedules do not include cisplatin and may be considered appropriate.

What factors influence the choice of surgery versus radiotherapy in older patients with MIBC?

The choice between surgery and radiotherapy depends on both clinical and patient factors. The clinical decision is based on the patient's PS and comorbidities (in particular those which contribute to perioperative risk, e.g. cardiac disease), and should be tailored to their specific circumstances, such as their ability to rehabilitate postoperatively. Patients who have complex comorbidities and/or geriatric syndromes and/or functional impairments should be medically reviewed and optimized prior to surgery.

Patient factors include the ability to manage a urinary diversion system, such as a stoma. Comorbidities such as significant arthritis or neurological weakness/numbness affecting the hands, significant tremor or cognitive impairment may affect a patient's ability to manage a stoma. These factors should be thoroughly assessed prior to surgery. Cardiopulmonary exercise testing has been shown to quantify a patient's risk of undergoing surgery.[14,15] Careful patient selection has been shown to enable good surgical outcomes in older patients. Clinical factors that would make surgery preferable to radiotherapy include a small bladder capacity with significant urinary symptoms, evidence of hydronephrosis on imaging, or widespread carcinoma *in situ*.

Radical radiotherapy is usually advocated in patients who are deemed medically unsuitable for cystectomy, or in those who opt for radiotherapy in order to preserve their bladder. Radiotherapy is not without its short- and long-term side effects, and the logistics regarding the number of visits required for treatment should also be discussed. Each case should be discussed by the MDT and with the patient, and decisions should be made on an individual basis.

Conclusion and learning points

- Age is not a contraindication to radical cystectomy. Each case should be taken on its individual merit. Good surgical outcomes in older patients depend on careful patient selection.

- Radical radiotherapy has been shown to have good outcomes in carefully selected patients; concomitant chemotherapy can reduce the local recurrence rate.

- Neoadjuvant cisplatin-based chemotherapy improves local control and OS and should be offered if there is no contraindication.

- Review medications if postural hypotension is identified. Cancer treatment may affect changes made to medications.

- Fear of falling is an important consequence of falls, affecting quality of life and contributing to social isolation.

References

1 National Institute for Health and Care Excellence (2013). *Falls: assessment and prevention of falls in older people. NICE clinical guideline 161.* Available from: www.nice.org.uk/guidance/cg161 (accessed 24 April 2015).

2 Svantesson U, Babagbemi B, Foster L, Alricsson M. Influences on modern multifactorial falls prevention interventions and fear of falling in non-frail older adults: a literature review. *J Clin Med Res* 2014; 6: 314–20.

3 Clemson L, Fiatarone Singh MA, Bundy A, *et al.* Integration of balance and strength training into daily life activity to reduce rate of falls in older people (the LiFE study): randomised parallel trial. *BMJ* 2012; 345: e5528.

4 Keall MD, Pierse N, Howden-Chapman P, *et al.* Home modifications to reduce injuries from falls in the Home Injury Prevention Intervention (HIPI) study: a cluster-randomised controlled trial. *Lancet* 2015; 385: 231–8.

5 Stensland KD, Galsky MD. Current approaches to the management of bladder cancer in older patients. *Am Soc Clin Oncol Educ Book* 2014: e250–6.

6 Froehner M, Brausi MA, Herr HW, *et al.* Complications following radical cystectomy for bladder cancer in the elderly. *Eur Urol* 2009; 56: 443–54.

7 Kouloulias V, Tolia M, Kollairakis N, *et al.* Evaluation of acute toxicity and symptoms palliation in a hypofractionated weekly schedule of external radiotherapy for elderly patients with muscular invasive bladder cancer. *Int Braz J Urol* 2013; 39: 77–82.

8 Munro NP, Sundaram SK, Weston PM, *et al.* A 10-year retrospective review of a nonrandomized cohort of 458 patients undergoing radical radiotherapy or cystectomy in Yorkshire, UK. *Int J Radiat Oncol Biol Phys* 2010; 77: 119–24.

9 Coppin CM, Gospodarowicz MK, James K, *et al.* Improved local control of invasive bladder cancer by concurrent cisplatin and preoperative or definitive radiation. The National Cancer Institute of Canada Clinical Trials Group. *J Clin Oncol* 1996; 14: 2901–7.

10 Shipley WU, Winter KA, Kaufman DS, *et al.* Phase III trial of neoadjuvant chemotherapy in patients with invasive bladder cancer treated with selective bladder preservation by combined

radiation therapy and chemotherapy: initial results of Radiation Therapy Oncology Group 89-03. *J Clin Oncol* 1998; 16: 3576–83.

11 Advanced Bladder Cancer Meta-analysis Collaboration. Neoadjuvant chemotherapy for invasive bladder cancer. *Cochrane Database Syst Rev* 2004; 1: CD005246.

12 Zaid HB, Patel SG, Stimson CJ, *et al.* Trends in the utilization of neoadjuvant chemotherapy in muscle-invasive bladder cancer: results from the National Cancer Database. *Urology* 2014; 83: 75–80.

13 Remuzzi G. Cigarette smoking and renal function impairment. *Am J Kidney Dis* 1999; 33: 807–13.

14 Tolchard S, Angell J, Pyke M, *et al.* Cardiopulmonary reserve as determined by cardiopulmonary exercise testing correlates with length of stay and predicts complications after radical cystectomy. *Br J Urol Int* 2015; 115: 554–61.

15 Prentis JM, Trenell MI, Vasdev N, *et al.* Impaired cardiopulmonary reserve in an elderly population is related to postoperative morbidity and length of hospital stay after radical cystectomy. *Br J Urol* 2013; 112: E13–19.

Further reading

- Chang JT, Morton SC, Rubenstein LZ, *et al.* Interventions for the prevention of falls in older adults: a systematic review and meta-analysis of randomized clinical trials. *BMJ* 2004; 328: 680–4.

- Wildes TM, Dua P, Fowler SA, *et al.* Systematic review of falls in older adults with cancer. *J Geriatr Oncol* 2015; 6: 70–83.

28 Early Prostate Cancer in an Asymptomatic Patient with Urinary Incontinence and History of Deep Vein Thrombosis

Vijay Bhagawati-Prasad, Satinder Jagdev, William Cross, Eileen Burns

Case history

An 80-year-old man presented to his GP with a long-standing history of urinary incontinence and nocturia. He reported no other symptoms and he described himself as 'fit and well' and independent in his activities of daily living. His past medical history included hypertension, type 2 diabetes mellitus and a left lower limb deep vein thrombosis treated with warfarin for 6 months, 3 years ago. His medications included metformin, amlodipine, simvastatin and lansoprazole.

A digital rectal examination (DRE) revealed an enlarged prostate with a smooth right-sided nodule. Apart from mild ankle oedema, his clinical examination was normal. Initial blood tests revealed raised prostate-specific antigen (PSA) 9.5 ng/ml and raised HbA_{1c} 82 mmol/mol. He was urgently referred to the local specialist centre where a staging MRI scan showed bilateral T2 organ-confined prostate cancer, slightly larger on the right with no evidence of metastatic disease. A transrectal ultrasound scan and prostatic biopsy revealed bilateral Gleason score 7 (3+4) prostate adenocarcinoma. In accordance with International Society of Geriatric Oncology guidelines, he was assessed to be 'vulnerable with reversible impairment' needing further medical intervention for his hypertension, diabetes and incontinence. The urology multidisciplinary team recommended that the patient should be counselled and potentially offered the following management options:

- Watch and wait approach.

- Radical prostate radiotherapy with 4–6 months of concurrent androgen deprivation therapy (ADT).

- Appointment with the incontinence clinic for management of his lower urinary tract symptoms.

At the specialist urology clinic, following urodynamic studies, his incontinence was ascribed to the following:

- Detrusor overactivity.

- Bladder outflow obstruction due to coexisting benign prostate enlargement.

- Peripheral oedema secondary to the dihydropyridine calcium channel blocker amlodipine, resulting in nocturnal diuresis.

- Polyuria due to poor diabetic control.

Amlodipine was stopped and he was referred back to his GP to be commenced on alternative antihypertensive medication under close supervision in view of tamsulosin's effect on BP. His incontinence improved on solifenacin, tamsulosin and support from the community diabetes team.

He was seen in the oncology clinic, where he reported significant enhancement in the quality of his life due to improvement in his incontinence. After considering the treatment options, he elected to embark on watchful waiting, as the radical treatment option could not further enhance the quality of his life and could potentially reduce it mainly due to recurrence of incontinence and androgen deprivation syndrome.

What factors should be considered in screening and evaluating an older patient with prostate cancer?

What is the role of hormonal treatment in the management of prostate cancer?

How should urinary incontinence initially be assessed in this older man?

What is the presentation and management approach of venous thromboembolism (VTE) in a cancer patient?

What factors should be considered in screening and evaluating an older patient with prostate cancer?

Prostate cancer is the most common malignancy and the second most common cause of cancer death amongst men in the UK. Below the age of 50 years, prostate cancer is relatively rare, accounting for only 1% of disease diagnoses. The age-specific incidence rate sharply rises from around the age of 50–54, peaking at nearly five times the rate by the age of 75–79 years.[1] By the age of 90, its prevalence dramatically increases to reach 50–60% of men. The widespread use of screening tools such as PSA has significantly contributed to increased levels of detection of early prostate cancer. Unlike other tumour types, the principles of early detection and improved cure rates must be cautiously applied to prostate cancer.

Early prostate cancer is usually slow growing and often produces no symptoms. The morbidity and mortality associated with invasive diagnostic procedures and treatment can exceed that of the cancer itself. Given the prolonged natural history of prostate cancer, most men will die with prostate cancer rather than because of it. Based on the Radical Prostatectomy Versus Observation for Localized Prostate Cancer (PIVOT) and the European Randomized Study of Screening for Prostate Cancer (ERSPC) trials, men with limited life expectancy and poor performance status (PS) are unlikely to benefit from screening with PSA.[2,3] Unless clinically indicated in influencing the management of the presenting symptom, opportunistic testing of PSA is not without significant difficulties. In older men it increases the possibility of overdiagnosis and can lead to overtreatment. As a consequence, patients may suffer troublesome side effects as well as potential psychological and financial burdens.

It is important to note that in some men, prostate cancer is unequivocally lethal. In a prospective cohort study of 3183 men with non-metastatic prostate cancer, Daskivich et al.[4] found that in men 75 years or older with three or more comorbidities, 71% died due to other causes rather than due to prostate cancer within 10 years of diagnosis. Death due to prostate cancer was minimal in patients with low-risk (3%) and intermediate-risk (7%) disease but appreciably higher in those with high-risk disease (18%).

The course of a newly diagnosed prostate cancer is hard to predict. Risk stratification therefore becomes all the more important. Localized prostate cancer can be stratified into a category of very low risk, low risk, intermediate risk, high risk and very high risk, based on the extent of disease (tumour, node, metastasis staging), histological grading (Gleason primary and secondary grades) and PSA measurements. Risk stratification combined with estimates of life expectancy, comorbidities, symptoms and patient preferences help derive individualized treatment options.

Broadly, early prostate cancer is managed with three standard treatment options: active surveillance, radiation therapy (brachytherapy or external beam radiation therapy [EBRT]) and radical prostatectomy. The advantages and disadvantages of these modalities are summarized in Table 28.1.

Active surveillance, which consists of closely monitoring the patient and delaying curative treatment until signs of progression to a more aggressive and potentially lethal cancer are detected, is recommended for low-risk, clinically insignificant cancer. It is important to appreciate how this differs from 'watchful waiting', where the aim of treatment, when offered, is to control the cancer in order to provide symptom palliation rather than to cure it.

Options for men with clinically localized intermediate- or high-risk prostate cancer include radical radiation therapy or radical prostatectomy with pelvic lymph node dissection. To benefit from radical treatment an assessment of the patient's expected life expectancy due to other factors, and the life expectancy from prostate cancer if left untreated, needs to be made. A large

Table 28.1 Advantages and disadvantages of treatment options available in early prostate cancer.

Treatment option	Advantage	Disadvantage
Active surveillance	Reduces overtreatment Avoids or postpones treatment-associated complications	Tumour may progress beyond the possibility of cure Late treatment may result in more side effects Living with an untreated cancer could cause severe anxiety
EBRT	Effective long-term control of disease Very low risk of urinary incontinence Option available even to those with comorbidities	Significant risk of impotence Temporary bowel and bladder symptoms during treatment and late rectal symptoms Information regarding microscopic metastasis to lymph nodes unavailable
Brachytherapy	Effective long-term control of disease Single treatment; thus quicker than EBRT Option available to those with multiple comorbidities	Significant risk of impotence Temporary bowel and bladder symptoms Information regarding microscopic metastasis to lymph nodes unavailable
Radical prostatectomy	Effective long-term control of disease Information regarding microscopic metastasis to lymph nodes available; thus predictions of prognosis can be more precise PSA failure easy to detect	Significant risk of impotence Risk of operative morbidity Risk of long-term incontinence

population-based cohort study of patients with prostate cancer aged 65+ and managed conservatively demonstrated that 10 year mortality from other causes was 59.8%, 57.2% and 56.5% in those with well-, moderately and poorly differentiated tumours, respectively. The 10 year prostate cancer-specific mortality was 8.3%, 9.1% and 25.6%, respectively. For high-risk disease, unless there are many or severe comorbidities, the risk from prostate cancer is significant. For intermediate risk, there is somewhat of a debate about the best treatment option; however, surveillance is a reasonable choice.[5]

What is the role of hormonal treatment in the management of prostate cancer?

ADT is the principal treatment option in the management of advanced or metastatic prostate cancer. Therapeutic depletion of androgens can be pharmacologically achieved by inhibiting their production in the primary sites, mainly the gonads and the adrenals. Testosterone depletion can be achieved medically by disrupting the hypothalamic–pituitary–gonadal axis (e.g. with luteinizing hormone-releasing hormone agonists or antagonists) or by surgical castration. Alternatively, androgen receptors can be directly blocked to further escalate androgen deprivation for additional therapeutic gain. In early prostate cancer, radiotherapy and concurrent ADT have been shown to improve outcomes in all parameters, including absolute and overall survival, especially in patients with high-grade tumours and Gleason scores of 8–10, compared with radiotherapy alone.[6,7]

Although, all of the above-mentioned methods of androgen deprivation have been proven to show clinical benefit in randomized trials in patients with prostate cancer, significant adverse symptoms are associated with the hypogonadal state. These include hot flushes, reduced libido, impotence, erectile dysfunction, anaemia, asthenia, weight gain, loss of muscle mass, bone loss, memory loss, reduced mental acuity, personality changes, low mood, insomnia and mood swings. These symptoms, which are grouped under the term 'androgen deprivation syndrome', can be ameliorated by exercise and other interventional measures.

Several studies have shown that ADT is associated with increased risk of diabetes, cardiovascular disease and myocardial infarction.[8] In patients with pre-existing cardiovascular disease, ADT has been linked with an increase in cardiovascular death.[9,10]

How should urinary incontinence initially be assessed in this older man?

Urinary incontinence, which can be defined as involuntary leakage of urine, increases with age and its prevalence ranges from 11% to 34% in men older than 65 years. Although urinary incontinence is twice as common in women as in men, men are half as likely as women to seek help for urinary incontinence. Urinary incontinence can lead to embarrassment, fear of stigmatization, perineal rashes, pressure ulcers, urosepsis, falls, fractures, depression, institutionalization and sexual dysfunction. Thus, treating incontinence can bring about significant improvement in the quality of life of the affected individual.

Incontinence could be due to factors which are outside the lower urinary tract (Table 28.2) or within the lower urinary tract. Factors affecting the lower urinary tract have been classically described as urge incontinence, stress incontinence and overflow incontinence. To help establish the factors that contribute to urinary incontinence and determine the diagnosis, a 3 day bladder diary and a thorough medical and drug history should be obtained. The initial assessment should also include examinations of the abdomen and external genitalia, a DRE, and a urine dipstick test to detect blood, glucose, protein, leucocytes and nitrites.

It is recommended that patients with complicated incontinence must be referred for specialist urological care. It is important to note that incontinence is treatable and often curable at all ages.

What is the presentation and management approach of VTE in a cancer patient?

The incidence of thrombosis is several folds higher in cancer patients than in patients without cancer. Certain cancers primarily originating from pancreas, stomach, brain, ovary, kidney, lung and haematological malignancies are strongly associated with VTE. Furthermore, the risk of acquiring VTE is two- to 20-fold greater in patients with metastatic disease. With the increasing sensitivity of scanners, greater numbers of 'incidental' pulmonary embolism are being diagnosed on routine staging scans. In addition, hospitalization further increases the risk of VTE. Intriguingly, about 10% of individuals diagnosed with sporadic VTE are diagnosed with cancer in the following months or years. Table 28.3 lists the predisposing prothrombotic factors associated with cancer.

Thrombosis was found to be the second leading cause of death in cancer patients receiving chemotherapy. Even after adjusting for disease stage, the risk of mortality is twofold or greater in cancer patients with VTE than in cancer patients without VTE. In a review of 8 million patients who were hospitalized for VTE, those with cancer had a threefold greater cumulative probability of death at 6 months compared with those who had VTE without cancer.[11]

Table 28.2 Urinary incontinence outside the lower urinary tract.

Cause	Mechanism	Agent
Delirium	Multifactorial causes	
Constipation	Stool impaction	
Drugs	Resulting in: Delirium Sedation Decreased mobility Urinary retention	Opiates Benzodiazepines Antihistamines Antipsychotics Anticholinergics Antidepressants Antiparkinson drugs
	Nocturnal diuresis due to fluid retention	Dihydropyridine calcium channel blockers NSAIDs Thiazolidinediones Dopamine receptor agonists
	Effect on sphincter	Alpha-adrenergic antagonists (relax sphincter) Alpha-adrenergic agonists (tighten sphincter)
	Excess urine output	Diuretics Hyperglycaemia Hypercalcaemia Theophylline Caffeine Alcohol
Neurological	Brain/spinal cord lesions	Brain injury Stroke Multiple sclerosis Neurodegenerative diseases such as dementia and Parkinson's disease
Functional	Affecting mobility	Arthritis affecting dexterity Dementia

NSAIDs, non-steroidal anti-inflammatory drugs.

Anticoagulant therapy is the principal treatment option for VTE. The goals, indications and contraindications of anticoagulation are the same in patients with or without cancer. The aim of the treatment is to prevent extension, embolization and recurrence of thrombus while minimizing the risk of bleeding. The annual risk of recurrence of VTE in a cancer patient is about 21% and the risk of major bleeds associated with long-term anticoagulation annually is about 12.4%. In patients without cancer, however, it was 6.8% and 4.9%, respectively.[12] Thus, patients with cancer are at a higher risk of recurrence of VTE, despite therapeutic anticoagulation, and experience serious bleeds even without excessive antithrombotic treatment.

Table 28.3 Predisposing prothrombotic factors associated with cancer and its treatment.

Patient–associated risk factors
  Race
    • Higher risk in African Americans, lower in Asians/Pacific Islanders
  Age
    • Risk increases with age
  Comorbidities
    • Previous history of VTE, ATE, poor PS, obesity, infection, pulmonary disease, renal disease, varicose veins, and inherited prothrombotic mutations such as Factor V Leiden and prothrombin gene mutation

Malignancy–associated risk factors
  Site of primary malignancy
    • Pancreas, stomach, brain, ovary, kidney and lung, and haematological malignancies such as multiple myeloma and lymphomas
  Histology
    • High-grade tumours and adenocarcinoma
  Stage
    • Metastatic disease

Treatment–associated risk factors
  Chemotherapy
  Hormonal therapy
    • Tamoxifen, aromatase inhibitors
  Antiangiogenic therapy associated with arterial events
    • Bevacizumab, sunitinib, sorafenib
  Immunomodulatory agents
    • Thalidomide, lenalidomide
  Major surgery
  Hospitalization
  Erythropoiesis-stimulating agent
  Central venous catheters
  Transfusions

Biomarkers indicating higher risk
  Pre-chemotherapy white cell count >11×10^9/l
  Pre-chemotherapy platelet count >350×10^9/l
  Hb <100 g/l
  Raised D-dimer
  C-reactive protein

ATE, arterial thromboembolism.

A number of meta-analyses of randomized controlled trials of low-molecular-weight heparin (LMWH) versus warfarin, a vitamin K antagonist, have assessed outcomes such as recurrence, complications and mortality. Based on its favourable efficacy, safety and convenience, treatment with LMWH is the preferred initial and long-term treatment option for VTE in patients with cancer. It is not uncommon to encounter circumstances where administration of LMWH treatment may not be a practical or clinically safe option. In patients who are averse to injections, treatment with oral anticoagulants such as vitamin K antagonists is preferred over no therapy. In patients with a contraindication to anticoagulants (for instance, in patients with serious or active bleeding), placement of vena cava filters is an alternative treatment option. The safety and efficacy of new oral anticoagulants that inhibit activated Factor X (e.g. rivaroxaban, apixaban, edoxaban) or thrombin (e.g. dabigatran) is not yet established in cancer patients and therefore their use is not recommended in patients with VTE and concurrent malignancy. Unpredictable gastrointestinal absorption, drug interaction with chemotherapy and altered metabolism due to renal/hepatic dysfunction in cancer patients may render oral anticoagulants inferior to LMWH.

Conclusion and learning points

- Early, low-risk prostate cancer is usually slow growing and often produces no symptoms.

- Men with limited life expectancy and poor PS are unlikely to benefit from screening with PSA. It should be avoided unless clinically indicated in influencing the management of the presenting symptom.

- Incontinence is treatable and often curable at all ages and can bring about significant improvement in the quality of life of the affected individual.

- The goals, indications and contraindications of anticoagulation are the same in patients with or without cancer.

- Because of unpredictable gastrointestinal absorption, drug interaction with chemotherapy and altered metabolism due to renal/hepatic dysfunction, treatment with oral anticoagulants may be inferior to LMWH treatment.

- Based on its favourable efficacy, safety and convenience, treatment with LMWH is the preferred initial and long-term treatment option for VTE in patients with cancer.

References

1 Cancer Research UK (2014). *Prostate cancer incidence statistics.* Available from: www.cancerresearchuk.org/health-professional/cancer-statistics/statistics-by-cancer-type/prostate-cancer/incidence (accessed 14 July 2015).

2 Wilt TJ. The Prostate Cancer Intervention Versus Observation Trial: VA/NCI/AHRQ Cooperative Studies Program #407 (PIVOT): design and baseline results of a randomized controlled trial comparing radical prostatectomy with watchful waiting for men with clinically localized prostate cancer. *J Natl Cancer Inst Monogr* 2012; 2012: 184–90.

3 Vasarainen H, Malmi H, Maattanen L, *et al.* Effects of prostate cancer screening on health-related quality of life: results of the Finnish arm of the European randomized screening trial (ERSPC). *Acta Oncol* 2013; 52: 1615–21.

4 Daskivich TJ, Fan K-H, Koyama T, *et al.* Effect of age, tumor risk, and comorbidity on competing risks for survival in a U.S. population-based cohort of men with prostate cancer. *Ann Intern Med* 2013; 158: 709–17.

5 Lu-Yao GL, Albertsen PC, Moore DF, *et al.* Outcomes of localized prostate cancer following conservative management. *JAMA* 2009; 302: 1202–9.

6 Bolla M, Van Tienhoven G, Warde P, *et al.* External irradiation with or without long-term androgen suppression for prostate cancer with high metastatic risk: 10-year results of an EORTC randomised study. *Lancet Oncol* 2010; 11: 1066–73.

7 Hanks GE, Pajak TF, Porter A, *et al.* Phase III trial of long-term adjuvant androgen deprivation after neoadjuvant hormonal cytoreduction and radiotherapy in locally advanced carcinoma of the prostate: the Radiation Therapy Oncology Group Protocol 92-02. *J Clin Oncol* 2003; 21: 3972–8.

8 Keating NL, O'Malley AJ, Freedland SJ, Smith MR. Diabetes and cardiovascular disease during androgen deprivation therapy: observational study of veterans with prostate cancer. *J Natl Cancer Inst* 2010; 102: 39–46.

9 Lu-Yao G, Stukel TA, Yao SL. Changing patterns in competing causes of death in men with prostate cancer: a population based study. *J Urol* 2004; 171 (6 part 1): 2285–90.

10 Nguyen PL, Chen MH, Beckman JA, *et al.* Influence of androgen deprivation therapy on all-cause mortality in men with high-risk prostate cancer and a history of congestive heart failure or myocardial infarction. *Int J Radiat Oncol Biol Phys* 2012; 82: 1411–16.

11 Levitan N, Dowlati A, Remick SC, *et al.* Rates of initial and recurrent thromboembolic disease among patients with malignancy versus those without malignancy. Risk analysis using Medicare claims data. *Medicine* 1999; 78: 285–91.

12 Prandoni P, Lensing AW, Piccioli A, *et al.* Recurrent venous thromboembolism and bleeding complications during anticoagulant treatment in patients with cancer and venous thrombosis. *Blood* 2002; 100: 3484–8.

Further reading

• Droz JP, Aapro M, Balducci L, *et al.* Management of prostate cancer in older patients: updated recommendations of a working group of the International Society of Geriatric Oncology. *Lancet Oncol* 2014; 15: e404–14.

• Fung C, Dale W, Mohile SG. Prostate cancer in the elderly patient. *J Clin Oncol* 2014; 32: 2523–30.

• National Institute for Health and Care Excellence (2010). *Lower urinary tract symptoms in men: assessment and management. NICE clinical guideline 97.* Available from: www.nice.org.uk/guidance/cg97 (accessed 14 July 2015).

• Laporte S, Bertoletti L, Romera A, *et al.* Long-term treatment of venous thromboembolism with tinzaparin compared to vitamin K antagonists: a meta-analysis of 5 randomized trials in non-cancer and cancer patients. *Thromb Res* 2012; 130: 853–8.

• Mottet N. *Guidelines on prostate cancer.* Arnhem: European Association of Urology, 2015.

29 A Blind Patient with a Large Gastrointestinal Stromal Tumour for Radical Surgery

Sebastian Trainor, Zuzanna Sawicka, Maria Marples

Case history

An 80-year-old woman presented to the accident and emergency department with a sudden collapse followed by large-volume melaena. Her past medical history included age-related macular degeneration, for which she was registered blind, drug-controlled type 2 diabetes, hypothyroidism, osteoporosis and hypertension, and she had a permanent pacemaker. Investigations revealed an Hb level of 40 g/l. She was supported with urgent red blood cell replacement. Her antihypertensive medication and bisphosphonate were stopped. An urgent upper gastrointestinal endoscopy revealed a large distal gastric tumour actively oozing blood from multiple locations. A CT scan showed a large 15 cm mass involving the distal stomach with five subcentimetre indeterminate liver lesions. The radiological appearances were of a gastrointestinal stromal tumour (GIST), which was confirmed by biopsy.

Her case was discussed by the specialist sarcoma multidisciplinary team. As the tumour was deemed operable, radical surgery was recommended pending anaesthetic review. The patient agreed to surgery and proceeded to an open laparotomy and partial distal gastrectomy. The surgery was complicated by an intraoperative acute myocardial infarction.

During a postoperative stay in the ITU she was reviewed by a cardiologist. An echocardiogram revealed moderate left ventricular systolic failure. She was commenced on an ACE inhibitor, beta-blocker, diuretic and an antiplatelet agent. Outpatient cardiology follow-up was arranged.

Four weeks later, at her initial oncology appointment, she was found to have New York Heart Association (NYHA) class III heart failure. She had returned home with extra home support following surgery. Her daughter had given up work to become her full-time carer. She had lost 6 kg in weight, despite developing bilateral lower limb oedema. Her diabetic control had become erratic due to poor nutritional intake, resulting in hypoglycaemic episodes. She complained of early satiety and diarrhoea after eating. The oncologist referred her for a Comprehensive Geriatric Assessment. This identified an increased risk of falls secondary to blindness, diuretic-related urinary frequency, weight loss and post-ITU muscle wasting resulting in generalized weakness and frailty. Her diuretics were increased and a downstairs and a bedside commode were provided to help manage her bladder and bowel. Antimotility medications were prescribed to reduce the diarrhoea. Gliclazide was discontinued, and her daughter was taught how to monitor blood glucose. A dietitian carried out a review and provided her with supplements and strategies to manage early satiety with frequent smaller meals. Home-based physiotherapy was arranged to increase strength and balance and she was referred to the community heart failure team.

Her tumour was found to be fully resected with negative microscopic margins and without rupture. The mitotic rate was high. Mutation analysis of the tumour showed a *KIT* exon 11 deletion. Arrangements were made for re-review in a further 4 weeks. At this appointment, her weight loss had stabilized, her heart failure had improved and she had had no further hypoglycaemic episodes. However, she had not recovered her preoperative performance status. Further treatment options were discussed, namely adjuvant imatinib for up to 3 years versus continued close surveillance with a plan to consider palliative imatinib treatment if the liver lesions proved to be metastases or the GIST recurred. Given the potential side effects of the drug (nausea, vomiting, diarrhoea and increased oedema), the patient made an informed choice for close surveillance and no adjuvant treatment.

Two years later, she reported progressive fatigue and weight loss. She was found to have multiple inoperable liver lesions with no change in the indeterminate lesions previously noted. A biopsy confirmed recurrent GIST. She commenced palliative low-dose imatinib 200 mg/day. Within 2 weeks she felt better. She developed worsening lower limb oedema that was managed with further alterations to the diuretics. She remains on imatinib with a partial response on the initial CT scan.

What are the goals of cancer treatment for this patient?

What is the evidence for her treatment options?

What is the implication of mutation analysis in this case?

What impact might this patient's blindness have on her postoperative care and the delivery of chemotherapy?

What are the goals of cancer treatment for this patient?

Initially the goals of treatment for this patient were curative surgery and to stop the bleeding. She was suffering from a life-threatening bleed from a large tumour in her distal stomach that could not be embolized. She was found to have a number of indeterminate subcentimetre liver lesions that were kept under surveillance.

The proposed care after the radical surgery depends on the tumour size, location and mitotic count. If she is considered to be at high risk of relapse after surgery, as defined by the Miettinen and Lasota 2006 criteria,[1] adjuvant imatinib will be considered in order to increase her chance of cure. Unfortunately, she presented 2 years later with advanced incurable disease with multiple liver metastases. At this point, the risk–benefit ratio of the drug changed and she commenced treatment with imatinib. The aim of treatment now changed from a curative approach to a palliative one with the aims to improve her symptoms, thus improving her quality of life, and to prolong her life.

What is the evidence for her treatment options?

Before the introduction of imatinib into clinical practice, disease-free survival following complete resection of GIST was as low as 45% at 5 years.[2] The landmark trials of adjuvant imatinib consistently showed a benefit in relapse-free survival. A trial by the American College of

Surgeons Oncology Group (ACOSOG Z9001)[3] included patients with a completely resected GIST of at least 3 cm in size that was found to be positive for the *KIT* mutation by immunohistochemistry. Patients were randomized to receive imatinib 400 mg/day or placebo for 1 year after surgical resection. At 1 year, the trial was stopped early following the finding that imatinib significantly improved recurrence-free survival (98% vs 83%; HR 0.35, 95% CI 0.22–0.53, one-sided *p*-value <0.0001). The benefit was later shown to be greatest in patients with high-risk disease.[4]

In a trial by the Scandinavian Sarcoma Group (SSG XVIII),[5] patients with high-risk resected *KIT* mutation-positive GIST were randomized to 36 versus 12 months of imatinib. Patients treated with 36 months of imatinib had a greater 5 year recurrence-free survival than those who received 12 months of treatment (65.6% vs 47.9%, respectively; HR 0.46, 95% CI 0.32–0.65, *p*<0.001). This set the standard of 36 months of adjuvant imatinib for high-risk resected *KIT*-positive GIST.

Although these trials were not specifically targeted to the older population, they both included large numbers of patients aged >65 years. The oldest patient in the SSG XVIII trial was aged 84. In both trials, patients with congestive heart failure of NYHA grades III and IV were excluded. There are case reports of patients developing decompensated heart failure following treatment with imatinib,[6] presumably from fluid overload or potentially as a direct cardiotoxic effect of the tyrosine kinase inhibitor (TKI) itself.

Based on the Miettinen and Lasota 2006 criteria,[1] it was clear that this patient's tumour was at high risk of recurrence and therefore warranted a discussion regarding the potential benefits of adjuvant imatinib.[7] She was given all the information and decided not to proceed with adjuvant imatinib, particularly considering her postoperative functional abilities.

In the advanced palliative care setting, clinical trials demonstrate that imatinib can benefit the majority of patients including older patients. In the earliest trials, the disease control rate was as high as 83%;[8] therefore, it was appropriate to re-offer this treatment to her in the context of metastatic recurrence 2 years later.

What is the implication of mutation analysis in this case?

The sensitivity of GISTs to imatinib and other TKIs depends on the driving mutations in the tumours. Mutations are found in the *KIT* gene in most patients' GISTs; the majority of the rest have mutations in *PDGFRA*, the platelet-derived growth factor receptor gene. A mutation in exon 11 of *KIT* predicts a high chance of response to imatinib, so it was appropriate to initiate treatment and to make an effort to persist with therapy. A mutation in exon 9 of *KIT* would have predicted a shorter duration of response to imatinib with evidence of better efficacy at higher doses, so there might have been an indication to try to increase her dosage to the standard 400 mg/day.[9] There are tumours with certain *KIT* and *PDGFRA* mutations that are not responsive to imatinib, including the D842V substitution mutation in exon 18 of *PDGFRA*.[10] In a study of 31 patients with this form of mutation, none had a beneficial response to imatinib.[11] Had this mutation been present in this patient, she might have had an early scan and early assessment for second-line therapy.

What impact might this patient's blindness have on her postoperative care and the delivery of chemotherapy?

Postoperative care

Adaptations to care delivery were made to accommodate the patient's blindness. Communication methods were adjusted so that she understood what was happening in the absence of visual clues. Her blindness contributed to an increased risk of delirium, which is common postoperatively (up to 80%), especially in the ITU.[12] Thus, particular care was taken to keep her orientated to time, place and person. Visiting hours were kept flexible to ensure regular contact with familiar voices of family and friends. Her call-bell was left in a consistent place where she knew how to reach it. Once mobile without assistance, her bay was kept clear of clutter so she could mobilize to the toilet through familiarity with the bay layout.

Postoperative nutrition

Her blindness may affect her access to food both in hospital and at home. In hospital, snacks and drinks were kept within reach at all times. She was assisted at mealtimes with prompting and verbally made aware when food was being presented to her. Out of hospital, blindness may affect her ability to leave the house to buy food and to cook or prepare food. Her daughter now supported this.

Management of diarrhoea and diuretic-related urinary frequency

Although prior to admission her blindness did not impede independent toileting, she now had postoperative weakness, weight loss and frailty. The provision of commodes, antimotility drugs and the assistance of her daughter with her care may mitigate her difficulties.

Diabetes control

She is unable to read the display of a regular blood glucose monitor. Routine monitoring can be effectively managed by others (e.g. district/practice nurse, or family members as in this case), or talking glucose meters are available for those who are otherwise able.

Delivery of chemotherapy

Blindness should be accommodated in the practicalities of delivering chemotherapy. For blind patients who are unable to travel independently and who do not have a family member/friend to support them, booking hospital transport should be offered (she may not be able to use a telephone without her sight). Extra time may be required to explain what interventions are being performed, as visual clues will be absent. As imatinib is given orally every day, it is important that it should be recognized and given safely: the packet has Braille labelling, and the drug can be presented in a dosette box. Appointment dates and times should not only be communicated via printed letters dependent on sight; alternative methods may be via telephone calls. Ensuring consistency of her appointments (e.g. always on a Monday at 11 am) may also be beneficial.

Conclusion and learning points

- Imatinib can increase recurrence-free survival in the adjuvant setting in GISTs with certain mutations in older patients.
- Imatinib can have high clinical benefit in the palliative setting for older patients and should be considered.
- Blindness can increase the complexity of delivering cancer treatment. Cancer teams should provide reasonable and individualized adjustments to deliver care effectively.

References

1 Miettinen M, Lasota J. Gastrointestinal stromal tumors: review on morphology, molecular pathology, prognosis, and differential diagnosis. *Arch Pathol Lab Med* 2006; 130: 1466–78.

2 DeMatteo RP, Lewis JJ, Leung D, *et al.* Two hundred gastrointestinal stromal tumors: recurrence patterns and prognostic factors for survival. *Ann Surg* 2000; 231: 51–8.

3 Dematteo RP, Ballman KV, Antonescu CR, *et al.* Adjuvant imatinib mesylate after resection of localised, primary gastrointestinal stromal tumour: a randomised, double-blind, placebo-controlled trial. *Lancet* 2009; 373: 1097–104.

4 Blackstein M. Risk assessment for tumor recurrence after surgical resection of localized primary gastrointestinal stromal tumor (GIST): North America intergroup phase III trial ACOSOG Z9001 (abstract). Presented at: 2010 ASCO Gastrointestinal Cancers Symposium, Orlando, FL, 23 January 2010.

5 Joensuu H, Eriksson M, Sundby Hall K, *et al.* One vs three years of adjuvant imatinib for operable gastrointestinal stromal tumor: a randomized trial. *JAMA* 2012; 307: 1265–72.

6 Ran HH, Zhang R, Lu XC, *et al.* Imatinib-induced decompensated heart failure in an elderly patient with chronic myeloid leukemia: case report and literature review. *J Geriatr Cardiol* 2012; 9: 411–14.

7 Joensuu H. Risk stratification of patients diagnosed with gastrointestinal stromal tumor. *Hum Pathol* 2008; 39: 1411–19.

8 Demetri GD, von Mehren M, Blanke CD, *et al.* Efficacy and safety of imatinib mesylate in advanced gastrointestinal stromal tumors. *N Engl J Med* 2002; 347: 472–80.

9 Gastrointestinal Stromal Tumor Meta-Analysis Group. Comparison of two doses of imatinib for the treatment of unresectable or metastatic gastrointestinal stromal tumors: a meta-analysis of 1,640 patients. *J Clin Oncol* 2010; 28: 1247–53.

10 Corless CL, Schroeder A, Griffith D, *et al. PDGFRA* mutations in gastrointestinal stromal tumors: frequency, spectrum and in vitro sensitivity to imatinib. *J Clin Oncol* 2005; 23: 5357–64.

11 Cassier PA, Fumagalli E, Rutkowski P, *et al.* Outcome of patients with platelet-derived growth factor receptor alpha-mutated gastrointestinal stromal tumors in the tyrosine kinase inhibitor era. *Clin Cancer Res* 2012; 18: 4458–64.

12 Girard TD, Pandharipande PP, Ely EW. Delirium in the intensive care unit. *Crit Care* 2008; 12 (suppl 3): S3.

Further reading

• National Institute for Health and Care Excellence (2014). *Imatinib for the adjuvant treatment of gastrointestinal stromal tumours (review of NICE technology appraisal guidance 196). NICE technology appraisal guidance 326.* Available from: www.nice.org.uk/guidance/ta326 (accessed 10 June 2015).

• National Institute for Health and Care Excellence (2004). *Imatinib for the treatment of unresectable and/or metastatic gastro-intestinal stromal tumours. NICE technology appraisal guidance 86.* Available from: www.nice.org.uk/guidance/ta86 (accessed 10 June 2015).

• National Institute for Health and Care Excellence (2010). *Imatinib for the treatment of unresectable and/or metastatic gastrointestinal stromal tumours. NICE technology appraisal guidance 209.* Available from: www.nice.org.uk/guidance/ta209 (accessed 10 June 2015).

• European Society for Medical Oncology (2014). *Gastrointestinal stromal tumours: ESMO clinical practice guidelines.* Available from: www.esmo.org/Guidelines/Sarcoma-and-GIST/Gastrointestinal-Stromal-Tumours (accessed 8 June 2015).

30 Use of Radical Radiotherapy in a Patient with a Brain Tumour and Deafness

Vinton Cheng, Nicola Turner, Susan Short

Case history

A 78-year-old woman presented following a sudden collapse with one witnessed seizure, on a background of increasing headaches over 1 week. Her past medical history consisted of type 2 diabetes and osteoarthritis. Her Mini-Mental State Examination score on admission was 26 out of 30. Initial investigations revealed an invasive ring-enhancing lesion in the left temporal lobe, consistent with a glioblastoma, with surrounding oedema and mild effacement of the left lateral ventricle. Following discussion with the oncologist, she was started on high-dose steroids and referred to the neuro-oncology multidisciplinary team (MDT), who recommended primary debulking surgery followed by radiotherapy. She was commenced on levetiracetam to prevent further seizures.

Two weeks following partial resection of the left temporal lobe, she attended clinic to discuss radiotherapy. During the consultation the oncologist noticed that she struggled to take in much of the information and therefore used a Comprehensive Geriatric Assessment screening tool, which revealed a significant hearing impairment. Concerned about the communication challenges, the oncologist arranged to see her again in 2 weeks with an urgent referral to the ENT clinic in the interim. Here, a thorough assessment identified several issues relating to her hearing:

- Conductive hearing loss secondary to excess earwax. After a week's treatment with olive oil ear drops, she visited the practice nurse to have her ears syringed, with immediate improvement in hearing.

- Age-related sensorineural deficit (presbycusis) in both ears, requiring a referral to the audiology department for bilateral fitted hearing aids.

- She had become increasingly withdrawn from her social network of family and friends due to difficulty in keeping up with conversation. She was also afraid of leaving her home and going to the shops on her own, as she could not hear the traffic very well.

On return to the oncology clinic, she was much brighter in mood and remained keen to engage in further treatment options. She had completed a course of tapering steroids. However, since then her blood sugar control had remained poor and so she was commenced on insulin by the community diabetes team. The oncologist explained the side effects of radiotherapy and recommended a course of 40 Gy in 15 fractions to the affected brain. She completed the treatment, the only toxicities being grade 2 fatigue, grade 1 scalp rash, and alopecia.

What was the goal of cancer treatment for this patient?

What impact can hearing loss have on the older cancer patient?

What toxicities are associated with her treatment?

What is the evidence base for her treatment?

How did comorbidities affect her cancer care?

How can hearing loss be identified and managed in cancer services?

What was the goal of cancer treatment for this patient?

Glioblastoma, or grade 4 astrocytoma, is the most common form of malignant primary brain tumour and has an annual incidence in the UK of around three new cases per 100,000 people. The peak age of incidence is 65–74 years; however, the number of people affected by glioblastoma is expected to rise, due to the ageing population.[1] Despite advances in its management, the prognosis for these patients remains poor: average life expectancy is 14.6 months even with maximal therapy.[2] Treatment goals therefore need to be balanced to maximize survival and quality of life by controlling symptoms and preserving functional capacity.

For this patient it is vital that the clinician elicits what are her motivating factors for seeking treatment. By understanding these driving forces the clinician can provide the appropriate information to her to support a shared decision-making process that meets the patient's goals.

What impact can hearing loss have on the older cancer patient?

Sensory impairment can impact heavily on a patient's everyday living. The MRC-funded UK National Study of Hearing carried out in the 1980s found that approximately three out of five people aged between 71 and 80 years had significantly impaired hearing.[3] Of those affected, the vast majority were not effectively managed by provision of a hearing aid.[4] Hearing loss has also been found to be associated with a host of other comorbidities, including cognitive decline, balance problems and falls.[5,6] As illustrated previously, hearing loss can result in social isolation and adversely affect psychological well-being. It is therefore important to manage the functional limitation through appropriate referral to specialist services, alongside the focus on anticancer treatment.

Impaired hearing acts as a barrier to effective communication and therefore can impede the building of a successful doctor–patient relationship. In this scenario, this concept is vital, as without it the consequences may include poor treatment adherence, inadequate management of toxicities and an overall negative experience of healthcare services. Hearing impairment can potentially be misinterpreted by clinicians or caregivers as cognitive impairment. It is also known that sensory impairment interferes with performance in cognitive assessment tools.[7] This is an important consideration for the healthcare provider, particularly when assessing mental capacity to consent to major treatment decisions, such as neurosurgery and radiotherapy.

What toxicities are associated with her treatment?

The toxicities that can result from cranial irradiation are outlined in Table 30.1. Of these, lethargy and alopecia are by far the most common acute or early delayed effects. Significant late neurotoxicities are uncommon and are related to the dose effect on specific organs at risk. Cranial irradiation is known to cause hearing loss if the radiation field includes the middle and inner ear. These effects can be divided into the following categories:

1. Early onset: usually linked to serous otitis media and radiation-induced Eustachian tube dysfunction, which result in conductive hearing loss. These are usually self-limiting and resolve with conservative management, including ear drops and adequate ear protection.
2. Late onset: sensorineural hearing loss is much less common and is dose-related.[8] If it occurs, hearing loss typically develops 6 months to 1 year following irradiation and is generally progressive, particularly at higher frequencies of hearing. Morbidity is greater in the older adult and in those with pre-existing hearing impairment.[9]

What is the evidence base for her treatment?

The landmark European Organisation for Research and Treatment of Cancer–National Cancer Institute of Canada study[2] demonstrated the effectiveness of concomitant and adjuvant temozolomide with radiotherapy in improving median survival by an additional 2.5 months compared with radiotherapy alone. This benefit was subsequently found to persist over a 5 year period of follow-up.[10] Patients over 70 years of age, however, were excluded from recruitment and the median age of participants was 56 years. As a result, how this benefit translates to the older adult is uncertain; therefore, application of the 'Stupp regimen' has been low in this population subset. In answer to this shortcoming, a global cooperative group phase III trial is currently underway to determine whether the addition of temozolomide to radiotherapy improves survival in the older adult; the results are expected in the near future.[11]

In contrast to chemotherapeutic agents, radiotherapy has been firmly established as being a safe, tolerable treatment that confers a survival advantage in adults aged 70 years and above. Keime-Guibert et al.[12] showed that focal fractionated radiotherapy improved median survival by approximately 12 weeks compared with best supportive care alone (median 29.1 vs. 16.9 weeks; HR 0.47, 95% CI 0.29–0.76, $p=0.002$). The trial also showed that radiotherapy did not significantly reduce quality of life or cognitive function whilst also highlighting the lack of severe adverse events. Two other prospective studies have shown that hypofractionated radiotherapy produces similar, if not superior, outcomes compared with standard radiotherapy (60 Gy in 30 fractions). In the Nordic trial,[13] hypofractionated (34 Gy in 10 fractions) versus standard radiotherapy was found

Table 30.1 Toxicity associated with cranial irradiation, categorized according to time of onset.

Acute (onset during treatment or weeks after)

• Headache	• Dizziness
• Lethargy	• Radiation dermatitis
• Nausea	• Alopecia
• Tinnitus/hearing loss	

Early delayed (onset weeks to months after completion of treatment)

• Somnolence syndrome	• Lethargy

Late delayed (onset months to years after completion of treatment)

• Optic neuropathy/cataracts	• Intracerebral haemorrhage/infarct
• Radiation necrosis	• Encephalopathy
• Cerebral atrophy	• Seizures
• Cognitive deficit	• Hypopituitarism
• Secondary brain tumour	• Sensorineural hearing loss

to be superior in terms of overall survival for those aged 70 years and above (median 7.0 vs. 5.2 months; HR 0.59, 95% CI 0.37–0.93, p=0.02). A Canadian study showed that there was no statistically significant difference in survival for hypofractionated (40 Gy in 15 fractions) compared with standard radiotherapy. There was, however, improved morbidity through reduction in toxicity, abbreviated treatment time and lower requirement for corticosteroids.[14]

More recently, two prospective trials have demonstrated the safety of single-agent temozolomide chemotherapy in the management of glioblastoma in the older adult: the Nordic trial[13] and a trial by the Neuro-Oncology Working Group of the German Cancer Society (NOA-08).[15] These trials also showed that temozolomide chemotherapy is not inferior to radiotherapy in terms of survival and highlighted the methylated O-6-methylguanine-DNA methyltransferase (*MGMT*) promoter status of tumour cells as a predictive biomarker for benefit from temozolomide.

How did comorbidities affect her cancer care?

Oral corticosteroid therapy is the mainstay in the initial management of malignant brain tumours to reduce intracranial pressure caused by vasogenic cerebral oedema. A typical regimen is dexamethasone 2–6 mg once daily. In some cases, however, this may need to be escalated to a maximum of 16 mg in 24 h, especially if a patient is severely symptomatic. It should be co-prescribed with gastric protection, such as a proton pump inhibitor or an H_2 receptor antagonist, due to the risk of peptic ulceration. Care should also be taken when prescribing high-dose steroids to check for interactions with coexisting medications. In particular there is much greater risk of upper gastrointestinal complications associated with concurrent use of non-steroidal anti-inflammatory drugs, which this woman may have been taking for her osteoarthritis.

This scenario highlights the challenge of maintaining diabetic control in a patient on steroid therapy. Although she completed a tapering course prior to commencing radiotherapy, steroids may need to be restarted during her treatment or shortly after to control any radiotherapy-induced side effects. This puts her at higher risk of hyperglycaemic complications. Figure 30.1 is an example of a hospital algorithm for the inpatient management of insulin-treated hyperglycaemia secondary to corticosteroid treatment. Where non-insulin therapy is preferred, gliclazide is the drug of choice for type 2 diabetes recommended by the Joint British Diabetes Societies for Inpatient Care.[16]

In known diabetes, steroid treatment should be discussed with the diabetic team at the start of treatment so that a pre-emptive plan for blood glucose control and monitoring can be made (including during a tapering course). Where insulin is recommended, consideration should be given to the practicalities of whether it is feasible or whether it requires additional support (e.g. can the patient self-inject insulin?). It is helpful to communicate the likely prognosis with other involved clinicians, as it affects therapeutic goals for comorbidities.

In the context of the patient's prognosis, the goal was to avoid hyperglycaemic symptoms rather than long-term diabetic complications. Tight glycaemic control would be inappropriate, as hypoglycaemia poses a higher risk to her. Thus, a pragmatic blood glucose target would be more sensible. Where possible, to limit adverse effects, the minimum dosage required to maintain symptom control should be used for the shortest possible period, taking into account the risk of adrenal suppression with prolonged administration of steroids. For those on steroids for prolonged periods, doses should be increased during an acute illness, due to the risk of adrenal crisis.

Contributing further to polypharmacy is the addition of an anticonvulsant as secondary prophylaxis, given the history of a witnessed seizure. Seizures occur in approximately 30–50% of

Management of hyperglycaemia secondary to corticosteroids

All adult patients prescribed systemic corticosteroids should have a 2 h post-lunch
(approx 2 or 3 pm) blood glucose test (even if not previously known to have diabetes)

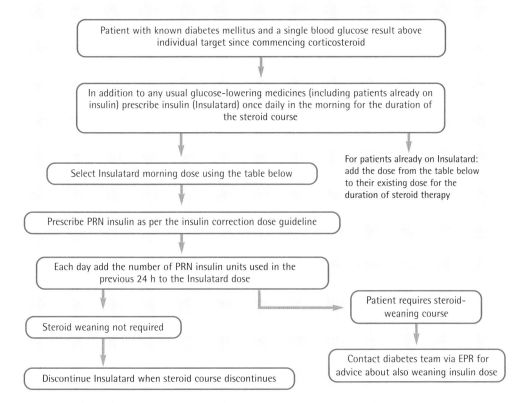

Table of Insulatard starting doses (once daily in the morning)

Prednisolone (or oral methylprednisolone) dose	Patient's actual body weight (kg)						
	44 or less	45–54	55–64	65–74	75–84	85–94	95 or more
40 mg or more	16 units	20 units	24 units	28 units	32 units	36 units	40 units
30 mg	12 units	15 units	18 units	21 units	24 units	27 units	30 units
20 mg	8 units	10 units	12 units	14 units	16 units	18 units	10 units
10 mg	4 units	5 units	6 units	7 units	8 units	9 units	10 units

Refer to inpatient diabetes team via EPR:
- Patients who develop hyperglycaemia secondary to corticosteroids who were NOT previously known to have diabetes
- Patient requires a steroid-weaning course
- Corticosteroid prescribed is not prednisolone or oral methylprednisolone
- Corticosteroid is prescribed more than once daily
- More than 40 units of Insulatard daily is required to achieve target blood glucose

Figure 30.1 Example hospital management algorithm for hyperglycaemia secondary to steroids (adapted from Guy's & St Thomas' NHS Foundation Trust). EPR, electronic patient records; PRN, as required.

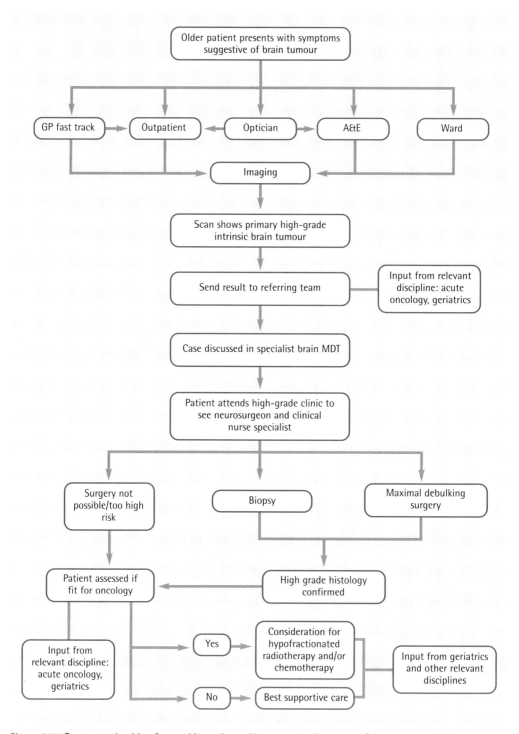

Figure 30.2 Treatment algorithm for an older patient with suspected glioblastoma (adapted from NHS Yorkshire Cancer Network guidelines for the management of brain and CNS tumours).

patients with glioblastoma.[17] Levetiracitam monotherapy has become the antiepileptic drug of choice for tumour-related seizures, given its favourable toxicity profile and minimal drug–drug interactions.

How can hearing loss be identified and managed in cancer services?

Because of the projected rise in the number of older people with impaired hearing it is imperative that cancer services adapt to meet the needs of this particular group. In the first instance, oncologists and other healthcare professionals must become culturally competent in communicating with people affected by hearing loss. There is a wealth of resources readily available in the NHS to aid communication with those who are hard of hearing, such as induction loop systems and Typetalk services. Specifically for this woman, who developed hearing loss later in life, the healthcare provider should also make use of a communication device, written information and non-verbal communication.

Having an understanding of the barriers faced by those with hearing loss and an awareness of the scale of the issue particularly in the older population will allow early identification of patients who require referral for specific intervention. Most UK hospitals and GPs have access to a local ENT or audiology clinic, where patients may receive a tailored assessment and treatment plan for their hearing loss. Some patients may have complex hearing needs: for example, those with tinnitus, balance problems or multiple comorbidities. In these situations, a referral to the geriatrician would be appropriate to ensure the patient engages with an integrated multidisciplinary service with access to physiotherapy, occupational therapy and medical expertise. Patients should be helped to access support through the voluntary sector and social services if it is required.

Finally, the oncologist must be aware of the potential ototoxicity of specific anticancer treatments, such as cisplatin chemotherapy and cranial radiotherapy, as well as co-prescribed medications. Where relevant, patients should be actively screened for deterioration in hearing during routine clinic reviews. Figure 30.2 provides a suggested algorithm for the investigation and treatment of an older adult with a suspected brain tumour. Here, specific opportunities are highlighted where involvement from non-oncological specialties, including geriatricians, may be mutually beneficial for the patient and treating team.

Conclusion and learning points

- Both primary brain tumours and hearing loss are predicted to become increasingly prevalent due to the ageing population.

- Post-resection hypofractionated radiotherapy is currently considered the standard of care for glioblastoma in the older adult; however, emerging evidence suggests single-agent temozolomide or concomitant treatment may become viable options in the future.

- Hearing loss can negatively impact on physical health and mental well-being and should be screened as part of the oncology assessment, including during and after cranial irradiation.

- Ensure patients on prolonged corticosteroid therapy are closely monitored for diabetic complications.

- Patients with complex hearing needs should be referred to specialist geriatric services (or a specialist audiovestibular service where available) for an MDT approach.

References

1   Williams M, Brodbelt A, Greenberg D, *et al*. Incidence and survival from glioblastoma in England, 2007–2011 (poster). Presented at: 10th NCRI Cancer Conference, Liverpool, 2–5 November 2014.

2   Stupp R, Mason WP, van den Bent MJ, *et al*. Radiotherapy plus concomitant and adjuvant temozolomide for glioblastoma. *N Engl J Med* 2005; 352: 987–96.

3   Davis A. *Hearing in adults*. London: Whurr, 1995.

4   Davis A, Smith P, Ferguson M, *et al*. Acceptability, benefit and costs of early screening for hearing disability: a study of potential screening tests and models. *Health Technol Assess* 2007; 11: 1–294.

5   Lin FR, Yaffe K, Xia J, *et al*. Hearing loss and cognitive decline in older adults. *JAMA Intern Med* 2013; 173: 293–9.

6   Lin FR, Ferrucci L. Hearing loss and falls among older adults in the United States. *Arch Intern Med* 2012; 172: 369–71.

7   Dupuis K, Pichora-Fuller MK, Chasteen AL, *et al*. Effects of hearing and vision impairments on the Montreal Cognitive Assessment. *Neuropsychol Dev Cogn B Aging Neuropsychol Cogn* 2015; 22: 413–37.

8   Jereczek-Fossa BA, Zarowski A, Milani F, *et al*. Radiotherapy-induced ear toxicity. *Cancer Treat Rev* 2003; 29: 417–30.

9   Kwong DL, Wei WI, Sham JS, *et al*. Sensorineural hearing loss in patients treated for nasopharyngeal carcinoma: a prospective study of the effect of radiation and cisplatin treatment. *Int J Radiat Oncol Biol Phys* 1996; 36: 281–9.

10 Stupp R, Hegi ME, Mason WP, *et al*. Effects of radiotherapy with concomitant and adjuvant temozolomide versus radiotherapy alone on survival in glioblastoma in a randomised phase III study: 5-year analysis of the EORTC-NCIC trial. *Lancet Oncol* 2009; 10: 459–66.

11 Perry JR, O'Callaghan CJ, Ding K, *et al*. A phase III randomized controlled trial of short-course radiotherapy with or without concomitant and adjuvant temozolomide in elderly patients with glioblastoma (abstract). *Neuro Oncol* 2014; 16: iii42–52.

12 Keime-Guibert F, Chinot O, Taillandier L, *et al*. Radiotherapy for glioblastoma in the elderly. *N Engl J Med* 2007; 356: 1527–35.

13 Malmström A, Grønberg BH, Marosi C, *et al*. Temozolomide versus standard 6-week radiotherapy versus hypofractionated radiotherapy in patients older than 60 years with glioblastoma: the Nordic randomised, phase 3 trial. *Lancet Oncol* 2012; 13: 916–26.

14 Roa W, Brasher PM, Bauman G, *et al*. Abbreviated course of radiation therapy in older patients with glioblastoma multiforme: a prospective randomized clinical trial. *Clin Oncol* 2004; 22: 1583–8.

15 Wick W, Platten M, Meisner C, *et al*. Temozolomide chemotherapy alone versus radiotherapy alone for malignant astrocytoma in the elderly: the NOA-08 randomised, phase 3 trial. *Lancet Oncol* 2012; 13: 707–15.

16 Joint British Diabetes Societies for Inpatient Care (2014). *Management of hyperglycaemia and steroid (glucocorticoid) therapy*. Available from: www.diabetologists-abcd.org.uk/JBDS/JBDS_IP_Steroids.pdf (accessed 3 June 2015).

17 van Breemen MS, Wilms EB, Vecht CJ. Epilepsy in patients with brain tumours: epidemiology, mechanisms, and management. *Lancet Neurol* 2007; 6: 421–30.

31 A Patient with Gastric Cancer and Problems with Vascular Access

Samantha Turnbull, Claire Scampion, Nicola Turner, Alan Anthoney

Case history

A 75-year-old woman presented to her GP with a 6 month history of weight loss and early satiety. She had previously been active at home and was the main carer for her husband who had advanced Parkinson's disease. The only past medical history of note was a non-ST elevation myocardial infarction, complicated by a transient episode of atrial fibrillation, 5 years previously. An echocardiogram at the time had shown a slightly decreased left ventricular ejection fraction (LVEF; 50%) but no valvular heart disease. She had no ongoing symptoms of angina and no signs or symptoms of significant heart failure.

Investigations, including gastro-oesophageal endoscopy and CT scan, showed a locally advanced gastric cancer with nodal disease but no distant metastases (T4N3M0). A biopsy confirmed adenocarcinoma with overexpression (3+ staining on immunohistochemistry) of human epidermal growth factor receptor 2 (HER2). Her estimated glomerular filtration rate (GFR) was slightly decreased at 75 ml/min. During her recent investigations there had been multiple problems with intravenous access (for blood sampling and contrast injection).

The patient's husband had regular geriatrician input, but he had had a number of falls at home, particularly at night, and had mild cognitive impairment. He mobilized unsteadily with a frame and his wife had adapted the home to single-level living. Her husband was completely dependent on her: she assisted him with all activities of daily living and helped him mobilize to the toilet three to four times every night, as his tremor precluded the use of urine bottles. He had a carer once daily for personal cares.

Through clinical history taking, the oncologist identified that her family were unable to assist with the care needs of her husband during a hospital admission or postoperative recovery. With the agreement of the patient and her husband, the oncologist asked their social worker to have an urgent discussion with the patient regarding what additional support could be offered during different treatment options. The oncologist provided the social worker with the likely timeframes for her treatment and the likely impact on her care-giving role. The social worker was able to offer an increase in the care package to bridge her husband's daytime needs but was unable to cover any night-time needs. The patient did not have the finances to cover the night-time needs privately. Respite placement was only available for a short period, and she felt this would be disorientating and would increase his likelihood of falls outside his own environment. Following discussion with her family, the oncology and surgical teams and the social worker, she decided against radical surgery, due to the effect of the recovery time and potential complications on her husband's care, particularly his needs at night.

Our patient underwent a full nutritional assessment prior to starting chemotherapy, including markers of nutritional status such as BMI and albumin levels. She commenced oral vitamin B supplements to prevent re-feeding syndrome. She also had a formal measurement of creatinine clearance prior to commencing cisplatin and a baseline echocardiogram to assess LVEF prior to starting trastuzumab.

As her Eastern Cooperative Oncology Group performance status (PS) was 0, her repeat LVEF remained >50% and her tumour was strongly HER2-positive, she commenced palliative chemotherapy with cisplatin, fluorouracil (5-FU) and trastuzumab via a peripherally inserted central catheter. She was able to continue living at home with her husband with the support of the community palliative care team, her GP and the district nurses. An increase in care package was arranged for her husband during her chemotherapy, and Age UK sitting services were arranged for him whilst she attended the chemotherapy day unit. Frank discussions were had around future expectations for her disease and treatment to allow her and her family to make pre-emptive plans for her husband for when her health deteriorated.

What should the intent of treatment be?

What are the risks of surgery?

What is the evidence base for cytotoxic chemotherapy?

How do her comorbidities affect treatment?

What are the options for (and complications of) alternative vascular access?

What should the intent of treatment be?

Patients who present with early-stage or locally advanced disease without distant metastases should be considered for potentially curative resection, although this surgery is extensive and involves subtotal or total gastrectomy and lymph node resection. Treatment may include perioperative chemotherapy with a view to reducing the likelihood of relapse after surgery. For patients undergoing surgery alone, 5 year survival may be in the region of 23%.[1] In another study it was found to be significantly lower in older age groups (although complicated by the fact that some patients received adjuvant chemotherapy).[2] In cases where radical surgery is not an option (excessive risk of surgical mortality or very advanced/metastatic disease), or where patients choose not to have surgery, there should be a discussion with the patient about palliative chemotherapy. This would aim to control symptoms whilst preserving quality of life and personal independence with a view to prolonging overall survival (OS). With triple-agent chemotherapy median survival can range from 8 to 12 months.[3] Where patients decline curative surgery, their rationale should be explored, as the reasons behind their concerns may be modifiable, e.g. care provision for a spouse.

What are the risks of surgery?

The risks and benefits of radical surgery were discussed in detail with the patient. Retrospective reviews of older Japanese patients who have undergone gastrectomy quote 5 year survival rates approaching 40%.[4,5] Survival was higher in female patients with less advanced disease who were able to have limited gastrectomy or lymph node dissection, but care needs to be taken when extrapolating these findings to other patient populations.

Following gastrectomy, 30 day mortality is just over 2%, with a total complication risk of nearly 20%. Advances in surgical techniques and the increasing number of preoperative medical clinics (specifically designed for the medical optimization of older people prior to surgery) mean that if there is a thorough assessment of comorbid conditions and physiological state, these risks can be minimized. Renal and respiratory complications are most common: for example, there is a >7% chance of respiratory complications following open gastrectomy.[6]

Risks of surgery are increased by comorbidities including cardiovascular and cerebrovascular disease, hypertension and renal impairment, which are more common in older people. Multivariate analysis in a large study of patients undergoing total or partial gastrectomy, predominantly for cancer, revealed, however, that the influence of pre-existing comorbid conditions on postoperative complications was not significant.[7] In this study, age was also not an independent risk factor for in-hospital mortality after gastrectomy. Complications may be related more closely to the stage of disease at presentation (which may be more advanced in older patients) than to age itself or to pre-existing medical conditions. There is evidence that surgery can have satisfactory outcomes in selected older patients.[4,5]

What is the evidence base for cytotoxic chemotherapy?

Adjuvant/neoadjuvant

In the phase III Medical Research Council Adjuvant Gastric Infusion Chemotherapy (MAGIC) trial,[1] patients (20% >70 years old; 100% PS 0–1) were randomized to receive either immediate surgical resection or perioperative chemotherapy with epirubicin, cisplatin and continuous infusional 5-FU in three cycles before surgery and three cycles after surgery. Five year survival was increased in the group receiving perioperative chemotherapy (36% compared with 23% in those having surgery only). There was also a suggestion that the benefit of perioperative chemotherapy was not as strong in older patients.

The Adjuvant Chemotherapy Trial of TS-1 for Gastric Cancer (ACTS-GC)[8] in Japan (using the oral fluoropyrimidine S-1) included 20% of patients aged 70 or older and showed a statistically non-significant trend towards improved OS in patients in this age group who received chemotherapy after surgery.

Palliative

If there is advanced disease and treatment is with palliative intent, chemotherapy can be given with drugs that include epirubicin, a platinum-based drug (cisplatin or oxaliplatin), and either continuous infusional 5-FU or capecitabine. The REAL-2 trial[3] evaluated the non-inferiority of substituting oxaliplatin for cisplatin and oral capecitabine for continuous infusional 5-FU in advanced gastro-oesophageal cancer. Median survival times varied between 9.3 months (epirubicin, oxaliplatin and 5-FU) and 11.2 months (epirubicin, oxaliplatin and capecitabine). The trial was conducted in a group of patients with a median age of less than 65 years, only 10% of whom had a PS >1.

The phase III Trastuzumab for Gastric Cancer (ToGA) trial[9] compared cisplatin-based chemotherapy with chemotherapy plus trastuzumab, a monoclonal antibody against HER2. Median OS was 11.1 vs 13.8 months, respectively: a finding which seemed to correspond to the over-60s group in the subgroup analysis. Median OS was increased to 17.9 months in the 3+ HER2-positive group.

Retrospective reviews of chemotherapy in older patients have shown that if triple-agent chemotherapy is given, as many as 50% of patients will need a dose reduction due to toxicity, and survival at 1 year can be less than one-third, reinforcing the importance of patient selection and consideration of quality of life. Poor PS and increased symptoms were associated with worse outcome.[10] This was supported by a pilot study (321-GO)[11] which showed that double-agent chemotherapy was tolerated better than triple-agent chemotherapy, with comparable treatment benefit. Median progression-free survival was, however, still less than 5 months. The results of a larger trial are awaited.

How do her comorbidities affect treatment?

Chemotherapy, whether given with radical or palliative intent, can cause significant toxicity. Epirubicin, 5-FU, capecitabine and trastuzumab can all cause cardiac complications. A thorough cardiac history and examination (including ECG) should be undertaken before commencing treatment. Evidence of ischaemic heart disease, especially unstable angina, would be a relative contraindication for 5-FU/capecitabine and should be discussed with the patient. The risk of epirubicin and trastuzumab cardiotoxicity increases with age and pre-existing cardiac damage (as indicated by decreased LVEF). A baseline echocardiogram is recommended before commencing trastuzumab: an LVEF <50% is a contraindication to treatment. In the ToGA trial only 6% of patients developed any cardiac toxicity and 5% of those on trastuzumab had a ≥10% reduction in LVEF. Although there are no set guidelines for monitoring cardiac toxicity, any symptoms of heart failure should warrant a repeat echocardiogram.

Cisplatin in the radical setting can result in non-reversible hearing loss and renal impairment. Borderline renal function does influence choice of platinum and fluoropyrimidine. For example, oxaliplatin can be substituted for cisplatin if GFR is less than 60 ml/min. Platinum-induced peripheral and autonomic neuropathy can also be debilitating, in terms of loss of daily function, and is exaggerated in patients with pre-existing comorbidities such as joint disease (rheumatoid or osteoarthritis) or autonomic dysfunction, and in those with pre-existing disorders of gait and balance. This was a significant consideration for this patient, who wanted to maintain her independence and continue caring for her husband.

Patients who develop severe diarrhoea, vomiting or stomatitis are at increased risk of renal impairment, which may be compounded by pre-existing malnutrition. Consideration should be given to the possibility that multiple or severe toxicities may leave the patient unfit for radical surgery.

Whether they are being considered for radical or palliative treatment, dietetic input is vital in patients showing symptoms of dysphagia, early satiety, weight loss and malnutrition. In the radical setting, preoperative nutritional support will help to prevent delayed wound healing and postoperative infection, and reduce recovery time.

For patients undergoing surgery, a thorough presurgical assessment, which may include a cardiopulmonary exercise test, is required to properly assess the risks of extensive surgery in those with multiple associated morbidities. Factors influencing risk should be modified where possible.

What are the options for (and complications of) alternative vascular access?

Vascular access can be an issue in all patients undergoing chemotherapy, whether with curative or palliative intent. Even if vascular access with a peripheral cannula is possible at the start of a treatment regimen, repeated venepuncture, coupled with potential thrombophlebitis following repeated infusions of chemotherapy, means that vascular access may become more troublesome as treatment progresses. Patients with gastric cancer receiving infusional 5-FU must have vascular access through a central venous line.

There are a number of options for central vascular access: peripherally inserted central catheter, tunnelled central venous line (Hickman line) or totally implanted venous device (subcutaneous portacath). While the first of these can be inserted at the bedside by an appropriately trained nurse using ultrasound guidance, Hickman lines and portacaths need to be inserted in theatre by a vascular or general surgeon.

Despite their advantages, a central venous catheter can have a number of potential complications. The commonest of these are venous thromboembolism and infections, but they can include pneumothorax (which would require a therapeutic chest drain), air embolism and blockage. There have also been reported cases of cardiac arrhythmias. These can lead to anxiety and stress for the patient and delays in treatment while the line is removed and replaced. There are some restrictions to activities with peripherally inserted central catheters and Hickman lines (such as not being able to swim), as well as body image issues, which can be avoided if a portacath is used, as it sits subcutaneously on the chest wall and is not readily visible.

Venous thromboembolism

Any indwelling vascular access device has an inherent risk of venous thromboembolism, which is compounded when using a prothrombotic chemotherapy regimen (such as cisplatin). A peripherally inserted central catheter line may confer a higher risk of deep vein thrombosis of the upper limb compared with other central venous catheters,[12] but there have been no prospective trials. This is due to this type of catheter being inserted into the cephalic vein, where the line occupies a greater proportion of the luminal diameter. There is no evidence for the use of anticoagulant prophylaxis. Diagnosis of upper limb deep vein thrombosis is not in itself an indication for line removal if the line is still functional and the venous thromboembolism does not become more extensive while the patient is being anticoagulated. In older patients, polypharmacy is more common and the risk of interactions with other medications may lead to unpredictable anticoagulation and risk of bleeding.

Infection

One of the major complications of indwelling lines is the risk of infection, which in neutropenic patients can confer even higher morbidity and mortality. Portacaths appear to have the lowest risk, followed by tunnelled Hickman lines and peripherally inserted central catheter lines.[13] Lines should be flushed and redressed regularly and removed when no longer necessary. Prophylactic antibiotics have not been shown to decrease the risk of line-related infections.[13] If patients present with signs of infection, both central and peripheral blood cultures should be taken prior to starting antibiotic therapy. Infections can be treated without having to remove the line, but removal may be necessary in cases of antibiotic resistance or fungal infections. Removing the line itself may be complicated in patients who are thrombocytopenic.

Conclusion and learning points

- Gastric cancer, even when treated with radical intent, is associated with poor prognosis. The balance of risk and benefit needs to be carefully considered given the modest 5 year survival, even with radical treatment.[1] Most trials have been done in populations of patients that do not represent the population we actually treat.

- For patients with difficult vascular access, a semi-permanent line offers a way of delivering chemotherapy, antibiotics and blood products, and is useful for the regular phlebotomy needed whilst on treatment. Whichever line is chosen, there can be significant associated risks including venous thromboembolism and potentially serious or life-threatening infection.

- Older patients with early or locally advanced disease should be considered for the same treatments as younger patients, i.e. curative resection and perioperative chemotherapy.
- Where patients feel unable to accept treatment options due to their care-giving role, or where the treatment planned will affect their ability to provide care, significant efforts should be made to facilitate provision of the necessary additional support.

References

1 Cunningham D, Allum WH, Stenning SP, *et al.* Perioperative chemotherapy versus surgery alone for resectable gastroesophageal cancer. *N Engl J Med* 2006; 355: 11–20.

2 Kunisaki C, Akiyama H, Nomura M, *et al.* Comparison of surgical outcomes of gastric cancer in elderly and middle-aged patients. *Am J Surg* 2006; 191: 216–24.

3 Cunningham D, Starling N, Rao S, *et al.* Capecitabine and oxaliplatin for advanced esophagogastric cancer. *N Engl J Med* 2008; 358: 36–46.

4 Endo S, Dousei T, Yoshikawa Y, *et al.* Prognosis of gastric carcinoma patients aged 85 years or older who underwent surgery or who received best supportive care only. *Int J Clin Oncol* 2013; 18: 1014–19.

5 Endo S, Yoshikawa Y, Hatanaka N, *et al.* Prognostic factors for gastrectomy in elderly patients. *Int Surg* 2014; 99: 166–73.

6 Lim JH, Lee DH, Shin CM, *et al.* Clinicopathological features and surgical safety of gastric cancer in elderly patients. *J Korean Med Sci* 2014; 29: 1639–45.

7 Karkar A, Patil S, Chamberlain RS. A population-based outcomes analysis of the impact of age on morbidity and mortality following gastrectomy: an analysis of 13,799 patients from the Nationwide Inpatient Sample Database. *J Cancer Ther* 2013; 4: 80–91.

8 Sasako M, Sakuramoto S, Katai H, *et al.* Five-year outcomes of a randomized phase III trial comparing adjuvant chemotherapy with S-1 versus surgery alone in stage II or III gastric cancer. *J Clin Oncol* 2011; 29: 4387–93.

9 Bang YJ, Van Cutsem E, Feyereislova A, *et al.* Trastuzumab in combination with chemotherapy versus chemotherapy alone for treatment of HER2-positive advanced gastric or gastro-oesophageal junction cancer (ToGA): a phase 3, open-label, randomised controlled trial. *Lancet* 2010; 376: 687–97.

10 Lord SR, Hall PS, McShane P, *et al.* Factors predicting outcome for advanced gastroesophageal cancer in elderly patients receiving palliative chemotherapy. *Clin Oncol* 2010; 22: 107–13.

11 Hall PS, Lord S, Collinson M, *et al.* Three, two, or one drug chemotherapy for frail or elderly patients with advanced gastroesophageal cancer (321-GO): a feasibility study. *J Clin Oncol* 2012; 30 (suppl): abstract 97.

12 Chopra V, Anand S, Hickner A, *et al.* Risk of venous thromboembolism associated with peripherally inserted central catheters: a systematic review and meta-analysis. *Lancet* 2013; 382: 311–25.

13 O'Grady N. Guidelines for the prevention of intravascular catheter related infections. *Clin Infect Dis* 2002; 35: 1281–307.

32 A Patient with Infectious Complications and Neutropenia on Chemotherapy

Gordon Urquhart, Claire Scampion, Nicola Turner, Tim Perren

Case history

A 75-year-old patient with early-stage breast cancer was admitted to the acute oncology assessment unit, having presented 3 months earlier with a symptomatic left-sided breast mass. A mammogram and breast ultrasound raised the suspicion of malignancy, which was confirmed on diagnostic biopsy. She proceeded to a left-sided mastectomy and axillary clearance for a 34 mm grade 3, node-positive (5/22), oestrogen receptor-positive (8/8), human epidermal growth factor receptor 2-negative, invasive ductal carcinoma. She had a past medical history of controlled hypertension, hypercholesterolaemia, vitamin D deficiency, constipation and mild asthma. Her concurrent medications were metoclopramide, ramipril, bendroflumethiazide, simvastatin, salbutamol inhaler, and calcium carbonate and vitamin D_3 tablets. She lived independently with her 76-year-old husband, who was well. Adjuvant chemotherapy was planned.

Ten days after commencing cycle 1 of adjuvant chemotherapy with epirubicin and cyclophosphamide, dosed according to body surface area, she presented to the acute oncology assessment unit complaining of feeling generally unwell and lethargic. She reported symptoms of nausea controlled with oral antiemetics in the absence of vomiting. Her husband reported that she had been withdrawn and more lethargic than usual. She had stopped going out and spent more time resting in a chair during the day. Her appetite and oral intake had reduced. Her husband was concerned that he was unable to get her to eat normally. It was noted that she had developed frequency of urine with one episode of urinary incontinence. Her temperature at home was 35.5°C.

Initial observations on arrival at the acute oncology assessment unit were: temperature 35.4°C, pulse rate 124 bpm, BP 100/56 mmHg, respiratory rate 18 breaths/min, oxygen saturations 98% on air. Examination revealed suprapubic tenderness. Her chest was clear and no other sources of infection were evident. An ECG demonstrated sinus tachycardia. Neutropenic sepsis was suspected and treatment was promptly initiated with intravenous antibiotic according to the local neutropenic sepsis guideline. Neutropenia was subsequently confirmed, along with an acute kidney injury and hyponatraemia. Urine and blood cultures grew *Escherichia coli* sensitive to amoxicillin and to piperacillin with tazobactam. She was treated with antibiotics and intravenous fluids. Her ramipril and bendroflumethiazide were withheld in light of the hypotension, hypovolaemia, hyponatraemia and acute kidney injury. A bladder scan demonstrated a 200 ml post-void residual volume. Further questioning identified that she had ongoing constipation.

During her hospital admission she was mobilized early with physiotherapy and had a nutritional assessment. Once her bowels opened with laxatives, her post-void volumes reduced to 10 ml. Her sodium and renal function normalized, her condition improved and she returned home after 5 days at her baseline functional abilities. Her ramipril was recommenced on discharge and bendroflumethiazide remained stopped. Repeat renal function tests were arranged for a few days' time.

She continued with chemotherapy with the addition of granulocyte colony-stimulating factor (GCSF) and was able to complete her chemotherapy schedule. She remained in remission at 12 months' follow up.

What was the goal of cancer treatment in this patient?

What assessments were made prior to the initiation of chemotherapy?

What is the risk of neutropenic sepsis in older patients?

Can we modify the risk of neutropenic sepsis?

What are the outcomes of neutropenic sepsis in older patients?

What was the goal of cancer treatment in this patient?

When opting for adjuvant chemotherapy treatment, the aim was to reduce the risk of breast cancer recurrence and improve overall survival from breast cancer. Adjuvant chemotherapy and hormonal treatment could improve her survival from breast cancer from around 50% to 70% at 5 years.

What assessments were made prior to the initiation of chemotherapy?

The treating oncologist reviewed the patient's clinical history, incorporating an assessment of her competing comorbidities, drug history, level of physical function and social circumstances. Serum haematological and biochemical parameters were checked. A baseline ECG demonstrated evidence of possible left ventricular hypertrophy. A subsequent echocardiogram showed preserved left ventricular function.

Her comorbidities were thoroughly assessed prior to chemotherapy for their relevance to expected toxicities. For risk of sepsis, her history of asthma and constipation were of particular importance. In this patient's case, her asthma was only mild and did not add additional risk of infection. However, in cases where patients have a history of infections/exacerbations related to respiratory disease such as bronchiectasis, asthma or chronic obstructive pulmonary disease, a review of these conditions is pertinent. It can be useful to review previous sputum cultures for patterns of organisms and sensitivities so that timely treatment can be planned. This patient had a history of constipation which predisposed her to incomplete bladder emptying (which in turn increases the risk of urinary tract infections). Identifying constipation and high post-void bladder volumes prior to chemotherapy may enable modifications to be made to reduce this risk, e.g. treatment with laxatives and using the double voiding technique. A thorough pretreatment assessment, using processes such as Comprehensive Geriatric Assessment (CGA), not only enables clinical optimization but can also inform cancer treatment decision making. The Elderly Cancer Patient (ELCAPA) study[1] incorporated CGA in the decision-making process in older patients with cancer. On the basis of CGA, around 21% of the study population had changes made to their initial cancer treatment plan. In a multivariate analysis, functional impairment and malnutrition were independently associated with changing cancer treatment.[1] A change in treatment most commonly involved a switch from chemotherapy to a supportive approach. How cancer outcomes were affected by the change in treatment decision was not reported.

What is the risk of neutropenic sepsis in older patients?

Clinical and experimental studies indicate that there is an age-related decline in the number of haematopoietic stem cells.[2] Furthermore, the bone marrow response to haematopoietic stress also appears to alter with increasing age. Barcenas et al.[3] identified around 3500 patients over the age of 65 years treated with chemotherapy for early-stage breast cancer. The risk of hospitalization for neutropenic infection was around 12% in these patients, but the risk varied by choice of chemotherapy regimen.[3] The risk of hospitalization for neutropenic fever and infections ranged from around 13% of patients treated with an anthracycline to 24% of those treated with a third-generation regimen, consisting of a taxane combined with an anthracycline and cyclophosphamide.[3]

A pooled analysis of patients older than 65 years with breast cancer treated with adjuvant taxane-based chemotherapy reported that the rate of febrile neutropenia associated with the use of docetaxel was around 9%.[4] A retrospective analysis of patients aged over 70 years treated with adjuvant or neoadjuvant docetaxel and cyclophosphamide chemotherapy demonstrated that around 8% suffered grade 3–4 neutropenia and 5% were treated for neutropenic sepsis.[5] When establishing the benefit of adjuvant cyclophosphamide, methotrexate and fluorouracil or cyclophosphamide and doxorubicin versus capecitabine, Muss et al.[6] reported a rate of febrile neutropenia in 8% of patients treated with cyclophosphamide, methotrexate and fluorouracil and 9% in patients treated with cyclophosphamide and doxorubicin.

Can we modify the risk of neutropenic sepsis?

A retrospective analysis of patients older than 65 years and treated for early-stage breast cancer with chemotherapy demonstrated a beneficial effect of primary prophylaxis GCSF in reducing the risk of patients hospitalized with neutropenic sepsis.[7] The administration of primary prophylaxis GCSF was associated with 16% fewer neutropenic hospitalizations within the first 3 months of starting chemotherapy.[7] In this case, local protocols restricted the use of GCSF to secondary prophylaxis.

What are the outcomes of neutropenic sepsis in older patients?

Kuderer et al.[2] demonstrated that the length of stay for the treatment of neutropenic sepsis was not longer in patients older than 65 years.[2] In a multivariate analysis, they demonstrated, however, that those older than 65 years had a greater risk of inpatient mortality from neutropenic sepsis compared with those younger than 65 years (OR 1.12, 95% CI 1.04–1.22). Barcenas et al.[3] demonstrated a less than 1% mortality rate in patients older than 65 years receiving adjuvant chemotherapy for breast cancer. The effects of neutropenic sepsis on physical function and independence are, however, not well defined. In general medical patients, Covinsky et al.[8] demonstrated that up to 35% of patients over the age of 70 who were acutely unwell on admission were discharged with poorer than baseline physical function.[8] It is important to minimize the risk of functional decline in hospitalized older patients, including those with neutropenic infections who are more likely to be accommodated in a side room with limited space to mobilize. Early multidisciplinary input is imperative.

Conclusion and learning points

- Older patients with breast cancer should be considered for adjuvant chemotherapy and hormonal treatment for the survival benefit.
- A thorough assessment of comorbidities prior to chemotherapy may identify factors that increase infection risk and enable interventions to be put in place.
- Older patients are at increased mortality risk from neutropenic sepsis.
- Primary prophylactic GCSF should be considered in vulnerable patients at risk of neutropenic sepsis.

References

1 Caillet P, Canoui-Poitrine F, Vouriot J, *et al.* Comprehensive geriatric assessment in the decision-making process in elderly patients with cancer: ELCAPA study. *J Clin Oncol* 2010; 29: 3636–42.

2 Kuderer NM, Dale DC, Crawford J, *et al.* Mortality, morbidity, and cost associated with febrile neutropenia in adult cancer patients. *Cancer* 2006; 106: 2258–66.

3 Barcenas CH, Niu J, Zhang N, *et al.* Risk of hospitalization according to chemotherapy regimen in early-stage breast cancer. *J Clin Oncol* 2014; 32: 2010–19.

4 Loibl S, Von Minckwitz G, Harbeck N, *et al.* Clinical feasibility of (neo)adjuvant taxane-based chemotherapy in older patients: analysis of >4,500 patients from four German randomized breast cancer trials. *Breast Cancer Res* 2008; 10: R77.

5 Freyer G, Campone M, Peron J, *et al.* Adjuvant docetaxel/cyclophosphamide in breast cancer patients over the age of 70: results of an observational study. *Crit Rev Oncol Haematol* 2011; 80: 466–73.

6 Muss HB, Berry DA, Cirrincione CT, *et al.* Adjuvant chemotherapy in older women with early-stage breast cancer. *N Engl J Med* 2009; 360: 2055–65.

7 Rajan SS, Lyman GH, Stearns SC, Carpenter WR. Effect of primary prophylactic granulocyte-colony stimulating factor use on incidence of neutropenia hospitalizations for elderly early-stage breast cancer patients receiving chemotherapy. *Med Care* 2011; 49: 649–57.

8 Covinsky KE, Palmer RM, Fortinsky RH, *et al.* Loss of independence in activities of daily living in older adults hospitalized with medical illnesses: increased vulnerability with age. *J Am Geriatr Soc* 2003; 51: 451–8.

Index